Principles for Evaluation of One Health Surveillance: The EVA Book

Marisa Peyre • François Roger
Flavie Goutard
Editors

Principles for Evaluation of One Health Surveillance: The EVA Book

Springer

Editors
Marisa Peyre
CIRAD, Deputy Head UMR ASTRE research unit
Campus International de Baillarguet
Montpellier, France

François Roger
CIRAD Resident Regional Director for Southeast Asia
Hanoï, Vietnam

Flavie Goutard
CIRAD, UMR ASTRE
GREASE network coordinator
Hanoï, Vietnam

ISBN 978-3-030-82726-7 ISBN 978-3-030-82727-4 (eBook)
https://doi.org/10.1007/978-3-030-82727-4

This Springer imprint is published by the registered company Springer Nature Switzerland AG
The registered company address is: Gewerbestrasse 11, 6330 Cham, Switzerland

Foreword

The surveillance of animal diseases has been of major importance to global trading markets and has gained even more importance with regard to public health issues due to incidents such as the SARS episode in 2003 and more recently the threat of influenza and the Covid-19 pandemics. Highly contagious animal diseases such as foot and mouth disease are a significant threat to trade and could lead to export barriers and major economic losses if not detected early enough. Moreover, zoonotic diseases (transmitted from animals to humans) account for 60% of human infectious diseases, while almost 100% of emerging infectious diseases in humans are of animal origin. This early detection of health events is critical to prevent their introduction and spread, and to limit their health and economic consequences especially with zoonotic risks as seen with the Covid-19 pandemic. National animal health surveillance systems are in place to ensure this early detection of the emergence and control of circulating diseases.

The OIE defines the surveillance of animal diseases as the systematic ongoing collection, collation and analysis of information related to animal health and the timely dissemination of information so that action can be taken. This definition includes critical elements relating to (i) the sustainability of activities in the long term, (ii) communication to relevant actors and (iii) the possibility of follow-up action. The quality of information generated by those systems provides the basis for global trade agreements and health risk prevention and control. Those systems need to be evaluated to ensure their performance and quality, and the optimal use of resources, especially in settings where resources are limited.

The surveillance of animal diseases is underpinned by a complex system essentially made possible by people sharing health information and making decisions based on it. In their decision-making on whether to share health information with other actors or not, each actor is influenced by his or her own context and constraints (socio-economic, cultural, religious, political): from the source (farmers) to policy-makers and vice versa; through to the entire chain of intermediary actors that comprise local Veterinary Services (veterinary paraprofessionals, public or private veterinarians, etc.) and political entities (e.g. village chief). The proper functioning of these networks therefore not only depends on the technical and economic constraints inherent to the organisation of the network and monitoring protocols (strategies), but also to the social issues generated by this network of contacts and information flows. However, until recently these aspects were not considered in the process due to the lack of tools and methodologies available. This book aims to provide key elements and methodological advances to address this gap.

International consensus and social acceptance has been achieved around the need to strengthen health surveillance, especially in regard to the Covid-19 emergence, yet the relevant definition of priorities and the appropriate allocation of resources remain major issues: where, when, how and with what funding?

The answers to these questions will vary depending on:

- the point of view: the priorities defined for a specific monitoring programme will be different for an individual (e.g. a poultry producer), society or state due to the different nature of the costs and benefits generated
- the geographical scale considered (local, national, regional or international)
- the time period chosen (short, medium or long term)

In many countries, according to the outcomes of the OIE PVS missions[1] carried out by OIE experts, the performance of animal health surveillance systems is perfectible. Nevertheless, conclusions on the epidemiology of diseases and decisions are made based on these findings. Evaluation is an essential step in the decision-making cycle to especially ensure the quality of the evidence used. The evaluation of surveillance can be envisaged in a global or targeted way by distinguishing on the one hand the operation of the network ('network process') and on the other its governance (national monitoring strategy, 'surveillance policy'). This distinction of scale will appeal to different methodological, socio-economic and institutional issues. The evaluation at the network level will try to answer the problem of social construction and the network's integration into this construction (what are the social issues related to the operation of the network?), by appealing to socio-economic issues, economic and political policies (is the strategy applicable?). At the level of governance, the issues will relate to the health and socio-economic contexts (is the strategy adapted?) and institutional issues (is the strategy applied?).

The transparent and objective interpretation of evaluation results allows for more objective decision-making and resource allocation, as well as a definition of more appropriate surveillance strategies and thus an improvement in the acceptability of the system by different stakeholders (local level: producers and veterinarians; national level: national veterinarians, reference laboratories, decision-makers). These aspects are essential when addressing underreporting issues and improving our understanding of the epidemiological cycles of animal and zoonotic diseases, including novel pathogen emerging risk.

The issues of priority, sustainability, social acceptance and communication are at the heart of the concerns of policy-makers when it comes to defining and implementing their strategies. Over the past decade, governments have seen their budgets dwindle, highlighting the need to evaluate the efficiency of their surveillance actions and to optimise actions to develop health surveillance at the global level. However, these assessments are not simple to implement, owing to both a lack of the

[1] https://www.oie.int/solidarity/pvs-pathway/

necessary data and conflicts of interest with other public actions and private actors of health surveillance.

Innovative methods and tools such as the ones presented in this EVA book are needed to overcome these shortcomings and to enable countries to optimise the management of their resources in terms of investment in animal health policy.

Monique Éloit
Director General, World Organisation for Animal Health (OIE)
Paris, France

EVA Book Sections Summary and Highlights

Needs for Evaluation of Health Surveillance

This section provides the baseline elements required to understand what is a health surveillance, how does it work and why it needs to be evaluated. It takes the reader through the definition and theoretical basis of surveillance, surveillance systems, evaluation and evaluation of health surveillance systems. The section also presents the different types of evaluation and how they could be applied to evaluate health surveillance systems.

Highlights:

- Health surveillance is critical to ensure early detection of emerging diseases.
- Timely evaluation is required to design and implement efficient and sustainable surveillance systems.
- Decision-makers are looking for scientific based evidence on how to best allocate resources for health surveillance—including comparing the cost and benefits of disease impact, surveillance and control.
- Practical and simple guidance on how to implement health surveillance evaluation—including economic evaluation of health surveillance systems—is required to better inform decision-making.

Evaluation Frameworks and Tools

This section provides an overview on the evaluation guidance available to account for the complexity of the surveillance systems under evaluation both in terms of diversity of objectives and diversity of actors. This section provides a step-by-step guidance on how to perform such evaluation and describe the current tools available to facilitate this process. Such tools could be used by technical advisers of health programme decision-makers to provide scientific based evidence on how to best design or improve health surveillance systems performances and process.

Highlights:

- Health surveillance systems are complex systems made of a diversity of actors addressing different objectives.

- Each actor of the system has its own needs and constraints which can impact the surveillance process—such aspects must be considered in the evaluation.
- Integrated evaluation is required to evaluate technical performances but also process and economic aspects of the surveillance systems.
- Integrated evaluation required interdisciplinary approaches combining epidemiology, social and economic sciences.
- An evaluation process can be split into three main phases: planning; framing and implementing (including reporting).
- The EVA Survtool promotes an integrated evaluation approach and can be used by decision-makers to facilitate the evaluation of health surveillance systems.
- The Eva tool includes a step-by-step guide on how to best perform the evaluation and provides a reference online platform for health surveillance evaluation methods.

Economic Evaluation

This section presents the basic principles behind economic evaluation of surveillance—highlighting its challenges linked to the close relationship between surveillance and intervention and the need to express benefits and cost in monetary terms for classical economic evaluation. This book presents methods applicable in both developed and developing countries to capture these elements and make meaningful recommendations to improve disease surveillance systems worldwide. The application of participatory approaches to capture social benefits and costs highlights the complexity of the surveillance process and the impact of social and cultural factors—not yet translated into monetary value—on individual decision-making which can also impact national disease surveillance and control policy if they are not considered in the evaluation and surveillance design processes.

Highlights:

- Perception of surveillance is affected by the socio-economic context.
- Disease impact and therefore surveillance benefits in avoiding those impacts are reduced by alternative options linked to the socio-economic context.
- People perception is strongly affected by surveillance consequences (= control actions).
- Some perceived costs do not have a market value (e.g. emotional distress, moral link to technical network, fear of conflict).
- It is necessary to characterize the contextual factors which affect surveillance function and performances and therefore its economic value.
- One Health approach can be taken to account for externality of zoonoses or environmental issues (e.g. AMR): how to measure the added value.
- One Health approach can generate intellectual capita that could better inform control measure and generate a measurable health effect.
- Gains in information and knowledge should be measured to assess the added value of One Health.

- Experimental economics can be used to describe, conceptualize and quantify non-monetary surveillance benefits.
  - Stated preference method can be used to assign value to benefits with non-market value and to estimate the willingness of farmers to accept different policy arrangement.
- Compensation levels are of secondary importance in the decision to report a health event—outstated by the uncertainty of receiving the compensation and the culling strategy.

Qualitative Evaluation Methods

As seen with the Covid-19 pandemic crisis, social acceptance, communication but also priority and sustainability are at the heart of concerns for decision-makers when it comes to define health surveillance and control strategies. Qualitative methods sometimes combined with quantitative ones are essential to capture such critical elements. This section presents an overview of existing qualitative methods to evaluate health surveillance systems including the added value of participatory approaches and the remaining challenges in this area. This section provides also detailed information on practical tools recently developed to assess qualitative attributes such as acceptability (AccePT method—Chapter 8) and degree of collaboration between partners (ECoSur tool—Chapter 9).

Highlights:

- Socio-economic and cultural constraints impact the decision of the actors of the surveillance system to postpone or not a case of illness.
- The types and responses to these constraints is not depending on the country development level; it depends strongly on the structure of the livestock sector concerned.
- The design of more effective and efficient surveillance systems, as well as their evaluation, requires the application of innovative methods and tools accounting for the perceptions, expectations and needs of the different actors.
- Participatory approaches are flexible enough to account for such socio-economic and cultural constraints.
- Acceptability refers to the willingness of individuals and organizations to participate in surveillance, as well as the extent of involvement of each of these users.
- The AccePT method is a standardized method to assess the acceptability of surveillance via participation of the network's actors.
- The AccePT method also leads to a better acceptability of the evaluation itself thanks to the direct involvement of the actors in the evaluation process.
- Collaboration means interactions between actors operating in different surveillance components and that improve the value of the surveillance system.
- ECoSur (Evaluation of Collaboration for Surveillance) evaluates the organization, functioning and functionalities of collaboration taking place in a multisectoral surveillance system such as One Health surveillance systems.

Quantitative Evaluation Methods

Surveillance data are often non-exhaustive, partially distorted and, also sometimes, non-representative because often generated by imperfect reporting, diagnosis, sampling and testing processes. Such ineffective surveillance can result in misjudging an epidemiological situation and adopting inappropriate intervention measures. These issues have been clearly highlighted during the Covid-19 pandemic crisis. There is a recognized need for more effective health surveillance which could be achieved by making sure regular and fit-to-purpose evaluations are performed. This section presents quantitative methods and tools to assess the performances of health surveillance systems—such as statistical (data-based) or mathematical simulation (process-based) modelling—to ensure quality of the data generated and to provide meaningful recommendations for improvement.

Highlights:

- Effectiveness is the ability of surveillance systems and strategies to reach their objectives.
- The evaluation attributes best reflecting effectiveness will depend on the surveillance objectives.
- Effectiveness attributes can be estimated by analysing the data directly produced by the surveillance system—when available—or by modelling surveillance processes.
- Data-based methods—such as multilist of unilist capture–recapture methods—rely on the availability of surveillance data and can only be applied ex post or in itinere (after or during the implementation).
- Process-based methods—such as mathematical modelling—depend on the surveillance types (passive or active)
- Passive surveillance requires reporting and confirmation process to be modelled.

Evaluation in the Policy Cycle

Surveillance strategies should be adapted to the local needs and constraints to be effective and implemented. It should also be translated into a legalized policy framework to ensure its sustainability. This section focuses on the role of health surveillance evaluation within the health policy cycle, to better inform decision-making. It presents key elements and challenges regarding the decision-making process behind health surveillance. It provides perspectives and means on how to best address decision-maker's needs—based on the innovative evaluation methods and tools presented in this book, including impact assessment of the evaluation process itself to inform policy decision—while designing effective and practical health surveillance strategies.

Highlights:

- Surveillance evaluation focuses on measuring the value of surveillance efforts to take meaningful actions and to inform policy decisions.
- The integration of surveillance evaluation into the policy cycle for animal disease mitigation is still in its infancy.
- Evaluation can help in bridging decision-making at practical and policy levels to promote positive and dynamic changes.
- Surveillance systems cannot be reduced to the technical and neutral operation of collecting, managing and analysing information; it includes decision-making in order to control risks.
- There is a gap between the "official" rules and norms (that are generally designed by centralized authorities) and their implementation in the field.
- Good governance is an ethical choice but is also the condition for a greater stakeholders' involvement and for surveillance effectiveness.
- Understanding how surveillance systems run in practice—real governance—is a powerful tool for designing more effective systems.
- Impact evaluation is increasingly requested for both donor and social accountability.
- Impact evaluation method can be used to assess the added value of evaluation to better inform health surveillance policies.
- Evaluation is critical to inform changes that needs to be adopted in public health policies at national level to ensure sustainability and impact of the actions.

About the Book

Over the past two decades, strengthening One Health surveillance has become a major issue to prevent emerging pandemic threats such as SARS Cov-1, animal influenza, Ebola and more recently SARS Cov-2 (covid-19). The emergence of infectious diseases remains a rare event, difficult to detect. Infectious disease information at the global level is based on national surveillance systems. The resources and reliability of these systems can vary widely, especially in countries with weak economies or political instability. In order to ensure the optimal use of resources, it is essential to evaluate the systems on a regular and appropriate basis. The issues of priority, sustainability, social acceptance and communication are at the heart of the concerns of policy-makers when it comes to defining and implementing health strategies. Over the past decade, governments have seen their budgets dwindle, highlighting the need to evaluate the efficiency of their surveillance actions and to optimise actions to develop health surveillance at the global level. However, these assessments are not simple to implement, both by the lack of necessary data and by conflicts of interest with other public actions and private actors of health surveillance. Innovative assessment tools are needed to overcome these shortcomings and to enable countries to optimise the management of their resources in terms of investment in animal health policy.

This book provides an overview along with detailed information on methods to evaluate health surveillance systems (animal health but also in a one health context), and more especially on the recent innovations in this field within the past 10 years.

Target Users

This book has been written for health surveillance and/or health evaluation specialists. But it will also be suitable for any health professionals or researchers with a growing interest for health surveillance and more especially health surveillance evaluation.

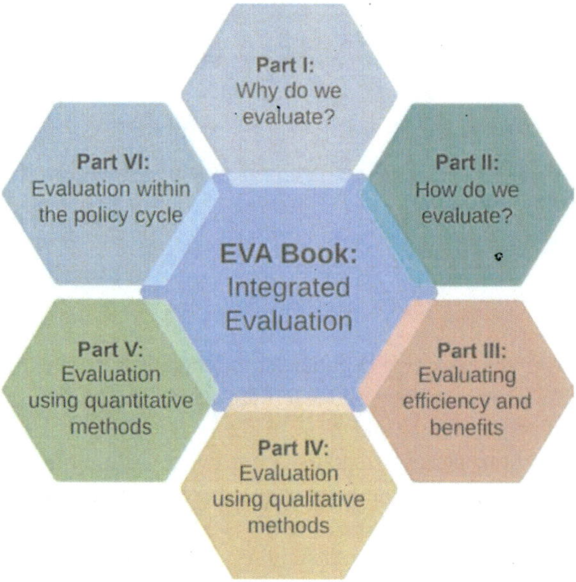

Fig. 1 The content of the EVA book promoting integrated evaluation of health surveillance systems

Overview of the Book Content

The book is divided in 6 parts and 16 chapters, which could be read independently and which provide a wide overview on health surveillance evaluation from theoretical roots to practical implementations using case study demonstration (Fig. 1). Through its different parts the book is promoting a practical and an integrated approach to health surveillance evaluation, considering technical but also process and socio-economic aspects, trying to address the following questions:

- What is evaluation of health surveillance systems and why do we need it? (**Part I**)
- How to evaluate health surveillance and what to take into consideration within the evaluation? (**Part II**)
- How to evaluate the efficiency and benefits of a surveillance system? (**Part III**)
- How to evaluate the process and technical efficacy of the surveillance systems using qualitative (**Part IV**) and quantitative (**Part V**) methods?
- How to ensure integration of the evaluation outputs within the policy cycle? (**Part VI**)
- What are the remaining challenges and needs for innovations in evaluation approaches? (**Chapter 16**)

Content Not Covered

Although the book gives basic information on what is surveillance and what is a surveillance system, it does not present in-depth information on surveillance nor methods on how to design surveillance systems. We recommend looking at other reference books regarding those aspects (presented at the end of the book).

Contents

Part I General Introduction on Health Surveillance Evaluation

1 Why Do We Need to Evaluate Health Surveillance Systems? 3
Marisa Peyre, Flavie Goutard, and François Roger

2 An Overview of the Different Types and Level of Evaluation: From Theory to Application in Health Surveillance 25
Marisa Peyre and Nicolas Antoine-Moussiaux

Part II What to Evaluate and How

3 Frameworks and Tools for Evaluating Health Surveillance Systems . . . 43
Marisa Peyre, Mo Salman, and Katie Steneroden

4 The EVA Survtool: An Integrated Framework to Plan Health Surveillance Evaluation 61
Marisa Peyre, Katja Schulz, Pham Thi Thanh Hoa, and Barbara Häsler

Part III Methods for Economic Evaluation

5 The Economics of Surveillance 95
Keith Howe

6 Applications of Principles to Case Studies Focusing on Non-Monetary Surveillance Values 117
Barbara Häsler, Alexis Delabouglise, Nicolas Antoine-Moussiaux, Thang D. Phan, Duan C. Dao, Thanh T. Nguyen, Hoa T. T. Pham, Bao D. Truong, Xuan N. T. Nguyen, Ton D. Vu, Khong V. Nguyen, Hien T. Le, D. Tatong, W. Phimpraphi, S. Kasemsuwan, Marisa Peyre, and Sara Babo Martins

Part IV Qualitative and Semi-Quantitative Methods for Process Evaluation

7 Qualitative Methods to Evaluate Health Surveillance Systems 149
Marisa Peyre and Flavie Goutard

8 The Use of Participatory Methods in the Evaluation of Health Surveillance Systems. 163
Flavie Goutard, Clémentine Calba, Sokha Chea, Nicolas Antoine-Moussiaux, Mathieu Pruvot, Katja Schulz, and Marisa Peyre

9 Evaluation of Collaboration in a Multisectoral Surveillance System: The ECoSur Tool 179
Marion Bordier, Camille Delavenne, Dung Thuy Thi Nguyen, Flavie Goutard, and Pascal Hendrikx

Part V Statistical and Modeling Approaches to Evaluate and Inform Surveillance Design

10 Quantitative Methods to Evaluate Health Surveillance Effectiveness 195
Vladimir Grosbois, Guillaume Fournié, Raphaël Duboz, Timothée Vergne, Marisa Peyre, and Flavie Goutard

11 Network Analysis for Surveillance Design and Evaluation. 219
Guillaume Fournié, Alexis Delabouglise, Raphaëlle Métras, Younjung Kim, and Raphaël Duboz

Part VI Evaluation in the Policy Cycle

12 Health Surveillance Evaluation in the Policy Cycle. 247
V. J. Del Rio Vilas, M. Arnold, and Marisa Peyre

13 Animal Health Surveillance: From Compliance to Real Governance 261
M. Figuié and A. Binot

14 Integrating Health Surveillance Evaluation Outputs in the Policy Cycle. 273
Katharina D. C. Stärk

15 Added Value and Impact of the Evaluation Process in Health Surveillance. 283
Marisa Peyre, Stéphanie Cong, Vu Dinh Ton, Guy Faure, Eugénie Baudon, Nguyen Viet Khong, Malik Peiris, Ben Cowling, and Flavie Goutard

16 Synthesis—Evaluate to Better Inform: A Way to Strengthening Health Surveillance Systems. 299
Marisa Peyre and Flavie Goutard

Glossary 309

About the Editors

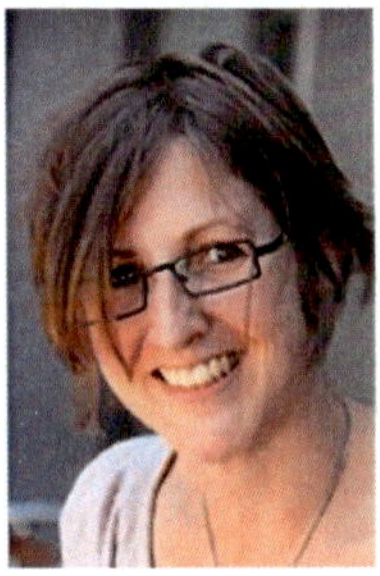

Marisa Peyre, Eng., PhD, HDR is an epidemiologist at CIRAD, French Institute for international agricultural research for development. She graduated in 1998 in biotechnology engineering (Bordeaux, France) and obtained her PhD in 2005 in Immunology (London, UK). She has worked for the past 15 years on the evaluation of animal health surveillance and control both in developed and developing countries and provides expertise for international organisations (OIE, FAO). Her key expertise is on evaluation of animal disease management systems (surveillance and control), animal health economics and participatory epidemiology. She is a professional trainer in health programme evaluation and in participatory evaluation and has been using this approach to improve animal health management strategies in South East Asia, Africa and Europe. She is currently the Deputy Head of ASTRE research unit (Animal, Health, Territories, Risk and Ecosystem) and is closely working with the World Animal Health Organization (OIE) to strengthen public-private partnerships in the veterinary domain and especially within the One Health approach. She coordinates for Cirad the PREZODE international initiative, to prevent and early detect emerging zoonotic risks.

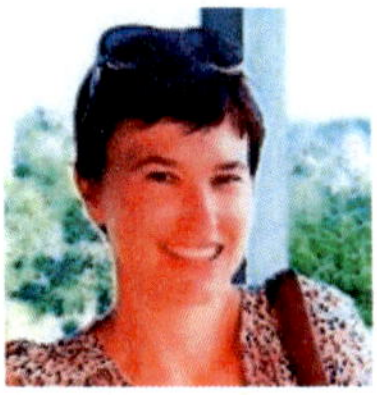

Flavie Goutard, DVM, Msc, PhD is a veterinarian and epidemiologist at CIRAD since 2005. She graduated in Veterinary Medicine from the National Veterinary School of Toulouse (France). She did her Master's in Epidemiology and Public Health (London, UK) followed by her PhD in 2015 in Health Risk (CNAM, France). She has 15 years of experience in the field of infectious diseases epidemiology in tropical countries, working mainly on the development of adapted surveillance and control strategies for animal diseases in rural settings. She was an adjunct professor at Kasetsart University, Bangkok,

Thailand, for 9 years where she directed a Master Program in the One Health field. She provides expertise for international organizations (OIE, FAO), and is currently coordinating the GREASE regional research platform on the management of emerging risks for Southeast Asia.

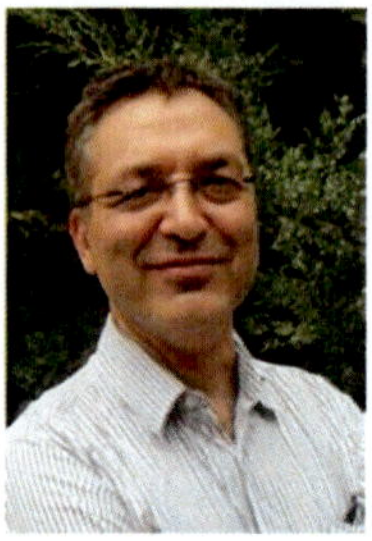

François Roger, DVM, Msc, PhD is a veterinarian and epidemiologist at CIRAD, where he was leading the AGIRs then ASTRE research units until 2020. He is currently the Regional Director for CIRAD in Continental South East Asia and based in Hanoi, Vietnam. After several years working in sub-Saharan Africa, the Indian Ocean and Europe, he developed research programmes in Southeast Asia and launched the GREASE platform for research and training on emerging risks in South East Asia (http://www.grease-network.org), which brings together different health sectors and disciplines according to the One Health approach.

About the Lead Authors

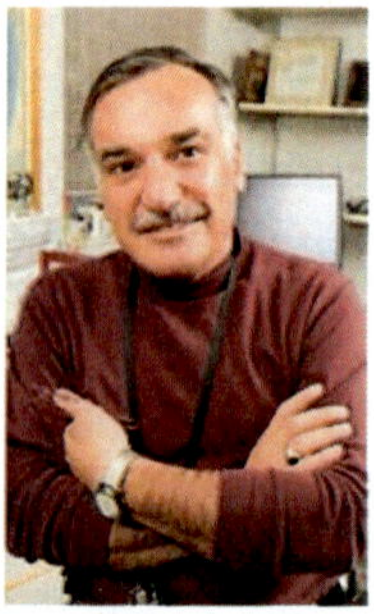

Mo Salman, DVM, MPVM, PhD, DACVPM, FACE For the last 36 years, Dr. Mo Salman is a professor in the Department of Clinical Sciences and is founder and director of the Animal Population Health Institute of College of Veterinary Medicine and Biomedical Sciences at Colorado State University. Dr. Salman's educational background is in veterinary medicine (BVMS), preventive veterinary medicine (MPVM) and comparative pathology (PhD). He is a Diplomate of the American College of Veterinary Preventive Medicine (ACVPM) and a Fellow of the American College of Epidemiology (ACE). His research interests focus on surveillance and survey methodologies for animal diseases with emphasis on infectious diseases. He is editor of a 2003 book entitled *Animal Disease Surveillance and Survey Systems: Methods and Applications*. For more than 25 years, Dr. Salman has been involved in training sessions and workshops both nationally and internationally in the field of epidemiology, surveillance, disease managements and risk assessment. Many of his research activities are engaged in stabilisation and reconstructions of national animal health programmes in countries such as Bosnia, Afghanistan, Iraq, Middle East, East Africa, Georgia and Armenia, among others. Dr. Salman had a position on the peer review of the European Union and the World Animal Health Organization (OIE). In 2013, he completed a year with US Department of State as a Jefferson

Science Fellow where he was the scientific advisor for the African Bureau. From Oct 1, 2015 to Sept 30, 2016, he was hired as the coordinator for the US Department of State: Biosecurity Engagement Program in Afghanistan. He is currently focusing on his role as an educator through building case studies for field training of public animal health officers across the world as well as active contribution to the conventional academic courses offered through CSU for undergraduate, graduate, and professional students.

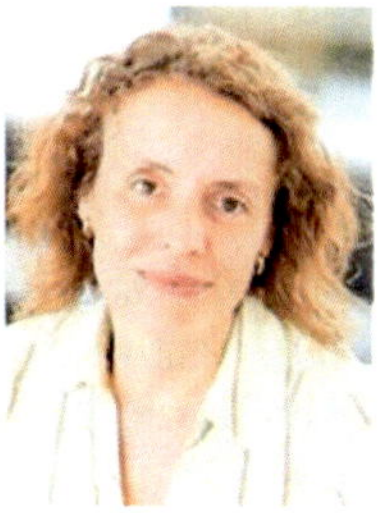

Barbara Häsler, DVM, PhD is a researcher and Professor in Agrihealth at the Royal Veterinary College London, United Kingdom, with expertise in animal health surveillance, economics applied to animal health and One Health, livestock food systems and evaluation. In her research she focuses on One Health and other interdisciplinary approaches to understand better how livestock food systems function and evolve and their impacts in terms of foodborne and zoonotic disease, nutrition and food security and environmental sustainability. She combines this with work on animal disease surveillance and control and how such mitigation measures can be made more efficient through improved resource allocation. She has been working on the economics of surveillance and practical evaluation approaches that allow users to assess surveillance characteristics including functionality, performance, value and One Health-ness.

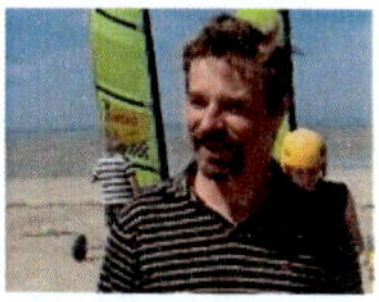

Vladimir Grosbois is a researcher in ASTRE: the animal health research group of CIRAD, the French research institute in agronomy for development. He worked for 10 years, as a quantitative ecologist, on the dynamics of wild animal populations in particular under the influence of climate changes before becoming a quantitative epidemiologist at CIRAD. His current research topics include the epidemiology of animal diseases at the interface of wild and rural areas, the surveillance of animal diseases and the interpretation and analysis of observational data on animal diseases. His main fields and research partners are located in South-East Asia and Southern Africa as well as in Europe. His approaches are quantitative, implying a great deal of statistical modelling. He also teaches general statistics and specific statistical modelling methods in master's programmes in France and in partner countries such as Zimbabwe and Thailand but also in training sessions for researchers and professionals from the animal health and environment management/conservation sectors.

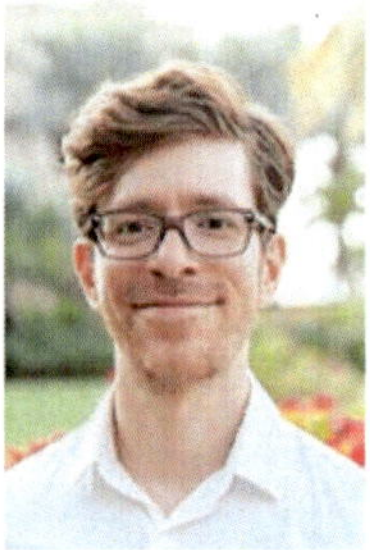

Guillaume Fournié, DVM, MSc, PhD is a veterinarian and an epidemiologist, currently working as a senior research fellow at the Royal Veterinary College (University of London, United Kingdom). With a strong interest in disease modelling and network analysis, Guillaume is exploring the way in which the configuration of livestock production systems shape the emergence, spread and maintenance of infectious diseases. He is experienced in conducting research at the interface between epidemiology and other disciplines, including virology, anthropology, neoclassical and behavioural economics, and archaeology. He has also a strong interest in the translation of science into policy.

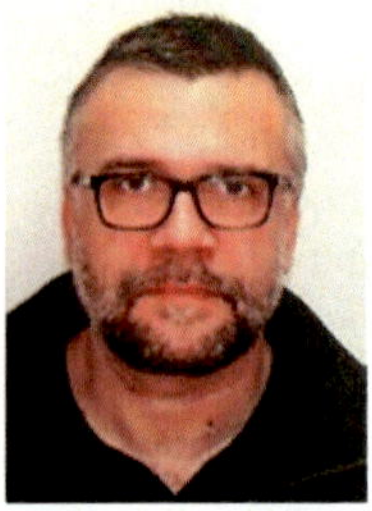

Victor Del Rio Vilas, DVM, MBA, MSc (Epi), PhD is currently at the World Health Organization (WHO), South East Asia Regional Office in New Delhi, India, where he coordinates the Global Outbreak Alert and Response Network (GOARN) in the region. He was previously at the Dept of Epidemiology, School of Veterinary Medicine, University of Surrey (UK), and at the Centre on Global Health Security at Chatham House, London. Until January 2018 he worked at the World Health Organization (WHO-Geneva) on the development of WHO's epidemic vulnerability evaluation framework. Until November 2016, Dr. Del Rio was a consultant with the Pan American Health Organization (PAHO/WHO), based in Rio de Janeiro (Brazil) with regional responsibilities. In that capacity, Dr. Del Rio advised Ministries/Departments of Health across the region on epidemiology, surveillance and control measures for a number of diseases such as rabies, leishmaniasis, yellow fever and on zoonoses programmatic issues. He also contributed to WHO's global response to the Ebola Virus Disease outbreak in Liberia in 2015; previously worked in Uzbekistan implementing the Biological Threat Reduction Program (Defence Threat Reduction Agency, US DoD), and as veterinary advisor and epidemiologist for UK's Department for Environment, Food and Rural Affairs (Defra) and the Veterinary Laboratories Agency.

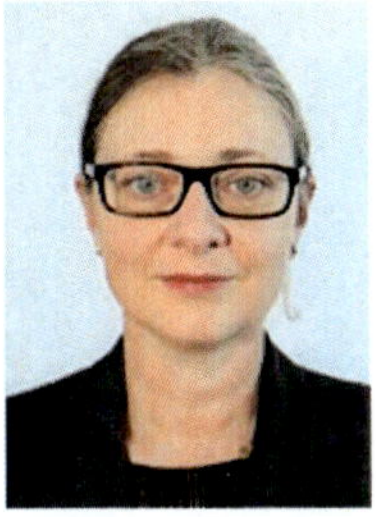

Katharina Stärk is an internationally recognised specialist in veterinary public health with over two decades of experience in the design, implementation and evaluation of animal health surveillance. She has worked in diverse environments including the private sector in Denmark and Switzerland as well as in academia in New Zealand, UK and Hong Kong. She is currently Head of Department of Animal Health at the Swiss Federal Office for Food Safety and Veterinary Affairs. Her professional passion is to translate science into practice with the aim to assure safe food for all.

Part I

General Introduction on Health Surveillance Evaluation

1 Why Do We Need to Evaluate Health Surveillance Systems?

Marisa Peyre, Flavie Goutard, and François Roger

Abstract

The need to set up efficient and sustainable surveillance systems has become a major concern particularly in recent years, following SARS, H1N1 influenza, and Covid19 pandemics. The recent crisis has highlighted the importance to early detect new emerging diseases, including zoonosis such as coronavirus, MERs-CoV, and Ebola. To ensure implementation of the best surveillance strategies and make optimal use of available resources, it is critical to perform timely and relevant evaluations of such systems both at planning and operational steps of the process. The evaluation must provide a robust scientific foundation to inform decision-makers and meet their demand for simple and practical evaluation guidance. The aim of this chapter is to provide a better understanding on the need and challenges for such evaluation of health surveillance systems to ensure quality and reliability of the data generated.

Keywords

Evaluation · Health · Decision making · Economics · Surveillance networks

M. Peyre (✉)
CIRAD, UMR ASTRE, Montpellier, France

ASTRE, CIRAD, INRAE, University of Montpellier, Montpellier, France
e-mail: marisa.peyre@cirad.fr

F. Goutard
CIRAD, UMR ASTRE, Hanoi, Vietnam

ASTRE, CIRAD, INRAE, University of Montpellier, Montpellier, France

F. Roger
CIRAD, DGDRS, Hanoi, Vietnam

ASTRE, CIRAD, INRAE, University of Montpellier, Montpellier, France

M. Peyre et al. (eds.), *Principles for Evaluation of One Health Surveillance: The EVA Book*, https://doi.org/10.1007/978-3-030-82727-4_1

1.1 Introduction

The need to set up efficient and sustainable surveillance systems has become a major concern particularly in recent years, following SARS, H1N1 influenza, and Covid19 pandemics, which have also highlighted the importance to detect new diseases [1], including emerging zoonosis, for example, MERs-CoV and Ebola. In the field of animal health, surveillance systems provide information for effective disease control, thereby improving productivity and food security, animal welfare, economic development, and access to international trade. Moreover, around 75% of emerging infectious diseases in humans are zoonoses [2, 3]. Therefore, the capacity of surveillance systems to accurately describe patterns of animal diseases is of public health importance. Information about infectious diseases at a global scale relies on government surveillance systems. And yet the resources and reliability of these systems can vary considerably, especially in countries characterized by weak economies or political instability [4]. To ensure implementation of the best strategies and make best use of available resources, it is critical to perform timely and relevant evaluations of surveillance systems [1]. Evaluation is one essential step in the policy cycle [5]. Evaluation, which implies a judgment on the surveillance systems and recommendations for improvement, is a critical part of surveillance in that it allows transparent interpretation of outputs, more objective decision-making and resource allocation, as well as improvements in system design and enhanced acceptance of system outputs by stakeholders [at local (e.g., farmers, veterinarians) and national levels (e.g., reference laboratory, veterinarians at central level)]. This is particularly important given the knowledge gaps in our understanding of many diseases, which leads to varying degrees of uncertainty and bias in generated outputs.

The aim of this chapter is to improve understanding on the need for evaluation of such surveillance systems to ensure the quality and reliability of the data generated.

All the notions described in this chapter are important to understand the importance and challenges of evaluation of animal health surveillance (AHS), along with the need to adapt the approach according to the different settings. Comparison between "north" [high-income countries (HICs)] and "south" [low- and middle-income countries (LMICs)] will be made throughout this section as differences between AHS in those settings have to be accounted for when planning and implementing an evaluation.

Reference books on animal health surveillance, providing definition and detailed information on what is surveillance, what is a surveillance system/networks, and how to design surveillance, are available, and elements from these books will be mentioned throughout this section without making systematic reference to them:

- Epidemiological surveillance in animal health, B. Dufour and P. Hendrikx (Ed); CIRAD, AEEMA, FAO and OIE edition. 2009.
- Guide to terrestrial animal health surveillance, OIE Ed. 2014.
- FAO. 2014. Risk-based disease surveillance—A manual for veterinarians on the design and analysis of surveillance for demonstration of freedom from disease. FAO Animal Production and Health Manual No. 17. Rome, Italy.
- Surveillance épidémiologique: principes, méthodes et application en santé publique, Astagneau et Ancelle Eds. Lavoisier publishing, 2011.

- RISKSUR consortium: Best practices for risk-based and cost-effective animal health surveillance in the European Union available at https://www.fp7-risksur.eu/progress/best-practice-document (accessed 14/11/2017).
- RISKSUR Glossary for definitions of the terms: https://www.fp7-risksur.eu/terminology/glossary (accessed 14/11/2017).

1.2 Part I: Surveillance

1.2.1 What Is Animal Health Surveillance?

Animal health surveillance (AHS) is the ongoing systematic collection, analysis, and interpretation of data and the dissemination of information to those who need to know in order to take action [6].

This definition comprises important notions about *sustainability* and long-term action, communication to relevant *stakeholders*, and perspectives for action.

1.2.1.1 Surveillance Networks

To ensure communication between relevant stakeholders, AHS has to be based on an organized structure called *network*. In LMICs, AHS often rely on the veterinary services organization network and do not target a specific disease (cf. Fig. 1.1: example of AHS networks). In HICs, AHS networks are often disease or *symptoms*-specific and numerous AHS networks could be mapped in one specific country (e.g. a mapping of the AHS activities in France in 2012 accounted for 109 networks and components) [7].

1.2.1.2 Surveillance Systems and Components

AHS could be implemented in different forms or activities, which are called "components." The main two types of components are

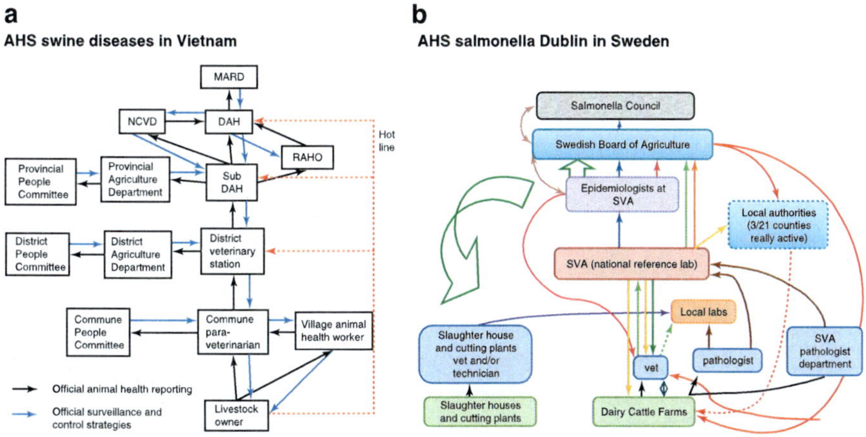

Fig. 1.1 Example of animal health surveillance network organization: in LMICs, (**a**) AHS network often relies on existing veterinary services structure; in HICs, AHS networks are often disease specific (**b**)

- Passive or scanned surveillance: observer-initiated provision of animal health related data (e.g. voluntary notification of suspect disease) or the use of existing data for surveillance. Decisions about whether information is provided, and what information is provided from which animals is made by the data provider.
- Active surveillance: initiated collection of animal health related data using a defined protocol to perform actions that are scheduled in advance. Decisions about whether information is collected, and what information should be collected from which animals is made by the investigator.

A range of surveillance components (and their associated networks) targeting a specific hazard is called a *surveillance system* (e.g., the avian influenza surveillance system in Vietnam encompass three main components: passive reporting of outbreaks, active surveillance in live bird markets, and active surveillance in farms) [8].

1.2.2 Surveillance Is Different from Epidemiological Surveys

- There is often confusion between epidemiological surveys (study design used in epidemiology research or development projects) and surveillance systems, and at this stage it is important to highlight the main differences between:
- Epidemiological surveys are methods used to describe a health event in human or animals populations (how, when, and where it occurred) or to identify risk factors' link with occurrence of diseases. A survey may be exploratory, descriptive, or explanatory. Surveys are time-framed, from a given point in time (cross-sectional survey) to a specific period of time (longitudinal surveys that can be implemented over years or even decades). Surveys can help to draw hypothesis on possible risk factors or to test these hypotheses.
- Surveillance systems are tools and networks used to ensure a continuous and systematic collection of data (with no limitation in time) leading to action. Surveillance can be used for diseases detections or disease trend monitoring. The data produced by the surveillance systems are regularly analyzed and interpreted to produce useful information for planning, implementation, or evaluation of control options. Surveillance systems are based on networks of actors and surveillance activities (or components). These activities may include the implementation of surveys (often longitudinal surveys) at one point in the life span of a surveillance system.

1.2.3 Why Do We Need Animal Health Surveillance?

There is a general context of increased risk of disease emergence and spread linked to a globalized world, and increased urbanization linked to an exponential increase of human population demography and needs for food supply and climatic changes. This general context leads to (i) increased contacts with wildlife because of losses of their natural habitats and food supply needs from poor communities, (ii) animal breeding intensification, (iii) increased resistance to drugs, and (iv) vectors [9] (Fig. 1.2).

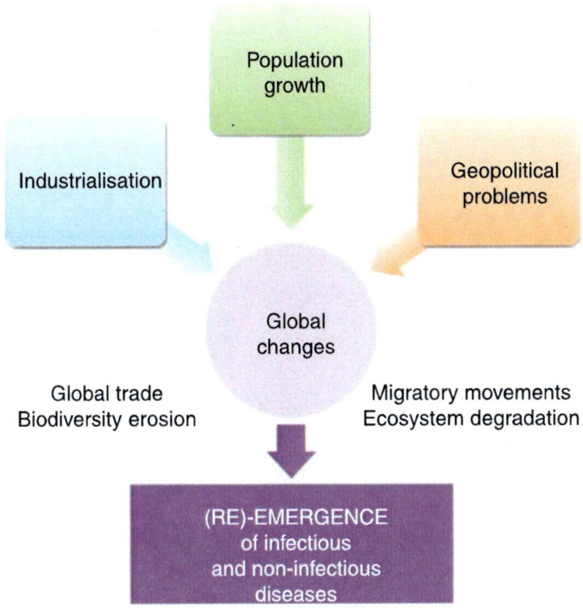

Fig. 1.2 Global factors and links leading to increased risks in animal/zoonotic disease emergence and spread. [10]

There are four main purposes of AHS:

- Detection of incursion of exotic, new (emerging), and reemerging diseases
- Declaration of freedom from specified diseases and infection
- Detection of cases of endemic diseases for control or eradication
- Monitoring of endemic disease for disease prevalence estimation (often to assess efficacy of control measures)

There is a global need to strengthen emerging diseases and transboundary animal disease surveillances to (i) protect the global human health and prevent potential pandemics, (ii) ensure commercial trade of animal products to protect national economies and food security, and (iii) prevent production losses to protect poorest communities' livelihood and reduce poverty.

1.2.4 Challenges in Animal Health Surveillance

1.2.4.1 Influence of the Animal Health Management Cycle and the Socioeconomic Contexts

AHS is integrated in the animal health management cycle in close connection to disease control (see Parts III and VI). This cycle is dynamic as disease situation will influence surveillance strategies that will influence control strategies and will in return influence the situation of the disease (Fig. 1.3). This cycle involves different types of

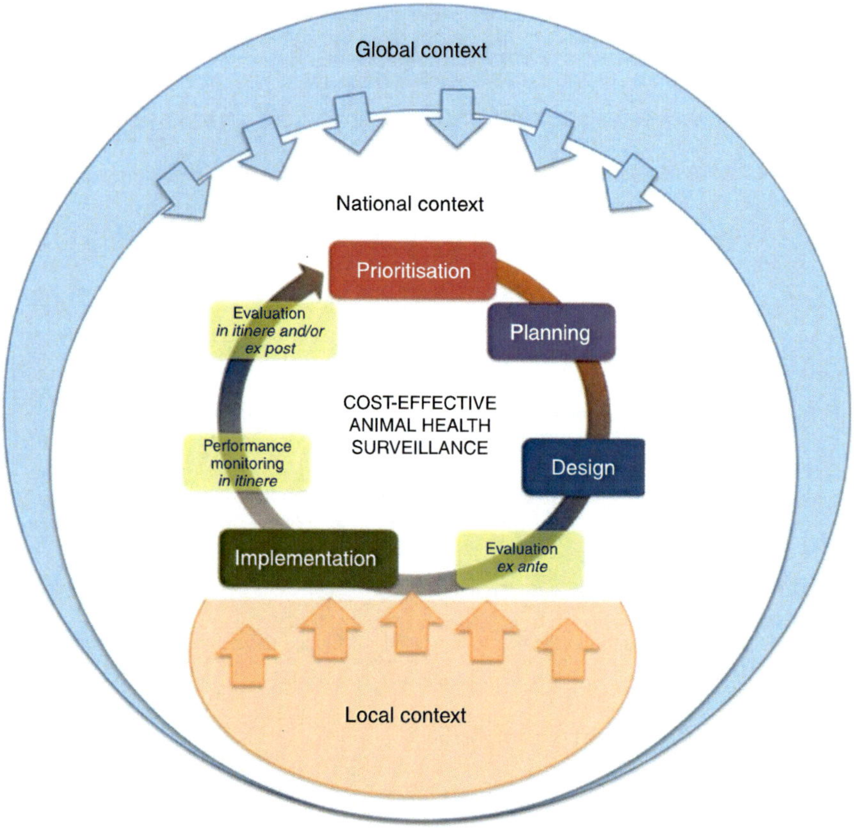

Fig. 1.3 Animal health management cycle embedded in local, national, and global socioeconomic contexts. (Adapted from [11])

actors (from the farmer to the decision-makers) who take decision and influence its outcome. Actors' decisions are influenced by their own socioeconomic, cultural, and political contexts, which vary from and between local, national, and global situations.

1.2.4.2 Which Priorities for Surveillance, Which Point of View?

There is an international consensus and social acceptance of the needs to strengthen surveillance; however, the main issue remains on how do we define priorities to ensure appropriate resource allocations to strengthen and implement surveillance but: where? when? and with which funds?

Answers to these questions will vary according to

- The nature of the point of view: the priorities set or a specific surveillance program will vary for an individual and the society as their costs and benefits will be different (Fig. 1.4)
- The scale taken into consideration (local, national, international)
- The time horizon considered (short term, mid-term, long term)

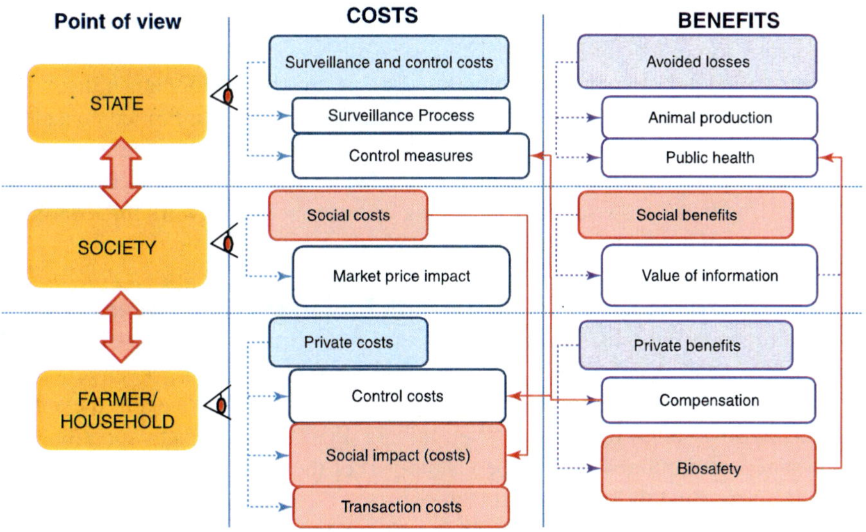

Fig. 1.4 Costs and benefits resulting for a surveillance program will vary according to the nature of the point of view (individual, societal, or state)

1.2.4.3 A Complex System of Information Sharing

Animal health surveillance is a complex system merging different types of actors with different expertise and different administrative levels. At each level, the actors hold the key to health information. Each category of actors has specific constraints driven by specific epidemiological but also economic and sociopolitics drivers and that influence their decision-making in terms of sharing health information and reporting or not reporting disease outbreak.

Moreover, health or animal priorities differ between different levels from the international to the national level but also from the national to the local level. We learn from social science and economics that

- Global stakes leading to surveillance implementation by governments are not shared by local actors. This is often linked to gap in perceptions and gap in expectations. (For example, in Southeast Asia, the surveillance of foot and mouth disease, which is endemic in the region, has become a priority for the local government in line with the global eradication strategies recently launched by the World Animal Health Organisation. However, the disease is not perceived as a priority by the local farmers).
- Every level of the system holds the key to the animal health information, which could lead to underreporting situation, local surveillance, and disease management, and therefore poor quality of the surveillance data generated by the system.
- The perception of the costs and benefits involved in animal health disease management process (including surveillance and control) will be different according to the different points of view. It is important in the evaluation process to identify

clearly the point of view taken (Fig. 1.4). When looking at the farmer and society, it is also important to understand that surveillance involves specific costs and benefits that are often not accounted for. This is mostly due to the fact that until recently there has been a lack of adapted methodology and a limited consideration of economic evaluation within the animal health surveillance evaluation process. Some of the work implemented in the RISKSUR project aimed at addressing these two issues by developing an integrated framework for economic evaluation of surveillance and specific methods.

1.2.4.4 Seeing the Unseen: Dealing with Underreporting Issues

It is well recognized that underreporting is the main limit of the scanned surveillance component of any health surveillance system and often active surveillance components are implemented to compensate for this issue. The iceberg metaphor (or paradigm) is often referred to when talking about animal health surveillance, with the reported outbreak being the visible part of the iceberg, and the active surveillance increasing this visible part (Fig. 1.5).

One of the main challenges of AHS is to know the real size of the iceberg (the real disease situation). Epidemiological conclusions are too often based on what is seen (parts A and B), with limited knowledge of any of the relative proportion of what is seen (A + B) over the total size of the iceberg (real disease situation). In other words, most epidemiological conclusions are often done without knowing the performances of passive and active surveillance components.

In many countries, the performances of AHS in terms of case detection ability (e.g., sensitivity; knowing the whole size of iceberg), representativeness, and coverage remain unknown; however, epidemiological conclusions are being drawn. But "a blind use of data without understanding the context and their provenance can generate surprisingly false results" (Simpson's paradox) [12]. However, things are changing, and evaluation is becoming increasingly important in health surveillance research to improve the epidemiological knowledge and control of animal and zoonotic diseases.

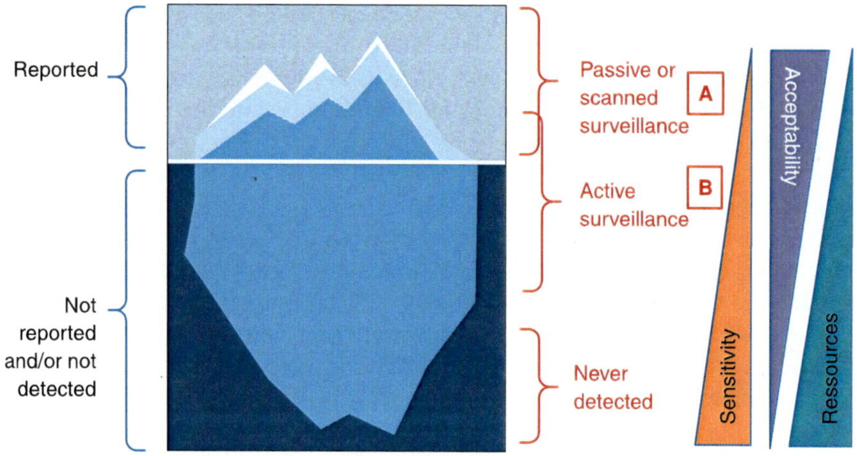

Fig. 1.5 The iceberg paradigm of animal health surveillance

1.3 Part II: Evaluation

1.3.1 What Is Evaluation?

Evaluation is a systematic determination of a subject's merit, worth, and significance using criteria governed by a set of standards.

- It can assist an organization, program, project, or any other intervention or initiative to assess any aim, feasible concept/proposal, or any alternative, to help in decision-making; or to ascertain the degree of achievement or value in regard to the aim and objectives and results of any such action that has been completed.
- The primary purpose of evaluation, in addition to gaining insight into prior or existing initiatives, is to enable reflection and assist in the identification of future change.
- The evaluation process is closely linked to the decision-making process and the need to advocate for changes (Fig. 1.6; see Part VI).
- Evaluation can come into many different scales and process according to the object and context under evaluation. It is of critical importance to tailor its definition to the specific object and context of the evaluation (e.g., the definition of animal health surveillance evaluation provided below).

The concept of evaluation is an entire field of research by itself and a specific discipline, with different schools and theoretical orientations, which will not be the object of this book [13]. To get more knowledge on the theoretical fundamentals of evaluation, please refer to specific literature.

Evaluation is different from assessment and performance monitoring:

- *Assessment* is the collection and analysis of data from a defined indicator. It is a technical step within the evaluation process.
- *Performance monitoring* is a day-to-day follow-up of the surveillance system operation, done in a continuous manner and whose results are used internally by the actors of the system. Performance monitoring is done using performance indicators.

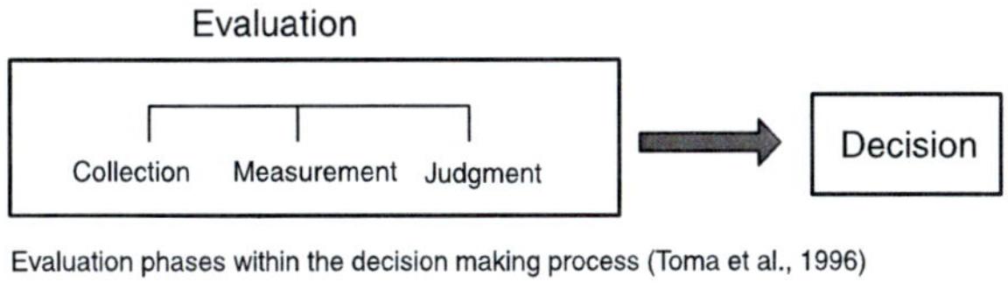

Fig. 1.6 Evaluation phases within the decision-making process. (From [14])

1.3.2 Historical Overview of Animal Health Surveillance Evaluation

Evaluation of animal health surveillance is a relatively recent but exponentially growing field of research and interest (Fig. 1.7).

Until recently, evaluation in animal health has mainly concentrated on the evaluation of effectiveness and cost–benefit of disease control, that is, the consequences of surveillance and not on the surveillance process by itself [15]. Animal health evaluation guides have been derived and driven by public health evaluation approaches; however, no harmonized approaches currently exist in both fields and most evaluations are performed on an ad hoc basis or based on empirical implementation. A review of the existing evaluation guides is presented in Chap. 3 of this book. Even though evaluation of public health surveillance systems is anterior from AHS evaluation, the methodological developments have been important in the animal health field in the past 10 years. Most of the methods developed and presented in this book could be adapted to and inform public health surveillance system evaluation.

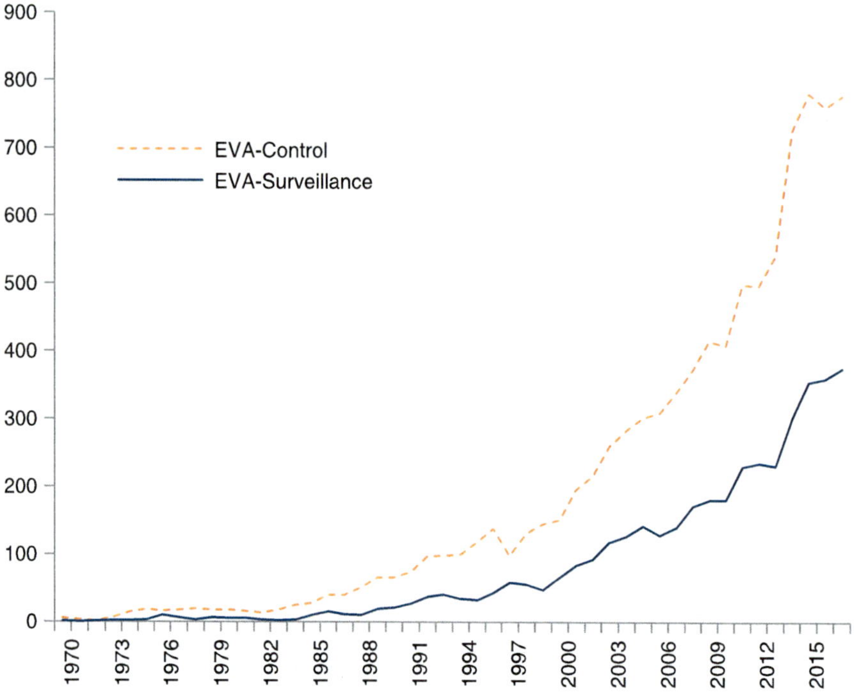

Fig. 1.7 Evolution of the number of scientific publications on AHS evaluation (MesH key terms) per year from 1970 to 2018

1.3.3 What Is Evaluation of Animal Health Surveillance?

The following definition was developed based on a literature review process of evaluation and evaluation of animal health terminology, and reviewed by experts in surveillance and evaluation within RISKSUR EU project.

> Evaluation is the determination of the merit of a surveillance system/component, by confronting the results of the assessment with standards targets, criteria or a counterfactual system. This process shall be transparent, objective and evidence-based. The outcome of an evaluation is a judgement and/or recommendations placed in the overall surveillance context. An evaluation can be performed at any development stage of the surveillance system. Ideally, an evaluation is conducted in regular intervals in line with the policy cycle, by internal and/or external evaluators. One, several or all components in the surveillance system and any number of attributes and/or criteria can be considered, depending on the evaluation question and the context.

What Do We Mean by "Merit of a Surveillance System"? The merit of a surveillance system represents its ability to perform and address its objective (i.e., the system is able to detect sufficient number of cases to control the disease; the system is able to prove disease freedom status with sufficient robustness). The performance of a surveillance system could be assessed at different levels, looking at

- *Technical effectiveness*: Looking at specific aspects of the system such as sensitivity, timeliness (cf. Part III).
- *Process effectiveness*: Looking at the system organization (e.g., data management, acceptability, cf. Part III) and its impact on its technical efficacy.
- *Efficiency*: Looking at the added value of the system versus a situation without any surveillance or another type of surveillance. This could be done by assessing economic criteria (e.g., cost-effectiveness or cost–benefit) (cf. Part III) or looking at the system impact (cf. Part VI).

Which Standard Targets/Criteria or Counterfactual System? In order to define the system merit, its technical effectiveness has to be compared to a standard target value; its process effectiveness or efficiency has to be compared to a counterfactual system; which would ensure that the system will be able to address its objective. Both could be defined according to a gold standard (the minimum value required to reach the objective or the ideal system process organization or components) or to a defined target value, which could vary according to the different socioeconomic and legislative contexts and epidemiological situations. Technical experts should define both based on scientific evidences, but the target value will be adapted to the specific context and could evolve with time.

- *Gold standard target value or counterfactual system examples*: To detect highly pathogenic avian influenza cases in order to control the disease in a given country, the system sensitivity should not be lower than 90% with timeliness (the time between case detection and control) lower than 1 day. The EU defines target prevalence for specific disease surveillance systems; so the system sensitivity should be sufficient to detect this prevalence within these requirements. The OASIS tool assesses the organization of a surveillance system based on how an « ideal » surveillance system should be organized to ensure its performance (Epidemiological surveillance in animal health, B. Dufour and P. Hendrikx (Ed); CIRAD, AEEMA, FAO and OIE edition. 2009).
- *Defined target value or counterfactual examples:* In Vietnam the sensitivity of HPAI surveillance system (passive surveillance) has been shown to be lower than 10%, a new system or component of the system should be developed to increase this sensitivity to a minimum of 60% in the first 2 years, and then subsequently adapted to detect 90% of the cases. In order to reduce the cost of classical swine fever surveillance in Germany, new surveillance system components were designed based on specific risk factors (seasonality; age of the animals) and used as a counterfactual to assess the efficiency of the system [16].

Why Do We Need Judgment and Recommendations? We need judgment and recommendations to advocate for changes implementation. Judgment on the merit of a surveillance system is the difference between a technical assessment and an evaluation. In order to ensure objectivity of the evaluation outputs, it is recommended that the (independent) evaluator make this judgment (cf. Annex XX on evaluator best practices and ethics). However, this could also be done in conjunction with the stakeholders or the system and the decision-makers to ensure understanding, adaptability, and acceptability of the judgment and recommendations.

Why Do We Need a "Transparent, Objective, and Evidence-Based" Evaluation? And how to ensure these elements? The evaluation should be transparent, objective, and evidence based to ensure trust in its outcome and promote implementation of the recommendations to generate changes. Changes could only be accepted and sustainable if they are perceived as in genuinely good to improve the surveillance system performances and not unfairly benefiting for some specific stakeholders. The evaluation process should therefore be clear and available for all stakeholders, along with the outputs and recommendations, especially the way they have been designed. Recommendations based on fact (evidences) and objective assessment will be perceived as fair. However, transparency, objectiveness, and evidence will not ensure acceptability as people make decisions based on their specific context (social, economic, cultural) (Chap. 7). These specific contexts should therefore be considered and understood during the evaluation. They will help in the design of the recommendations (Chap. 14).

Why Do We Need to Define an Evaluation Context and an Evaluation Question? The evaluation context provides the background information that will help to make choices about how the evaluation needs to be carried out (Why? What? How?). Any evaluation is bound to a specific context (i.e., the surveillance system; the nature of the disease; the decision-makers' need; the cost requirements, legal requirements, etc.). The choice of type, level, and elements to be included in the evaluation process will depend on the broader socioeconomic context within which the evaluation is being performed. Some elements of the context are essential to frame the evaluation and define the evaluation question and also to analyze and discuss the outputs of the evaluation by setting them back in their context (cf. Sect. 2, Chap. 4).

Why Do We Need to Define an Evaluation Question? Evaluation comes with a cost, the process will be resources demanding (both in terms of human and financial resources) according to the type and level of evaluation performed. An evaluation should be therefore done with a clear objective, which comes with one or multiple clearly formulated questions. This will ensure framing the evaluation process exactly to the needs and ensuring saving resources. It is impossible to make a judgment and recommendation without a clearly defined question to address.

1.3.4 What Is Economic Evaluation?

Economics is a discipline focused on the efficiency criteria for making choices between alternative uses of limited resources. It provides robust criteria to assess how decisions about the allocation of resources impact on the well-being of different groups of people in society and for society as a whole. Economics is not only about finance (what is the cost?). Economics is about social behaviors for resource allocation (which decisions do I need to make?).

Economic evaluation of surveillance systems/components should be required as an aid to decision-making in surveillance to inform the allocation of scarce resources. It shows the consequences of alternatives and helps to identify which of these are to be preferred from an economic point of view.

A unifying underlying principle of economic analyses is to provide a measure of the relative value attached to competing alternative strategies and thereby facilitate decisions about the allocation of resources. Economic evaluation of surveillance system including its principles, methods, and tools is described in Part III of this book.

1.3.5 Why Do we Need to Evaluate AHS?

Perceptions are diverse regarding the primary purpose of evaluation, but the common ground lies in the fact that evaluators aspire to construct and provide the best possible information that might bear on the value of whatever is being evaluated (Fig. 1.9):

- Bettering products, personnel, programs, organizations, governments, consumers, and the public interest
- Contributing to informed decision-making and more enlightened change.
- Precipitating needed change
- Empowering all stakeholders by collecting data from them and engaging them in the evaluation process.
- Experiencing the excitement of new insights

As described earlier, we need surveillance to detect disease cases in order to control, prevent introduction, and document freedom or effectiveness of disease control measures. What we detect is only a fraction of cases happening and that active surveillance can increase this visible fraction (the iceberg paradigm). We need to know the real disease situation (the true size of the iceberg) to ensure that the response is adapted to the real situation and that epidemiological analysis is based on robust surveillance data. Evaluation of AHS allows us to understand the limits of the surveillance and conclude on the quality of the data generated by the system. This provides information on the bias of the epidemiological analysis and could better inform decision-making by trying to minimize those biases. AHS evaluation helps to provide information on the unseen by assessing the performance of the surveillance systems and components to estimate true disease prevalence and circulation patterns (e.g., assessing surveillance system acceptability to estimate the underreporting; using capture–recapture methods to estimate system sensitivity) [17, 18]. AHS evaluation would promote technical improvements (better design; improved effectiveness/efficiency) but also qualitative criteria such as trust, acceptability, and behavioral changes (Fig. 1.8).

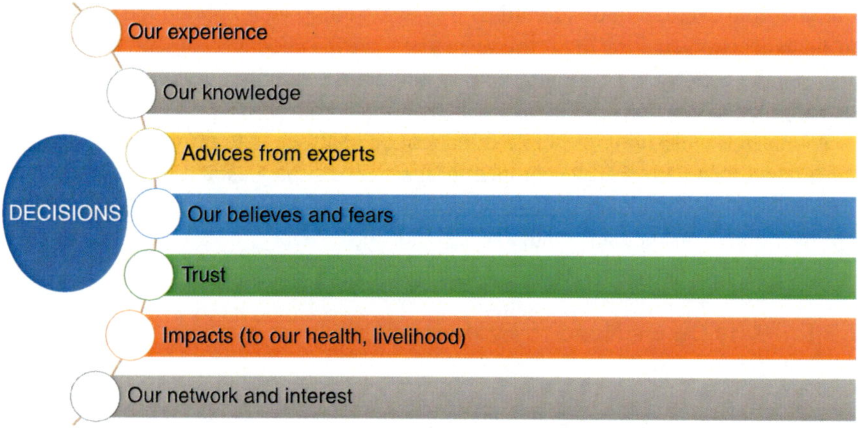

Fig. 1.8 The different factors that influence how individuals make decision

1.3.6 Brief Overview of the Evaluation Process

Going through a rigorous evaluation process also helps generating trust:

(i) Between all the actors of the system and across the different administrative levels (e.g., national coordinators; local user; beneficiaries); by improving understanding of the perception of the system by the beneficiary and implementing changes to improve this perception; the use of qualitative approaches such as participatory evaluation, which involves all the actors in the evaluation process itself (see Part IV), could also contribute to improving trust and involvement of the system users and beneficiaries.
(ii) Between the international and national actors, demonstrating the quality of the data generated by the AHS and therefore providing increase assurance in the true disease situation in the country. This could have an impact on trade market and funds accesses. The evaluation outputs could also support the countries in their advocacy to generate development and/or research funds to improve their sanitary situation by providing documented evidences on strengths and limits of the surveillance and interventions to improve it.

Evaluation process and outputs will help promoting changes by demonstrating the needs to generate changes for improvement and providing robust information on adapted and relevant corrective actions/intervention to implement. The decisions we make are highly influenced by social, cultural, political, religious, or economic drivers (Fig. 1.8); to be sustainable, any behavioral changes required should be adapted/take into consideration those drivers (see Parts III and VI for more information about social aspects of surveillance process and decision-making process).

Surveillance systems are complex and need to be adapted to epidemiological systems driven by epidemiological, economic, social (including political, cultural), and environmental factors. To allow the design of cost-effective surveillance systems, there is a need to design comprehensive, practical, and affordable evaluation frameworks for timely evaluation of not only the benefits and costs of a surveillance and control program but also the factors required for local acceptance, which itself is crucial for the effectiveness and viability of the system at national and international scale [19] (Fig. 1.10). Moreover, an assessment of system efficiency has to take account of each country's specific needs and resources, and it has to be quantitative as much as possible to minimize the impact of subjectivity. In order to control diseases, institutional constraints must be considered together with technical aspects.

1.3.6.1 Limits of the Existing Evaluation Frameworks

A review of the *evaluation methods of surveillance systems and current practices* performed by Calba [20] highlighted the importance and need to develop an

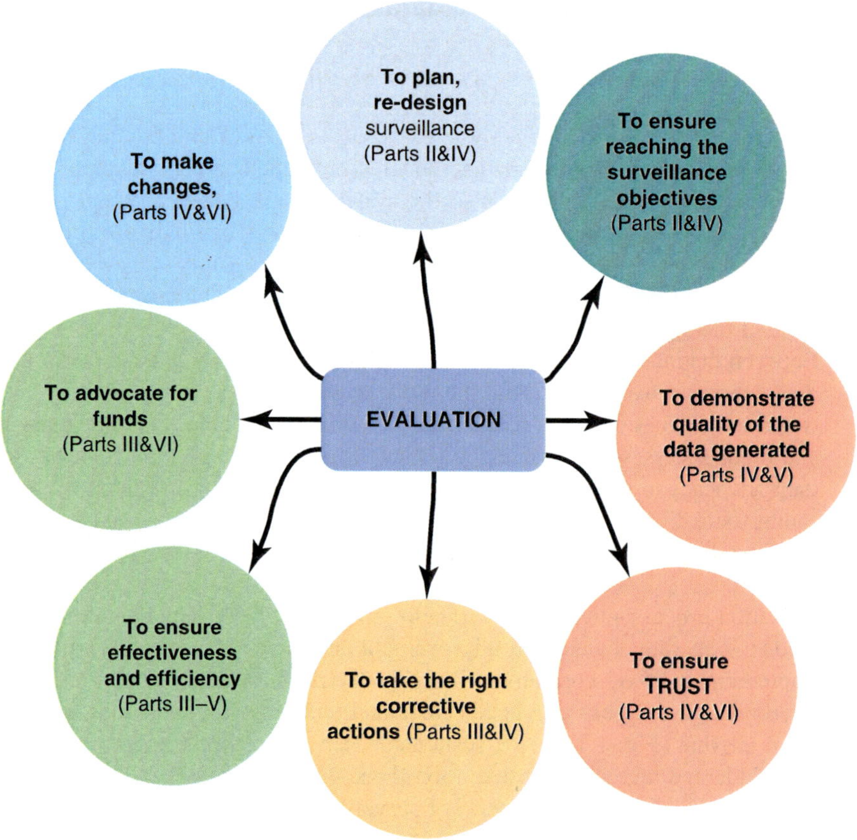

Fig. 1.9 The multiple objectives of animal health surveillance evaluation

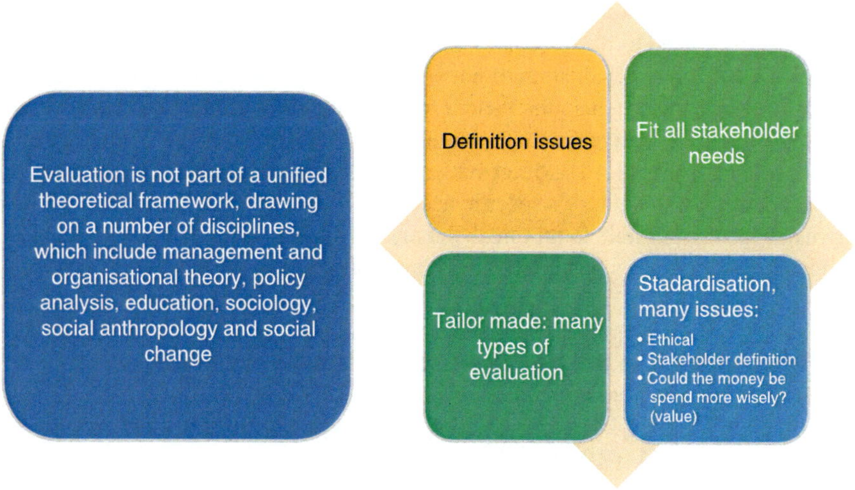

Fig. 1.10 The current challenges in animal health surveillance evaluation

integrated evaluation approach including not only the epidemiological aspects of the evaluation but also the social and economic aspects (Part III, Chap. 6) [20]. This review showed that

(i) Most of the evaluation frameworks and guidelines have been so far developed based on empirical situation, on an ad hoc basis, each providing different levels of detail for implementation and usually targeting only partial aspects of the surveillance system characteristics; specific evaluation of surveillance (as opposed to the evaluation of disease interventions) has been performed only on limited occasions and a variety of approaches and methods are used without a generally agreed protocol [21].
(ii) A set of generic guidelines were available (CDC, WHO) but covered also partial aspects each and were highly complementary.
(iii) The terminology used was not standardized, generating some confusion for the users.
(iv) There was no rationale in the use of evaluation attributes and often a lack of methods or information on the methods to assess them; more than 25 attributes have been described for the evaluation of animal health surveillance systems, making a complete evaluation—if all attributes are used—time-consuming and expensive. In some cases, no methods have been described for the measurement of these attributes and only a fraction of these evaluation attributes are included in the evaluation guidelines and applied in case studies ([21–23], RISKSUR D1.2).
(v) Economic evaluation activities currently focus mainly on disease control programs and economic impact of diseases in populations and only a small proportion of published studies focused on economic evaluation of surveillance.
(vi) There is no standardized gold standards or effectiveness targets for animal health surveillance; in animal health, there is no index of an effectiveness measure available as it exists in the human health system evaluation process [e.g., disability-adjusted life-years (DALYs) and quality-adjusted life-years (QALYs)] [24].

Some of these challenges have been addressed in the past decade, and the methods are described in this book.

Peyre et al. developed an integrated evaluation framework and tool (part of the SurvTool surveillance design and evaluation decision tool) that built on from existing recognized frameworks and remains adapted to any particular epidemiological and surveillance system context (in terms of attribute evaluation selection and relevance), providing guidance in relation to suitable methods for attribute assessment [25] (see Part II).

A glossary of evaluation terms to complement the existing "surveillance glossary" [23] has been developed as part of the RISKSUR project (https://www.fp7-risksur.eu/terminology/glossary) and is further consolidated in this book (see Glossary) to develop a set of internationally recognized and standardized effectiveness metrics for economic evaluation of animal health surveillance.

1.3.6.2 The Need for an Effectiveness Measure and the Benefit Issue

When considering the start, end, or change of a surveillance program, policymakers need to know if and how much surveillance is worth. Animal disease creates two sources of lost well-being for people. First, the monetary value of losses linked to the negative effects of disease itself (e.g., losses in production, mortality, etc.); second, the additional resource costs incurred in the attempt to limit those losses (such resources could have been used to generate other outputs elsewhere in the economy). In assessing the rationality of any resource-usage decision, the key criterion is whether the value of recovered outputs is sufficient to at least cover the additional resource costs [26].

In some instances, decision-makers may not require explicit quantification of the (monetary) benefit, but may be interested in the costs of the surveillance options related to selected performance indicators, which can act as proxies for a benefit. In an economic analysis, these performance indicators (i.e., effectiveness measures) would be compared to the costs of surveillance in a cost-effectiveness analysis (CEA) (see Part III). Cost-effectiveness analysis, commonly used to assess human health interventions, has rarely been applied to animal health decision-making problems (Babo Martins and Rushton, in press). In human health economics, the effectiveness often refers to the avoidance of illness or death, but the outcome of any objective can—in theory—be measured in various technical terms, for example, reduction of abortions or detection of cases of disease. However, it is important that the value of the effect in question reflects a (nonmonetary or monetary) benefit.

Unlike in health economics, where attempts have been made to harmonize CEA methodologies and encourage comparability of studies [27], there are no specific guidelines available yet for its application in animal health. The key is to select effectiveness measures that are meaningful; otherwise, they will not inform the allocation of scarce resources (see Part III). Ideally, they can be compared against some predefined standards or values that have been established in studies in the past. For example, if previous studies established that each day of earlier detection of a highly pathogenic avian influenza (HPAI) outbreak resulted in the avoidance of losses worth £100,000, a cost-effectiveness ratio of a surveillance system to early detect HPAI expressed as costs/days of earlier detection can be easily interpreted. However, without this information, effectiveness measures like time of introduction of disease until detection or the probability of detecting an outbreak are not informative in a CEA.

Further, surveillance generates other benefits that cannot be easily measured, but nonetheless have a value. Examples include consumer confidence, reputation, feelings of safety, contentment, peace of mind—all these have perceived values that are generally not converted to monetary values by the price system of the market. Therefore, indirect methods of valuation such as willingness-to-pay or stated choice preference approaches need to be adopted [28] (see Part III).

1.3.6.3 The Decision-Makers' Point of View (See Part VI)

Current world trade patterns and the globalization in general terms favor the rapid movement of people, animals, and material, resulting in increased risks of introduction of new diseases in a given territory. Animal health surveillance is an essential tool to detect disease or infection, to monitor disease trends, to facilitate the control of disease or infection, to support claims for freedom from disease or infection, to provide data for use in risk assessment, for animal, and/or public health purposes, and to substantiate the rationale for sanitary measures. Today, animal health surveillance programs play a key role in animal health policy (at national level and for EU, ASEAN, and other communities of countries of economic interests). They are fully integrated into most livestock industries, food production systems, and rural economies.

Priority setting, affordability, sustainability, social acceptance, and communication remain issues that policymakers have to consider when drafting and implementing their policy (Box 1.1: example of DM needs in France). In the spirit of the "prevention is better than cure," the policymaker wishes to promote the early identification of problems before they emerge while being ready to manage outbreaks and crises is a major objective. This approach leads on to reinforcing of biosecurity measures in all areas in which animals are found (farms, markets, border posts, transport vehicles, etc.).

Regulating animal surveillance as part of the animal health policy allows for coordinated and in the long run (hopefully) cheaper action on priorities, making it more effective and less expensive than actions by individual. For example, border controls for differing national lists of animal diseases are often inefficient and ineffective, given the movement of commodities (legal or illegal) that often overtake the limited resources for surveillance. Therefore, diseases of significance need to be addressed jointly within a same region. An action in one MS may however result in dissemination to others. Trade partners might also implement restrictions on imports if an outbreak is not properly controlled in one of the countries of the region.

During the last decade, all national administrations have seen their budgets severely reduced, resulting in the need to assess cost-effectiveness of their surveillance actions. These assessments are not that easy as the data available to quantify investments in surveillance and monitoring activities are very limited at both national and international levels. Secondly, surveillance activities overlap with multiple other public interventions and private management of the supply chains, both in terms of personal and resources. As a consequence, it is very difficult to define and allocate partial cost to a surveillance budget and very few attempts have been made to achieve this. Tools are required to help countries to perform a technical and budgetary optimization of their resources as a key instrument for the definition of their national policy for animal surveillance as part of the animal health policy (Box 1.1: example of DM needs in France).

Box 1.1 Limits of Economic Evaluation of Animal Health Management in Terms of Decision-Making: Example of Results from a Rapid Appraisal in France (Adapted from [29])

- Importance of political issues at stakes that are unlinked to scientific, technical, or economic-based evidence:
- Limited use of economic evaluation in decision-making process, in part due to the lack of tools.
- Lack of adapted and comprehensive economic evaluation tool that will account for
  - The multiplicity of actors and decision-making logics that result in a large diversity of behaviors
  - The complexity of the links between the actors
  - The lack of baseline situation knowledge.
  - The specific impact of one policy versus the others
  - The differences between programs implemented under the same policy.
  - The multiple objectives for one action

These data link back to the following questions that will be addressed within the RISKSUR project:

- What is the logic behind decision-making in animal health management?
- How to build up a practical and comprehensive tool to address decision-makers' needs?
- How to account for multiple objectives situation?

1.4 Conclusion on the Need for Animal Health Surveillance Evaluation

Setting up AH surveillance programs is becoming increasingly challenging as globalization, changing livestock trade patterns, and climate change impact on animal disease risks and create increasingly complex patterns of disease transmission and spread. In addition, public authorities and decision-makers, who are responsible for planning and implementing surveillance programs, are facing budget cuts, which makes it increasingly difficult to maintain and promote efficient and effective animal health surveillance. Decision-makers are looking for evidence on how to best use resources to establish fit-for-purpose surveillance, and effective evaluation is necessary to achieve this goal. Ideally, this should be done by providing a simple and practical guide for decision-makers.

Economic evaluation of health management programs implies to compare different policies to identify a solution that maximizes public welfare or at least generates a net benefit for society. Indeed, technical achievements are only a part of decision-making in the policy-formulation process. Economic evaluation of animal health surveillance is technically challenging because of its complex link to intervention, the technical capacity and data requirements needed to assess epidemiological and economic performance, and the lack of standardized metrics and practical tools for economic appraisals. These technical challenges stand in stark contrast with decision-makers' demand for a simple and practical guidance for performing systematic evaluation of existing or planned animal health surveillance systems, which in turn should result in the development of more effective policies.

The evaluation thus must provide a robust scientific foundation for the decision-making process while still presenting the findings in a user-friendly and applied format. There is a need for guidance on how to select appropriate evaluation questions (according to the context of surveillance), which method to use, and how feasible the evaluation is in a given time frame and available resources. This book aims to address this need.

References

1. Shahab S. Finding value in the evaluation of public health syndromic surveillance systems from a policy perspective. K. u. Search Canada, Alberta Health Services. 2009:24.
2. Granger LM. Global surveillance: suggestions for a strategic approach. FAO animal production and health proceedings. 2011; ISSN 1810-0732;14.
3. Taylor LH, Latham SM, and Woolhouse ME. Risk factors for human disease emergence. Philos Trans R Soc Lond B Biol Sci. 2001;356(1411):983–9.
4. Jebara KB. Surveillance, detection and response: managing emerging diseases at national and international levels. Rev Sci Tech. 2004;23(2):709–15.
5. Jann W, Wegrich K. Handbook of public policy analysis, untag-smd.ac.id; 2007.
6. World Animal Health Organisation (OIE). Animal Health Surveillance, in: Terrestrial Animal Health Code. OIE; 2019.
7. Häsler B, Garza M, Bisdorff B, Léger A, Tavornpanich S, Lindberg A, van Schaik G, Alban L, Stärk KD. Assessment on the adoption of recommended standards, novel approaches and best practices for animal health surveillance by decision makers in Europe 30; n.d.
8. Duteurtre V, Delabouglise A, Goutard F, Nguyen Viet Khong K, Duteurtre G, Roger F, Peyre M. Influenza aviaire au Vietnam: état des lieux et complémentarité des activités de surveillance et des études épidémiologiques (2007–2011). Rev D'élevage Médecine Vét Pays Trop. 2016;68:175. https://doi.org/10.19182/remvt.31165.
9. Jones KE, Patel NG, Levy MA, Storeygard A, Balk D, Gittleman JL, Daszak P. Global trends in emerging infectious diseases. Nature. 2008;451:990–3. https://doi.org/10.1038/nature06536.
10. Destoumieux-Garzón D, Mavingui P, Boetsch G, Boissier J, Darriet F, Duboz P, Fritsch C, Giraudoux P, Le Roux F, Morand S, Paillard C, Pontier D, Sueur C, Voituron Y. The one health concept: 10 years old and a long road ahead. Front Vet Sci. 2018;5:14. https://doi.org/10.3389/fvets.2018.00014.
11. Best Practices for risk-based and cost effective animal health surveillance, p. 110; n.d.
12. Julious SA, Mullee MA. Confounding and Simpson's paradox. BMJ. 1994;309:1480–1. https://doi.org/10.1136/bmj.309.6967.1480.
13. Alkin MC. Evaluation roots: a wider perspective of theorits' views and influences. 2nd ed. Washington DC: SAGE Publications Ltd; 2013.
14. Toma B, Dufour B, B2net JJ, Sanaa M, Shaw A, Moutou F, 2099. Epidemiologie appliquée à la lutte collective contre les maladies animales transmissibles majeures (3e éd.). Association pour l'étude de l'épidémiologie des maladies animales, Maisons-Alfort, 600 p.
15. Drewe JA, Hoinville LJ, Cook AJC, Floyd T, Stärk KDC. Evaluation of animal and public health surveillance systems: a systematic review. Epidemiol Infect. 2012;140:575–90. https://doi.org/10.1017/S0950268811002160.

16. Schulz K, Peyre M, Staubach C, Schauer B, Schulz J, Calba C, Häsler B, Conraths FJ. Surveillance strategies for Classical Swine Fever in wild boar – a comprehensive evaluation study to ensure powerful surveillance. Sci. Rep. 7, 43871; 2017. https://doi.org/10.1038/srep43871.
17. Schulz K, Calba C, Peyre M, Staubach C, Conraths FJ. Hunters' acceptability of the surveillance system and alternative surveillance strategies for classical swine fever in wild boar—a participatory approach. BMC Vet Res. 2016;12. https://doi.org/10.1186/s12917-016-0822-5.
18. Vergne T, Grosbois V, Jobre Y, Saad A, El Nabi AA, Galal S, Kalifa M, El Kader SA, Dauphin G, Roger F, Lubroth J, Peyre M. Avian influenza vaccination of poultry and passive case reporting, Egypt. Emerg Infect Dis. 2012;18:2076–8. https://doi.org/10.3201/eid1812.120616.
19. Antoine-Moussiaux N, Binot A, Chaudron M, Goutard F, Roger F, Peyre M. Socio-economic evaluation of animal health surveillance: principles and prospects. CIRADAFD Report, 41pp. Online access; 2011. http://revasia.cirad.fr/publications/rapports.
20. Calba C, Goutard FL, Hoinville L, Hendrikx P, Lindberg A, Saegerman C, Peyre M. Surveillance system evaluation: a systematic review of the existing approaches. BMC Public Health. 2015;15. https://doi.org/10.1186/s12889-015-1791-5.
21. Drewe JA, LJ. Hoinville, et al. Evaluation of animal and public health surveillance systems: a systematic review. Epidemiology and Infection. 2012;140(4):575–90.
22. Hoinville L. Animal Health Surveillance Terminology Final Report from Pre-ICAHS Workshop December 2011 (version 1.0).
23. Hoinville LJ, Alban L, Drewe JA, Gibbens JC, Gustafson L, Häsler B, Saegerman C, Salman M, Stärk K.D.C. Proposed terms and concepts for describing and evaluating animal-health surveillance systems, Preventive Veterinary Medicine. 2013;112:1–2. http://dx.doi.org/10.1016/j.prevetmed.2013.06.006.
24. Dehove A, Commault J, Petitclerc M, Teissier M, & Mace J. Economic analysis and costing of animal health: a literature review of methods and importance. Rev. Sci. Tech. 2012;31: 605–604.
25. Peyre M, Hoinville L, Njoroge J, Cameron A, Traon D, Goutard F, Calba C, Grosbois V, Delabouglise A, Varant V, Drewe J, Pfeiffer D, Häsler B. The RISKSUR EVA Tool (Survtool): a tool for the integrated evaluation of animal health surveillance systems. Prev Vet Med. 2019:104777. https://doi.org/10.1016/j.prevetmed.2019.104777.
26. Mclnerney JP, Howe KS, Schepers JA. A framework for the economic analysis of disease in farm livestock. Prev Vet Med. 1992;13:137–54.
27. Murray CJ, Evans DB, Acharya A, Baltussen R.M.P.M. Development of WHO guidelines on generalized cost-effectiveness analysis, Health Economics. 2000;9:235–51.
28. Antoine-Moussiaux N, Delabouglise A, Vu DT, Nguyen VK, Goutard F, Roger F, Peyre M. Social impact of HPAI surveillance network: Participatory evaluation at the community level in Vietnam 13th ISVEE conference, Maastricht, Netherlands, August. 2012:20–4.
29. Chaudron M. French only. Rentabilité de la surveillance épidémiologique des maladies animales dans les pays en développement: Contribution de l'évaluation économique et perspectives de recherche (Revue bibliographique et entretiens d'acteurs). Rapport de stage Master CEAV-SPV. AFD-CIRAD; 2010.

2 An Overview of the Different Types and Level of Evaluation: From Theory to Application in Health Surveillance

Marisa Peyre and Nicolas Antoine-Moussiaux

Abstract

Evaluation is a systematic assessment against standards, which can ascertain the degree/value of achievement, help in decision-making, enable reflection, and enable future changes. Different levels of evaluation may be considered including technical, process, economic, social, and political elements according to the needs and purpose of evaluation. In any evaluation process, one should always consider the point of view taken, the timing of evaluation, the period under evaluation, and the level of evaluation. This chapter presents some theoretical concept of evaluation ideology and reviews the different types of evaluation available in the literature and how they can be applied to evaluate animal health surveillance systems.

Keywords

Evaluation · Typology · Health surveillance

M. Peyre (✉)
CIRAD, UMR ASTRE, Montpellier, France

ASTRE, CIRAD, INRAE, University of Montpellier, Montpellier, France
e-mail: marisa.peyre@cirad.fr

N. Antoine-Moussiaux
Fundamental and Applied Research for Animals and Health (FARAH), University of Liège, Liege, Belgium

M. Peyre et al. (eds.), *Principles for Evaluation of One Health Surveillance: The EVA Book*, https://doi.org/10.1007/978-3-030-82727-4_2

2.1 Introduction

2.1.1 Evaluation Ideology and Classification Attempts

As developed by House [1], current evaluation models are based on a common liberal ideology. Hence, evaluation responds to fundamental features of liberalism: freedom of choice, individualism, and empiricism [1]. First, freedom of choice must be understood as conditioning the meaningfulness or usefulness of evaluation. Evaluation is indeed supposed to make sense with respect to one's decision-making, might it be that of the person under evaluation, of the evaluator, or the client of the evaluation. Second, individualism, which considers the individual to preexist to society, deeply influenced the methods of evaluation. Derived from economics, sociology, psychology, and often termed as methodological individualism, these methods consider the individual as the relevant unit to understand decision-making and the performance of a human system. Third, empiricism defines a mode of enquiry and knowledge, a relation to reality that is mediated through senses. Current evaluation methods may refer to objectivist ethics, when evaluation is founded on information that is congruent between independent observers or sensors (otherwise stated, information that can be verified). On the opposite, evaluations may follow subjectivist ethics, when considering any information derived from unique personal experiences, disregarding the need for or accepting the impossibility for cross-checking that information.

Evaluation approaches have been developed following two major disciplinary schools based on different ethical considerations: (i) *the utilitarian models*, where "the good" is determined by what maximizes some single, explicit interpretation of happiness for society as a whole; (ii) *the intuitionist or pluralist models*, which considers that there is no single interpretation of "the good" and these interpretations need not be explicitly stated nor justified (Table 2.1) [1, 3]. The utilitarian model is essentially based on objectivist methods that are used to acquire knowledge capable of external verification (intersubjective agreement) through publicly inspectable methods and data (e.g., experimental research). The intuitionist or pluralist models are mainly based on subjectivist methods used to acquire new knowledge based on existing personal knowledge and experiences that are (explicit) or are not (tacit) available for public inspection (e.g., accreditation).

Within these two main options, utilitarian and objectivist or pluralist and subjectivist, House [1] further distinguishes between eight types of evaluation (Fig. 2.1):

- *System analysis*, where evaluation looks at few quantitative measures (e.g., performance levels) and compares the differences in programs with different performance levels [1].
- *Behavioral objectives*, where program objectives are defined according to specific performance level that are linked to specific behaviors or actors in the system (Tyler model) [3].

Table 2.1 A taxonomy of major evaluation models (adapted from [1])

Type	Model	Major audiences	Assumes consensus on	Methodology		Outcomes		Typical questions	References
Utilitarian	System analysis	Decision makers, managers	Goals: Known cause and effect; quantified variables	Cost–benefit analysis	Objectivity	Efficiency	Social efficiency	Are the expected effect achieved? Can the effects be achieved more economically? What are the most efficient programs?	Rivlin [2]
	Behavioral, objectives		Prespecified objectives; quantified outcomes and variables	Attributes assessment		Productivity; accountability		Are the objectives achieved? Is the program producing?	Alkin [3]
	Decision-making		General goals; criteria	Surveys, questionnaires, interviews; natural variation		Effectiveness; quality control		Is the program effective? What parts are effective?	Vedung [4]
	Goal free	Consumers (mass)	Consequences; criteria	Bias controls, logical analysis; modus operandi		Consumer choice, social utility		What are *all* the effects?	Vedung [4]

(continued)

Table 2.1 (continued)

Type	Model	Major audiences	Assumes consensus on	Methodology		Outcomes		Typical questions	References
Intuitionist/ pluralist	Art criticism	Practitioners, consumers (elite)	Critics; standards	Critical review	Subjectivity	Improved standards	Personal understanding	Would an expert approve the program?	Mathison [5]
	Accreditation		Criteria, panel, procedures	Review by panel; self-study		Professional acceptance		How would professional rate this program?	Stufflebeam and Coryn [6]
	Adversary	Practitioners, consumers (mass)	Procedures and judges	Quasi-legal procedures		Resolution		What are the pros and the cons of the program?	Alkin [3]
	Transaction		Negotiations, activities	Case studies; interviews; observations		Understanding; diversity		How is the program perceived for different actors and people involved?	House [7]

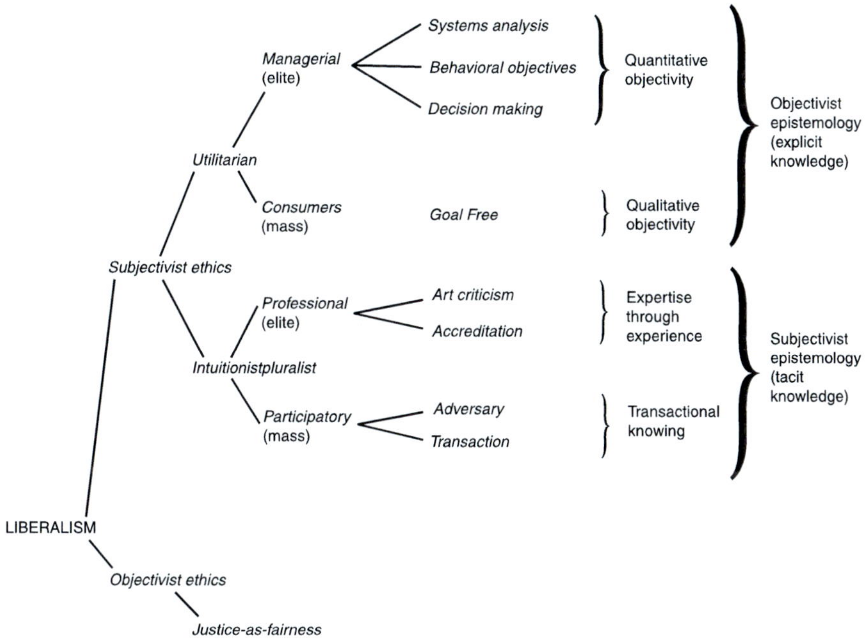

Fig. 2.1 A scheme relating major evaluation models to the philosophy of liberalism [1]

- *Decision-making*, which structures the evaluation by the decision to be made. Recommendations on these decisions have to be made by the evaluator (Stufflebeam model) [4].
- *Goal free*, which reduces the bias of the evaluation process by not informing the evaluator of the initial goal of the programs, the evaluator must explore all outcomes (Scriven's model) [4].
- *Art criticism*, where the evaluator has sufficient experience and training to make judgment on the program under evaluation (Eisner's artistic evaluation model) [5].
- *Accreditation*, which reviews pre-collected information by people who run the programs. The reviewers make comments approving or disapproving the program [3].
- *Adversary*, which is used to present the pros and cons of a program (quasi-legal procedures, often in the form of trial by jury) [3].
- *Transaction*, which concentrates on the process itself. It uses informal investigation methods based on empirical case studies (Stake's model) [7].

The type of evaluation implemented will also differ according to its target beneficiaries: *elite evaluation* focuses on the interests of managers and professionals (e.g., connoisseur studies), whereas *mass perspective evaluation* focuses on consumers and participatory approaches (e.g., consumer perception studies).

Evaluation may also be classified according to its objectivity level and its external influences:

- Pseudo-evaluation: Promotes a positive or negative view of an object regardless of what its value actually is and might be politically controlled (selected information), public relation (positive image).
- Quasi-evaluation: The questions orientation includes approaches that might or might not provide answers specifically related to the value of an object. For example, focusing only on questions of knowledge without addressing any questions of value (e.g., experimental research).
- *True evaluation*: The values orientation includes approaches primarily intended to determine the value of an object (e.g., decision-oriented, consumer-oriented studies).

2.1.2 Methodological Specificities

Objectivist methods will work on defining techniques others could use. The intuitionist relies on training and experience to ensure that truth is served (Table 2.2). The subjectivist approaches are less interested in the absolute truth than in relating the evaluation to the particular experience of the audience (their truth) in order to obtain valid insight from the group for whom the evaluation is done (which are the basic principles underlying participatory approaches). The evaluation is intentionally context-bound and findings are interpreted in context. Because of its greater experience of the context, "*the audience interpretation of an event may be superior to that of the evaluator*" [1]. Managerial utilitarian models (e.g., system analysis; behavioral, objectives; decision-making) require a common goal, a consensus on the goal of a particular program is reached, and this consensus defines the purpose of evaluation and the evaluation information generated is "scientifically objective" (because of based on quantitative facts rather than qualitative observations). These

Table 2.2 Main differences between the objective and subjective approach in current evaluation models

	Utilitarian approach—objective	Intuitionist/ pluralist approach—subjective
Validity	Predicting one observable category from another	Relative to the condition of the human mind. "What is valid for one person may not be valid for others."
Method	Defining techniques other could uses Prediction is the goal One individual perception is regarded as being subjective, objectivity comes with a number of congruent observations (intersubjective agreement)	Training and experience. Multiple perspectives. Qualitative emphasis rather than quantitative.
Utility	Maximizing society interest Rigid separation between observers and facts Single standard of social utility to be compared to	Maximizing the observer interest. Based on personal judgment and personal desire. Each individual is the best judge of event for himself.

models also rely on the cause and effect relationship. For example, Scriven model consists in reaching objectivity by controlling bias using a set of organizational and social approaches and relying on the intersubjectivity principle (Table 2.2).

2.1.3 Decision-Making in Evaluation Models

Classic liberalism sees society as an association of self-determining individuals who cooperate with others for self-interest ends [8]. Mills considers the individual best to judge of its own interest (internal sphere) and that the government (external sphere) should only interfere to maximize satisfaction (utility concept based on the utilitarian model: estimate of future consequences of various alternatives) (Fig. 2.2a). Mills recognized, however, that if the individuals are not the best judge then the state might legitimately interfere (Table 2.3, Fig. 2.2a). In modern liberalism and utilitarian models [2], the government provides the effectiveness standards to base the judgment and make the choices in the public interest (Table 2.3, Fig. 2.2b). Intuitionist/pluralist models rely on professional authority (e.g., art criticism; accreditation and adversary models) or a combination of scientific authority and participation in evaluation (Table 2.3). Only democratic pluralism based on groups rather than individual diversity sets the grounds for getting the government to act in a certain direction ("balance-of-power" theory) [1]. Stake states that the evaluator "must remain responsive to any legitimate interest" but is not obliged to represent any specific point of views. Only active involvement will push representation of a

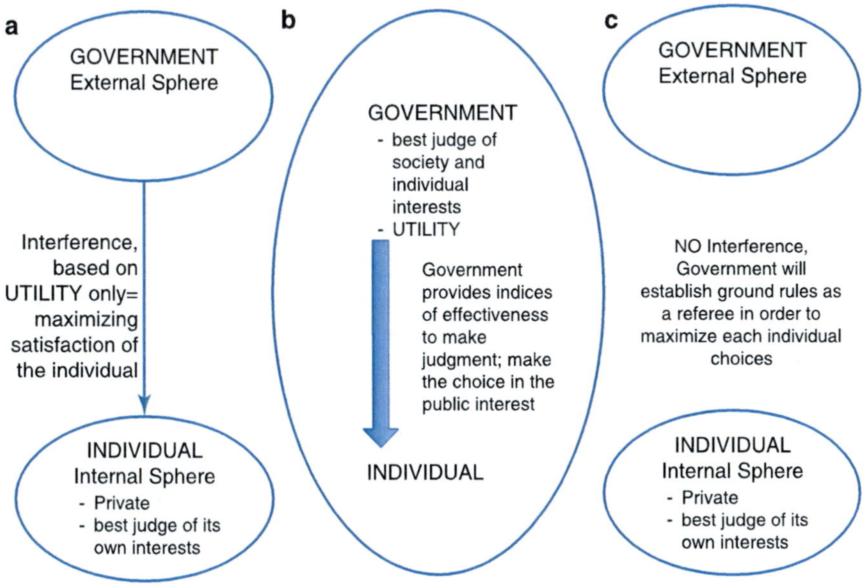

Fig. 2.2 Classical liberalism (Mills) (**a**); modern liberalism (Rivlin) (**b**); pluralism (Stakes) (**c**)

Table 2.3 Decision-making in evaluation models

Utilitarian evaluation models	Intuitionist/pluralist evaluation models
Relegate decision-making to the government. The government evaluates, defines the problems, and takes action to maximize social utility.	Rely on participatory decision-making to maximize local and individual choices rather than social utility. Problems are best solved directly by local people.

group point of view in the evaluation. In this way, legitimate groups define issues and only a few issues are to be explored.

2.1.4 Revisiting the Main Evaluation Models to Animal Health Evaluation

We have revisited the evaluation model typology presented in the previous section and developed by House in the 1970s and widely used until now, in line with the new developments in evaluation approaches in the field of animal and public health (Table 2.4).

All the models described in the previous section rely on the freedom of speech principle, which believes that only the competition of ideas will strengthen the truth. Under House typology, the managerial evaluation "has something of a watchdog function" and tends to be based on "scientifically objective information." Scientifically objective information is based on using objective methods such as tests or questionnaires to ensure reproducibility of the results. The data are analyzed using objective quantitative techniques in the sense that they can be verified by logical inspection regardless of who uses the techniques. In its extreme form, it entirely excludes nonquantitative data.

Until recently, health surveillance approach has followed a modern liberalism approach [2] (Fig. 2.2b), considering the government as the best judge of society interest and making choices in health surveillance strategies in the public interest. Mainly utilitarian objective evaluation approaches based on technical assessment of the effectiveness or efficiency have been implemented to follow this model.

Since a rising interest in improving animal health surveillance to prevent pandemics (see Chap. 1), evidence has shown that such models require either strong acceptability by the people implementing the action and/or strong regulation and/or strong enforcement and control. In any case, this requires high-level resources (human and financial). Low reporting or detection of disease is a major challenge in animal health surveillance. This could be reduced by active surveillance implementation, which also requires high level of resources. Moreover, recent work has highlighted issues beyond technical and resource ones, linked to social acceptability of the actions [15, 16]. Even in high-resources settings (e.g., industrial countries), it has become clear that other issues were at stake beyond regulation, control, and active implementation [17, 18].

Till now, evaluation in animal health has mainly also followed similar objective utilitarian models, which aims to ensure reliability of the outcomes; using methods

Table 2.4 Revisiting major evaluation model taxonomy, applied to animal health evaluation current approaches

Main evaluation question and objective	Evaluation type	Type of method		Decision-making	Examples	References
Is my system/component working? Evaluation of technical performances of the surveillance system	Technical effectiveness	Quantitative	Objective	Common goal/ target effectiveness	Capture/recapture method; new effectiveness rational	Grosbois et al. [9], Vergne et al. [10] (see Part V)
	Functional effectiveness	Qualitative (semi-quantitative)	Reduce bias of subjectivity	Individual perceptions	AccePT	Calba et al. [11] (see Part IV)
How, why, and under which conditions is my system/component working? Evaluation of surveillance system process and qualitative criteria	Process	Qualitative (semi-quantitative), expert consensus	Reduce bias of subjectivity	Common goal, standard ("ideal system")	OASIS, expert opinion	Hendrikx et al. [12] (see Part IV)
What is the value of my system/ component? Which option is the most relevant? Comparing alternatives, socioeconomic evaluations	Efficiency/ value	Quantitative	Objective	Maximizing society benefits	Cost–benefit analysis	Truong et al. [13] (see Part III)
	Efficiency/ value	Quantitative Multiple observer consensus	Reduce bias of subjectivity	Maximizing individual benefits for society benefit	Willingness to pay/ contingent valuation, choice experiments	Pham et al. [14] (see Part III)

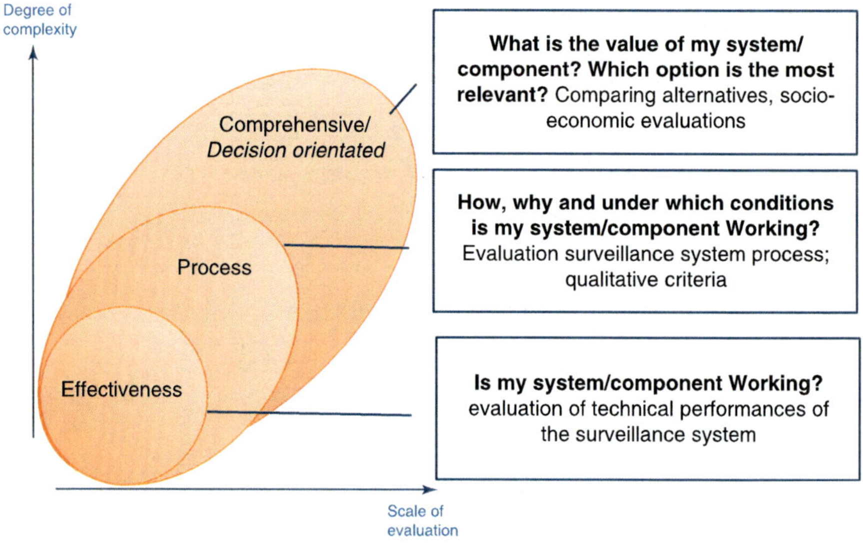

Fig. 2.3 Health surveillance evaluation scale, purpose, and degree of complexity

that will achieve high-observer agreement as opposed to procedures that may have much greater validity (Table 2.1, Fig. 2.1). As argued by House [1], utilitarian evaluation, even if based on quantitative or qualitative objectivity, could not guarantee performances of the programs in practice. Indeed, reliability is not a guarantee of validity.

In the past 10 years, we and other research groups have developed approaches to account for the individual perceptions following objective methodological approaches to benefit social efficiency (using personal understanding to improve social efficiency; ensuring that individual understanding will benefit to social efficiency), mixing up the different evaluation models to promote developmental evaluation approaches that do not advocate for any particular evaluation content, model, or method: such as *context evaluation, utilization-focused evaluation,* and *empowerment* (Box 2.1, Table 2.4, Fig. 2.3) [3].

Box 2.1 Developmental Evaluation Approaches [3]

Context evaluation: A "bottom-up" approach to (1) framing the questions and use the context; (2) negotiating agreement on acceptability of design, measures, and procedures; (3) data collection and reporting; and (4) interpretation and facilitation of use.

Utilization-focused evaluation: "The evaluation focus on the intended use of the evaluation outcomes by the intended users; it should be judged by its utility and actual use: looking at how real people in the real world apply evaluation findings and experience the evaluation process."

Empowerment evaluation: "Aims to increase the likelihood that programs will achieve results by increasing the capacity of program stakeholders to plan, implement, and evaluated their own programs."

2.2 The Different Types of Evaluation

2.2.1 The Different Purposes of Animal Health Surveillance Evaluation

The main objective of evaluation of animal health surveillance system is to promote changes and reflect on the system in place. Six main specific objectives have been identified related to design/planning, optimization of resource allocation, decision-making, quality of data, ensuring trade, and ensuring stakeholder trust (Fig. 2.4).

Evaluation provides advocacy elements for ad hoc changes of the system (fine tuning) and (re-)planning and (re)design, to terminate the activities (exit strategy) or to generate good practices information [19].

Evaluation of animal health surveillance system can have a different focus that will influence the evaluation question, the methods used, and the type of recommendations (Box 2.2).

Box 2.2 Different Evaluation Focus

Focus on facts and value judgment: A study designed to assist some audience to assess an object's merit and worth; for example, what are the strengths and weaknesses of my surveillance system process?

Focus on reaching objectives and quantitative measurement: A critical assessment, in an as objective manner as possible, of the degree to which a service or its component parts fulfill stated goals; for example, is the level of detection of disease cases sufficient to control the disease?

Focus on process and results (e.g., *M&E):* A systematic, rigorous, and meticulous application of scientific methods to assess the design, implementation, improvement, or outcomes of a program, based on predefined indicators; for example, what is the level of the specific performance indicators defined in my surveillance system.

Technical (or effectiveness) evaluation: Is about assessing the performances of a surveillance system (e.g., sensitivity, timeliness) to evaluate its capacity to reach its objective (e.g., disease control).

Process (or functional) evaluation: Is about assessing the conditions in which the system is performing and the elements of the system organisation and function that will affect its performances to make corrective actions to improve the system performances. Evaluation of the system process will allow to better understand the reasons behind limited performances. This will allow meaningful, adapted, and therefore more sustainable recommendations for effectiveness improvement, linked to the specific context of the system itself (see Part VI). Process evaluation will also allow to identify direct or indirect impact of a change in the surveillance activities, which will inform a cost-analysis (see Sect. 2.3)

OBJECTIVES OF THE EVALUATION OF SURVEILLANCE SYSTEMS[1]:

1. To inform the design and re-design: to facilitate choice between different options; to identify alternative options. E.g. to improve the system, to compare different design.
2. To inform local decision makers optimisation of resource allocation: balance between performances/improvement of the system and resources involved.
3. To inform local decision makers choice between different animal health management programmes: benefit of the system for the society.
4. To provide information on the quality of the surveillance data generated, and real disease situation.
5. To inform trade regulation authorities: quality of the surveillance data and real disease situation.
6. To ensure stakeholder trust is obtained: at local and global level; effect on sustainability and efficiency of the system; "to ensure trust and keep trust"

[1]Workshop results SVEPM 2015 Belgium

Fig. 2.4 Objectives of the evaluation of surveillance system [19]

Comprehensive or integrated evaluation: Is about integrating evaluation of system effectiveness and process to ensure all elements affecting the system performances are considered; this will improve sustainability and impact of the actions (e.g., assessing the system sensitivity and the acceptability of the actors of the system, which impacts the sensitivity level in order to promote changes to improve reporting and increase sensitivity) and could include economics (understanding decision-making in resource allocation by the system actors to improve its efficiency).

2.2.2 When to Evaluate

Evaluation can be performed *ex ante* (i.e., before the implementation of the system), *in itinere* (i.e., while the system is in place and running), or *ex post* (after the end of the system). Surveillance systems are rarely terminated; therefore, *ex ante* and *in itinere* are the most commonly applied moments for evaluation in animal health surveillance. Table 2.5 provides a link between timing and surveillance objectives. Figure 2.6 provides the list of potential trigger points that will motivate the need to evaluate.

- *Ex ante evaluation* is meant to be formative, that is, to provide essential elements to improve the value of the proposal, project, organization—could be performed to provide essential elements for the design and planning of the surveillance system. For example, epidemiological models could be used to evaluate which sampling protocol will ensure highest effectiveness of the system and therefore inform on the sampling design; *participatory* studies to assess the local constraints and the acceptability of surveillance could be implemented to select between different organization options (Fig. 2.5).

Table 2.5 Links between evaluation timing and objectives

Steps of the object under evaluation	*Ex ante*	*In itinere*	*Ex post*
Planning	Expected outputs, incomes, expected impact		
Design	How to reach the outputs, outcomes, impact		
Implementation	What to do to reach the outputs, outcomes, impact	Which outputs, outcomes, and impacts were reached and/or required outputs and outcomes to reach the impacts	
Redesign; replanning		What to implement to reach the missing/new outputs, outcomes, and impacts	Which outputs, outcomes, and impacts were reached What went wrong/right; what should be done/ corrected in a new process (lessons learnt)

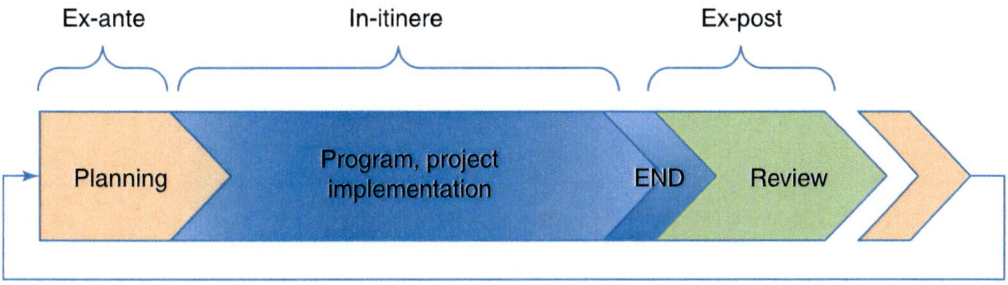

Fig. 2.5 The different timing of evaluation

- *In itinere* evaluation is meant to be corrective, that is, to adjust the value of the proposal, project, organization—implies either regular evaluation moments of the surveillance system (components), for example, annually, every 2 years, as needed. The timing for evaluation will depend on the purpose of surveillance, objective of the surveillance system (component), and on specific trigger points such as the evolution of the disease situation. It can be done to assess its performances and its added value. When done with regular intervals, it provides information on process efficacy and data output. Already when planning the system and its evaluation, it is good to include those elements that will trigger undertaking evaluation (Fig. 2.5).
- *Ex post* evaluation is meant to be assumptive, that is, drawing lessons from completed action, project ...—is very rare but can be implemented to identify lessons to be learned from the implementation and running of the surveillance system (component). The surveillance system (component) could have been exited due

DIRECT OR INDIRECT[1] TRIGGER POINTS FOR EVALUATION OF A SURVEILLANCE SYSTEM[2]

- Change in local disease situation, e.g. increase in outbreaks number, incursion of disease
- Change in disease control options
- Change in surveillance design, e.g. introduction of novel surveillance component
- Public health issue
- Change in neighbouring countries, international disease situation, e.g. increase in risk of introduction
- History of surveillance and timing since last evaluation
- Political request, legislative requirement
- Risk awareness perception issue; society perception
- Trade requirements
- Socio-economic context, e.g. reduction in budget triggers need for improve resources allocations and cost optimisation

[1]Those points could be interlinked
[2]Workshop results SVEPM 2015 Belgium

Fig. 2.6 Trigger points for evaluation in animal health

to sustainability issues or because the disease was eradicated (e.g., rinderpest surveillance) (Fig. 2.5).

2.3 Best Evaluation Practices

The American Evaluation Association has defined specific criteria for evaluators to ensure best practices in evaluation (source: American Evaluation Association; http://www.eval.org/p/cm/ld/fid=51):

- Implement systematic enquiry
- Adhere to highest technical standards
- Explore strengths and shortcomings of evaluation questions and approaches
- Communicate approaches, methods, and limitations accurately
- Hold appropriate competences to undertake the evaluation
- Show appropriate respect
- Take responsibilities in the implementation and reporting of the evaluation
- Ensure integrity/honesty including
  - Independence: no conflict of interest
  - Impartiality: considering all stakeholders; links between findings and recommendations
  - Transparency: all relevant stakeholders' needs to be aware of the evaluation aim and detail process: take into account general and public interests; include

all relevant stakeholders in the process; balance client and stakeholder needs; examine assumptions and potential side effects; present results in understandable forms

2.3.1 Evaluation of Best Practices Initiatives

- UN Evaluation Group: to establish UN norms and standards for evaluation (http://www.uneval.org/)
- OECD-DAC Evaluation Group: to improve development evaluation standards.
- MDB Evaluation Cooperation Group: to share lessons from MDB evaluations and promote evaluation harmonization and collaboration.
- BetterEvaluation initiative: to share information to improve evaluation (http://betterevaluation.org):
- "An international collaboration to improve evaluation practice and theory by sharing and generating information about options (methods or processes) and approaches."

2.4 Conclusion

We have seen that until recently evaluation in animal health had mainly been based on quantitative or qualitative objective approaches that could not guarantee performances of the programs in practice. It is therefore recommended to mix different evaluation approaches to take into consideration the specific context and needs of the users of the evaluation outcomes. This book aims to promote the use of such an integrated evaluation approach, under best evaluation practices, to account for technical, process, and socioeconomic aspects of surveillance systems. Specific methods to do so are presented through the different following parts of this book.

References

1. House ER. Assumptions underlying evaluation models. Educ Res. 1978;7:4–12. https://doi.org/10.3102/0013189X007003004.
2. Rivlin AM. Systematic thinking for social action. Brookings Institution Press; 2015.
3. Alkin MC. Evaluation roots: a wider perspective of theorits' views and influences. 2nd ed. Washington, DC: SAGE Publications Ltd; 2013.
4. Vedung E. Public policy and program evaluation. Transaction Publishers; 2009.
5. Mathison S. Encyclopedia of evaluation. SAGE; 2005.
6. Stufflebeam DL, Coryn CLS. Evaluation theory, models, and applications. John Wiley & Sons; 2014.
7. House ER. Evaluating with validity. IAP; 2010.
8. van de Haar E. Classical liberalism and international relations theory: Hume, Smith, Mises, and Hayek. Cham: Springer; 2009.

9. Grosbois V, Häsler B, Peyre M, Hiep DT, Vergne T. A rationale to unify measurements of effectiveness for animal health surveillance. Prev Vet Med. 2015;120:70–85. https://doi.org/10.1016/j.prevetmed.2014.12.014.
10. Vergne T, Del Rio Vilas VJ, Cameron A, Dufour B, Grosbois V. Capture–recapture approaches and the surveillance of livestock diseases: a review. Prev Vet Med. 2015;120:253–64. https://doi.org/10.1016/j.prevetmed.2015.04.003.
11. Calba C, Goutard FL, Vanholme L, Antoine-Moussiaux N, Hendrikx P, Saegerman C. The added-value of using participatory approaches to assess the acceptability of surveillance systems: the case of bovine tuberculosis in Belgium. PLoS One. 2016;11:e0159041. https://doi.org/10.1371/journal.pone.0159041.
12. Hendrikx P, Gay E, Chazel M, Moutou F, Danan C, Richomme C, Boue F, Souillard R, Gauchard F, Dufour B. OASIS: an assessment tool of epidemiological surveillance systems in animal health and food safety. Epidemiol Infect. 2011;139:1486–96. https://doi.org/10.1017/S0950268811000161.
13. Truong DB, Goutard FL, Bertagnoli S, Delabouglise A, Grosbois V, Peyre M. Benefit–cost analysis of foot-and-mouth disease vaccination at the farm-level in south Vietnam. Front Vet Sci. 2018;5:26. https://doi.org/10.3389/fvets.2018.00026.
14. Pham HTT, Peyre M, Trinh TQ, Nguyen OC, Vu TD, Rukkwamsuk T, Antoine-Moussiaux N. Application of discrete choice experiment to assess farmers' willingness to report swine diseases in the red River Delta region, Vietnam. Prev Vet Med. 2017;138:28–36. https://doi.org/10.1016/j.prevetmed.2017.01.002.
15. Delabouglise A, Antoine-Moussiaux N, Tatong D, Chumkaeo A, Binot A, Fournié G, Pilot E, Phimpraphi W, Kasemsuwan S, Paul MC, Duboz R, Salem G, Peyre M. Cultural practices shaping zoonotic diseases surveillance: the case of highly pathogenic avian influenza and Thailand native chicken farmers. Transbound Emerg Dis. 2017;64:1294–305. https://doi.org/10.1111/tbed.12506.
16. Masumbuko Claude K, Underschultz J, Hawkes MT. Social resistance drives persistent transmission of Ebola virus disease in eastern Democratic Republic of Congo: a mixed-methods study. PLoS One. 2019;14:e0223104. https://doi.org/10.1371/journal.pone.0223104.
17. Calba C, Antoine-Moussiaux N, Charrier F, Hendrikx P, Saegerman C, Peyre M, Goutard FL. Applying participatory approaches in the evaluation of surveillance systems: a pilot study on African swine fever surveillance in Corsica. Prev Vet Med. 2015;122:389–98. https://doi.org/10.1016/j.prevetmed.2015.10.001.
18. Schulz K, Calba C, Peyre M, Staubach C, Conraths FJ. Hunters' acceptability of the surveillance system and alternative surveillance strategies for classical swine fever in wild boar—a participatory approach. BMC Vet Res. 2016;12:187. https://doi.org/10.1186/s12917-016-0822-5.
19. Risksur Consortium. Best Practices for risk-based and cost effective animal health surveillance. p. 110; 2015.

Part II

What to Evaluate and How

Frameworks and Tools for Evaluating Health Surveillance Systems

3

Marisa Peyre, Mo Salman, and Katie Steneroden

Abstract

Health surveillance systems are complex as they can target different types of objectives—early disease detection to prevent introduction and case detection to ensure disease control or demonstration of freedom from disease. Such systems are designed as networks of multiple actors with different needs and constraints. To allow for the design of cost-effective systems, timely evaluation is required. In 2015, Calba et al. reviewed the existing animal health evaluation frameworks, highlighting their limits and the need to develop an integrated approach to epidemiological and economic evaluation of surveillance systems. This work emphasized the need to build from current evaluation approaches and also the importance of promoting assessment of attributes covering the social and economic aspects of animal health surveillance. All surveillance systems require continuous evaluation to improve effectiveness, expected outcomes, and impact. The aim of this chapter is to build on the past 10 years of work in this area and propose a step-by-step framework to facilitate the evaluation of animal health surveillance systems.

Keywords

Evaluation · Health surveillance · Evaluation framework · Decision making · Process evaluation

M. Peyre (✉)
CIRAD, UMR ASTRE, Montpellier, France

ASTRE, CIRAD, INRAE, University of Montpellier, Montpellier, France
e-mail: marisa.peyre@cirad.fr

M. Salman (✉) · K. Steneroden
College of Veterinary Medicine and Biomedical Sciences, Colorado State University, Fort Collins, USA
e-mail: m.d.salman@colostate.edu

M. Peyre et al. (eds.), *Principles for Evaluation of One Health Surveillance: The EVA Book*, https://doi.org/10.1007/978-3-030-82727-4_3

3.1 Introduction

Animal disease monitoring and surveillance systems have been used by many to summarize the concepts and approaches involved in effective disease surveillance [1]. The term monitoring describes a continuous, adaptable process of collecting data about diseases and their determinants in a given population in the absence of immediate control activities. The term surveillance is used to describe a specific type of monitoring where control or eradication measures are implemented on the reference population whenever certain threshold levels related to adverse health status have been exceeded. Surveillance is usually directed at a specific disease or problem and implies that there are actions to be taken when thresholds occur, and therefore by definition surveillance is an active part of a disease control program [2]. For the purpose of this chapter, a surveillance system will include elements of both monitoring and surveillance activities.

An animal disease surveillance system is composed of various objectives with the overall aim of systematic collection, analysis, and interpretation of animal health-related data needed for the planning, implementation, and evaluation of animal disease mitigation strategies.

The objectives of the system are

- Early detection and early warning activities with the aim *to reduce the impact of underlying animal diseases.*
- Monitoring and verification of disease events in their natural environment to *mitigate the specific levels of these events as they occur.*
- Evaluation and ranking of disease events to *assign priority for plan of action according to the collected data.*
- Assessing the various mitigation strategies for effectiveness with the aim to implement these strategies assessing? With the required *modifications and/or policy to the surveillance system.*

As a system, the above objectives are required for a comprehensive and functional program. The majority of current surveillance systems, however, do not contain all the necessary objectives, and depending on the program's specific aim, may only focus on one or more of them. Nevertheless, long-term success of a comprehensive surveillance system depends on inclusion of all the above objectives.

Surveillance systems are complex and need to consider the principles of epidemiology driven by epidemiological, economic, social (including political, cultural), and environmental factors in interactive ways. To allow for the design of cost-effective systems, the plan needs to consider practical and affordable assessment frameworks for timely evaluation of the benefits and costs of the system. Additionally, the assessment must be accepted by the local users and providers of the system [3–5].

In 2015, Calba et al. reviewed the existing animal health evaluation frameworks, highlighting their limits and the need to develop an integrated approach to epidemiological and economic evaluation of surveillance systems. This work emphasized the need to build from current evaluation approaches and also the importance of promoting assessment of attributes covering the social and economic aspects of animal health surveillance (AHS).

All surveillance systems require continuous evaluation to improve effectiveness, expected outcomes, and impact. The aim of this chapter is to propose a step-by-step framework to facilitate the evaluation of animal health surveillance systems. This chapter will build on previous suggested methods [1] and provide detailed steps in conducting animal health surveillance system evaluation methods.

3.2 Evaluation Vs. Assessment

The terms "assessment" and "evaluation" are interrelated. Assessment is the systematic process of documenting and using empirical data on the knowledge, skills, attitudes, and beliefs of the users and providers of the system. The evaluators attempt to improve the operation of the system. For example, an assessor will measure the sensitivity of a system and compare it to a target value to assess if the system is sensitive enough. If the sensitivity is below the defined threshold, the assessor suggests a procedure to increase the overall sensitivity, for example, by broadening the case definition of the required reported health event for the underlying disease.

Evaluation, on the other hand, focuses on the output and performance of a system in relation to achieving its stated aim. Evaluation is a comprehensive or a quality review of the system. Evaluation processes normally involve some standards, criteria, measures of performance, or objectives that describe the value of the system outcome. Evaluation can identify criteria for success, lessons learned, things to achieve, ways to improve the work, and the means to move forward. Thus, evaluation is product-oriented specifically to respond to the question: "What's been achieved or impacted?" The aim of evaluation is to help the decision makers and reviewers of the progress determine the success or effectiveness of a system. It provides a comprehensive description of a system including insight into its operation. The evaluation may be subjective or objective depending on the performance indices or the matrices that are used in the evaluation. To follow up on the above example for assessment, the evaluation of a surveillance system indicates that the system as in its current operation is *not* adequate to be used for early detection of the underlining disease. It does not, however, mean the system is not efficient in other objectives of its surveillance activities.

3.3 Overview of Current Animal and Human Health Surveillance Evaluation Guides: Advantages and Limits

Many evaluation guides are available in the literature to undertake an evaluation process. In 2015, those guides were reviewed to identify the gaps and needs of current methods and provide elements to help the user select the most appropriate approach [6] (Table 3.1). Sixteen evaluation approaches have been reported, mainly developed in the area of public health (PH) (10 approaches) but also in animal

Table 3.1 Health surveillance evaluation guides (adapted from [6])

Reference	Name	Year	Topic of surveillance	Type
Peyre et al.	Survtool (EVA)	2017	AH	Integrated framework
Drewe et al.	SERVAL	2013	AH	Framework
El Allacki et al.	Conceptual evaluation	2012	AH and PH	Method
Hendrikx et al.	OASIS	2011	AH	Tool
Dufour	CCP	1999	AH	Method
Malecki et al.	–	2008	EPH	Framework
WHO	IPCAT	2011	PH	Tool
WHO	HMN assessment and monitoring tool	2008	PH	Tool
Meynard et al.	–	2008	PH	Framework
ECDC	–	2006	PH	Framework
WHO	–	2006	PH	Guidelines
HSCC	–	2004	PH	Framework
KTL	–	2004	PH	Tool
Buehler et al. (CDC)	–	2004	PH	Framework
German et al. (CDC)	–	2001	PH	Guidelines
WHO	–	1997	PH	Framework

health (AH—4 approaches) one approach in both PH and AH and one approach in environmental health (Table 3.1). Although several technical reports and publications were produced under the topic of animal health programs, none to our knowledge have proposed a framework for a comprehensive evaluation of animal health surveillance systems until 2012. Building upon an existing framework, an innovative framework was developed within the RISKSUR project to fill in these gaps and allow for both design and evaluation of animal health surveillance systems (Survtool EVA) [7, 8].

Peyre et al. [8] highlighted the need for standardization of the terminology used in these evaluations and a requirement for the definition of gold standards, efficiency, and effectiveness measures. The absence of these required components reduces the ability to compare different systems, and therefore, the identification of systems that are most efficient would be difficult. Indeed, several evaluation approaches are available, and most of those have been developed and used on an ad hoc basis. The criteria considered by each approach are usually organized into a template structure, which controls the logical flow of the evaluation process. Various terms have been used to describe these processes (e.g., guidelines, method, framework, tool).

In animal health, there is not a single performance index to measure the effectiveness such as disability-adjusted life-years (DALYs) and quality-adjusted life-years (QALYs) that exist in public health. Specific evaluation of surveillance has been performed only on limited occasions, and a variety of approaches and methods are used without generally agreed upon protocols [9]. Indeed, more than 25 attributes have been described for the evaluation of animal health surveillance systems, making a complete evaluation time-consuming and expensive [7, 9, 10]. Economic evaluation activities currently focus mainly on disease control programs and economic impact of diseases in populations [11]. The work performed within the RISKSUR consortium also highlighted the relatively small number of papers published on the subject of economic evaluation of surveillance.

The main recommendations of the review were (i) the need for a structured evaluation process for animal surveillance systems that allows for flexibility in the selection of evaluation attributes and attribute assessment methods to make it context specific (this has been developed as part of the Survtool framework (see Chap. 4); (ii) the need to design a glossary of evaluation terms (to complement the existing "surveillance glossary"; [10])—such a glossary is available at the end of this book and here: https://www.fp7-risksur.eu/terminology/glossary; and (iii) to develop a set of internationally recognized and standardized effectiveness metrics for economic evaluation of animal health surveillance (see Sect. 3.3).

3.4 The Evaluation Process

The evaluation process could be represented as a cycle of seven main steps organized in three different phases (Fig. 3.1):

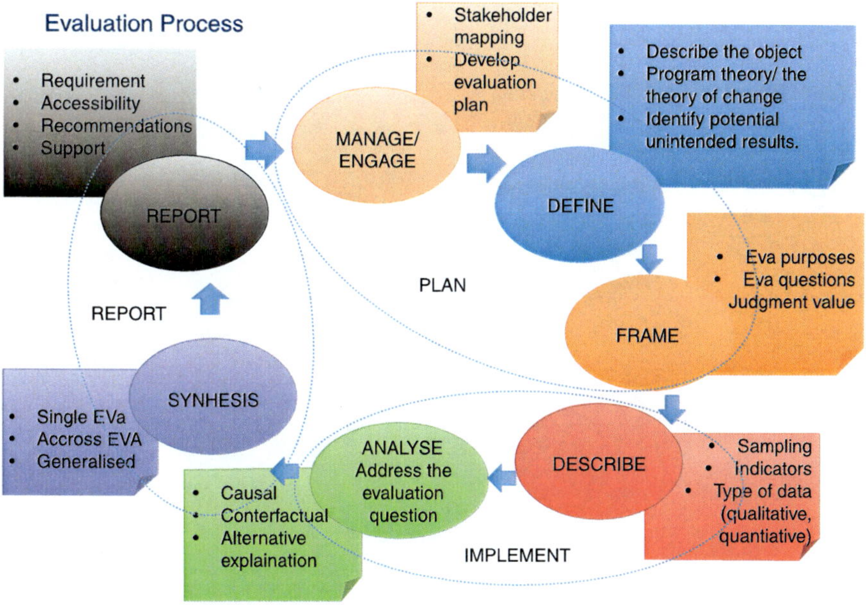

Fig. 3.1 The evaluation process cycle

- Phase I is *to plan* the evaluation and define the aim (underlying questions), required resources, and needs of the evaluation. This involves engaging with the decision makers via stakeholder mapping and workshops to identify, together, the gaps and frame the evaluation plan.
- Phase II is *to implement* the evaluation with a description of the detailed methods used to achieve the evaluation aims, including the use of analytical tools.
- Phase III is *to report* on the evaluation: The reporting step is essential to ensure that the results will be taken over by the relevant stakeholders or the decision makers. The initial requirements of the evaluation should be answered along with accessibility of the results to nonscientific audiences and the provision of meaningful recommendations.
- The outcomes of the evaluation will inform the next evaluation cycle; this will ensure lessons are learned and that the planning of the next evaluation is based on evidence generated by the first one.

3.4.1 Planning Phase

The planning phase includes three main aspects: managing/engaging, defining, and framing (Fig. 3.2).

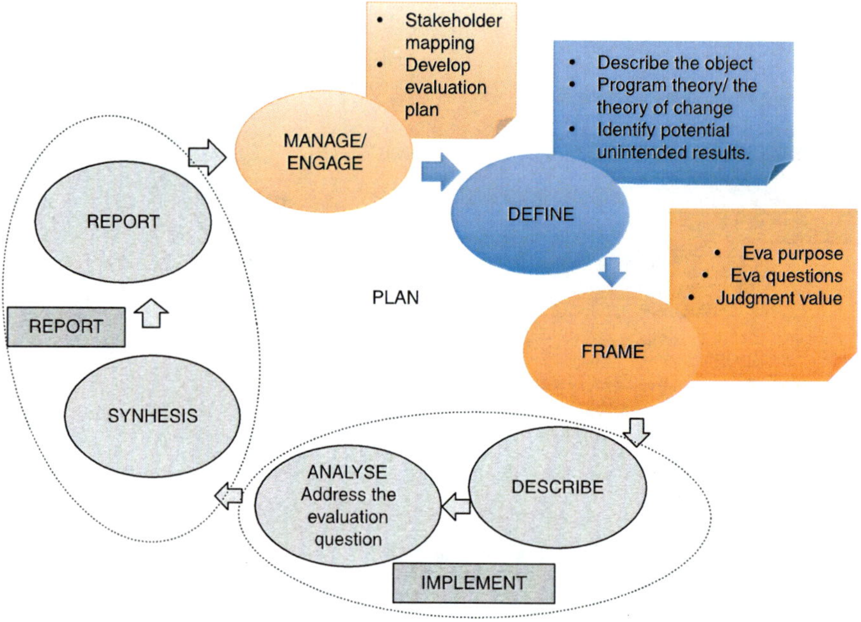

Fig. 3.2 The planning phase of the evaluation process

3.4.1.1 Engaging Stakeholders

The first step in the evaluation process is to plan the evaluation and define the object and context of the evaluation. This involves engaging with the decision makers via a stakeholder mapping and workshop to identify, with them, the gaps and needs required to frame the evaluation plan. This will contribute to ensuring uptake of the recommendations by the people that implement and therefore impact the evaluation activity (see Part VI).

Determine the stakeholders: Data collection is the main activity of a surveillance system. Providers of the data are essential streams to ensure both reliability and accuracy of the data. The collected data should, as much as possible, serve the aim of the system including the users of the findings. Both providers and users are involved in making decisions, participating in program activities, or are affected by those activities. The program may have both primary and secondary stakeholders. The primary stakeholders are those who are directly involved in or directly affected by the program's outcomes. Secondary stakeholders are those who are less involved and less affected by the program but may have some either short- or long-term involvement or could influence the program outcomes, which could still be important to include (e.g., the Ministry of Health for surveillance programs not related to zoonotic diseases). The implementers of the program will be the starting point to determine a list of stakeholders.

3.4.1.2 Needs and Required Resources for the Evaluation

When engaging with stakeholders, needs and resources for the evaluation must be identified. The following list of essential items can be used to determine the resources and needs including gaps in the system (Table 3.2):

- The official name/title of the system and its program. The program is usually the official public designation of the system, and the system is the technical procedure or the protocol to be administrated by the program.
- The list of the people and their credentials that are involved in the execution of the protocol. This list may include previous and currently involved people if there is a long history of the ongoing surveillance system.
- The aim(s) of the program in both technical and governance format (e.g., all the legislative documents that formalize the program or specify its framing).
- Outputs, or at least some recent results of the program, particularly communiques with users and providers of the program.
- The proposed protocol to meet the expected outcomes.

The above items provide the background information that will help to make choices about how the evaluation needs to be carried out (Why? What? How?). Evaluation is bound to a specific context (i.e., the surveillance system, the nature of the disease, the decision maker's needs, the cost requirements, legal requirements, etc.). It is essential to define the evaluation question(s) and determine the required analytical tools (Table 3.2).

Table 3.2 Essential elements of context to frame the evaluation process

Context elements	Relevance
Surveillance objective	Impacts on the selection of evaluation attributes
Hazard name	Provides information on the disease under evaluation, which will impact the complexity of the evaluation (e.g., between animal disease and zoonotic diseases)
Geographical area	Provides information on the scale of evaluation
Legal requirements	Provides information on the need to meet an effectiveness target or not
Strengths and weaknesses about current approach	Provides summary information on the rationale behind the decision to evaluate
Stakeholder concerns about current approach	Provides information on the involvement and interest of decision makers in the evaluation process
Alternative strategies to consider	Provides information on the type of evaluation required (based on a counterfactual or not)
Do you want to evaluate or change the system or some components in the system?	Provides information on the level of evaluation
How many components will you include in this evaluation?	Provides information on the number of counterfactual considered
Are you considering risk-based options?	Relevant for the inclusion of the attribute risk-based criteria definition in the evaluation plan
Will you consider the costs of surveillance in your evaluation?	Provides information on the interest of economic evaluation
Do you know the current cost of your system and/or components?	Provides information on the data required
Do you have a budget constraint?	Provides information to define the economic evaluation (meeting a budget target or not)

3.4.2 Framing the Evaluation

3.4.2.1 Define the Purpose of the Evaluation

The evaluation process should include a clear statement of the type of evaluation undertaken. Such statement should be shared with the implementers of the system and program prior to the initiation of the evaluation process so that there is an agreement on the expected outcomes. The type and complexity level of evaluation performed will be framed according to its purpose and expected outcomes to ensure efficient use of resources. Specific processes may be required if the purpose of the evaluation is to demonstrate how the program is satisfying its proposed surveillance stream(s), using its resources, and whether any modifications in its process are required. In contrast, a different process using outcome and impact evaluation may be required if the purpose is to assess the extent to which the surveillance system has affected its participants or the environment. Following agreement on the evaluation purpose, clear evaluation question(s) should be formulated to help in the selection of evaluation tools and methods. The evaluation statement may require revision until all of the technical staff of the surveillance system agree.

3.4.2.2 How to Define the Evaluation Question(S)?

The evaluation questions could be of multiple natures: *descriptive* (e.g., what is the current situation, how is the system organized?); *causal*, trying to understand the factors that contribute to the results of the surveillance (e.g., what are the system organization aspects that affect the effectiveness of the system?); *technical*, trying to understand what could be done better and which alternatives will be best (e.g., is the system/component cost-effective?); and *functional*, related to identifying changes that should be made to improve the system (e.g., what are the strengths and weaknesses of the system). It is important to notice that those questions could be interlinked and more than one type of question could be asked during an evaluation process. For example, if someone wants to know how the surveillance system is performing, what factors are influencing its effectiveness and which corrective action should be implemented to improve it.

The important elements to consider when defining evaluation questions are

- Which evaluation level—system or component?
- Which element of evaluation to include—process, effectiveness, economic?
- Which economic evaluation question—cost-optimization, cost-effectiveness, cost–benefit?

A list of 11 evaluation questions have been defined by experts to account for diverse evaluation needs (Table 3.3) [8]. A decision tree pathway was also developed to assist the user with the choice of the evaluation questions. In this pathway, the users are guided through a series of questions (11 in the longest pathway) to define their evaluation priorities (e.g., system or component evaluation; previous knowledge of effectiveness; need for economic analysis) and identify the most relevant evaluation question. This guidance pathway to assist with the choice of the evaluation questions can also be found in Survtools (Table 3.3) [8].

3.4.3 Which Evaluation Attributes Should Address the Question(s)?

The evaluation of a surveillance system and its components will look at different aspects of the system according to the purpose and evaluation questions. A set of evaluation attributes to assess these aspects have been previously defined and are presented in Table 3.3 [8, 10].

The following attributes that influence the overall quality of the system have been characterized according to the following criteria [1, 13].

Simplicity, acceptability, and practicality of the surveillance system: The execution of the system should be as much as possible simple in its operation and practical in its approach in order to obtain reliable data and information. A critical evaluation of the system requires engagement of the stakeholders (providers and users of the system) using, for example, participatory approaches and focus group discussions. Appropriate, constructive sets of questions to determine their

Table 3.3 Evaluation attributes (adapted from [10, 12])

Category	Attribute name	Attribute definition
Organizational	Risk-based criteria definition	Validity and relevance of the risk criteria selected and the approach/method used for their identification.
	Surveillance system organization	An assessment of the organizational structures and management of the surveillance system including the existence of clear, relevant objectives, the existence of steering and technical committees whose members have relevant expertise and clearly defined roles and responsibilities, stakeholder involvement, and the existence of effective processes for data management and dissemination of information.
Functional	Availability and sustainability	The ability to be operational when needed (availability) and the robustness and ability of system to be ongoing in the long term (sustainability).
	Acceptability and engagement	Willingness of persons and organizations to participate in the surveillance system, the degree to which each of these users is involved in the surveillance. Could also assess their beliefs about the benefits or adverse consequences of their participation in the system including the provision of compensation for the consequence of disease detection.
	Simplicity	Refers to the surveillance system structure, ease of operation, and flow of data through the system.
	Flexibility, adaptability	The ability to adapt to changing information needs or operating conditions with little additional time, personnel, or allocated funds. The extent to which the system can accommodate collection of information about new health hazards or additional/alternative types of data; changes in case definitions or technology; and variations in funding sources or reporting methods should be assessed.
	Compatibility	Compatibility with and ability to integrate data from other sources and surveillance components, e.g., one health surveillance (part of data collection and data management).
	Multiple hazard	Whether the system captures information about more than one hazard.
Effectiveness	Coverage	The proportion of the population of interest (target population) that is included in the surveillance activity.
	Representativeness	The extent to which the features of the population of interest are reflected by the population included in the surveillance activity; these features may include herd size, production type, age, sex, or geographical location or time of sampling (important for some systems, e.g., for vector-borne disease).
	False alarm rate (inverse of specificity)	Proportion of negative events (e.g., nonoutbreak periods) incorrectly classified as events (outbreaks). This is the inverse of the specificity but is more easily understood than specificity.
	Bias = accuracy	The extent to which a prevalence estimate produced by the surveillance system deviates from the true prevalence value. Bias is reduced as representativeness is increased.

	Precision	How closely defined a numerical estimate is. A precise estimate has a narrow confidence interval. Precision is influenced by prevalence, sample size, and surveillance approach used.
	Timeliness	Timeliness can be defined in various ways: • This is usually defined as the time between any two defined steps in a surveillance system; the time points chosen are likely to vary depending on the purpose of the surveillance activity. • For planning purposes, timeliness can also be defined as whether surveillance detects changes in time for risk mitigation measures to reduce the likelihood of further spread. The precise definition of timeliness chosen should be stated as part of the evaluation process. Some suggested definitions for the RISKSUR project are *For early detection and demonstrating freedom* • Measured using time—Time between introduction of infection and detection of outbreak or presence by surveillance system • Measured using case numbers—Number of animals/farms infected when outbreak or infection detected *For case detection to facilitate control* • Measured using time—Time between infection of animal (or farm) and their detection • Measured using case numbers—Number of other animals/farms infected before case detected *For detecting a change in prevalence* • Measured using time—Time between increase in prevalence and detection of increase • Measured using case numbers—Number of additional animals/farms infected when prevalence increase is identified
	Sensitivity (detection probability and detection fraction)	Sensitivity of a surveillance system can be considered on three levels. • *Surveillance sensitivity (case detection probability)* refers to the proportion of individual animals or herds in the population of interest that have the health-related condition of interest that the surveillance system is able to detect. Sensitivity could be measured in terms of *detection fraction* (number of cases detected divided by the coverage level) in a context of nonexhaustive coverage. • *Surveillance sensitivity (outbreak detection)* refers to the probability that the surveillance system will detect a significant increase (outbreak) of disease. This may be an increase in the level of a disease that is not currently present in the population or the occurrence of any cases of disease that are not currently present. • *Surveillance sensitivity (presence)* refers to the probability that disease will be detected if present at a certain level (prevalence) in the population.
	PPV	The probability that health event is present given that health event is detected.

(continued)

Table 3.3 (continued)

Category	Attribute name	Attribute definition
	NPV	The probability that no health event is present given that no health event is detected.
	Robustness	The ability of the surveillance system to produce acceptable outcomes over a range of assumptions about uncertainty by maximizing the reliability of an adequate outcome. Robustness can be assessed using info-gap models.
Value	Cost	The concept of economic cost includes (1) the losses due to disease (e.g., reduced milk yield, mortality) and (2) the resources required to detect the disease by a system (e.g., time, services, consumables for surveillance). In economic evaluation, the resources used to detect disease are compared with the disease losses with the aim to identify an optimal balance where a higher economic efficiency is achieved. Estimation of the total economic cost stemming from losses and expenditures is called a disease impact assessment. Estimation of the resource expenditures only is called a cost analysis.
	Benefit	The benefit of surveillance quantifies the monetary and nonmonetary positive direct and indirect consequences produced by the surveillance system and assesses whether users are satisfied that their requirements have been met. This includes financial savings, better use of resources, and any losses avoided due to the existence of the system and the information it provides. These avoided losses may include the avoidance of • animal production losses • human mortality and morbidity • decrease in consumer confidence • threatened livelihoods • harmed ecosystems • utility loss Often, the benefit of surveillance estimated as losses avoided can only be realized by implementing an intervention. Hence, it is necessary to also assess the effect of the intervention and look at surveillance, intervention, and loss avoidance as a three-variable relationship. Further benefits of surveillance include maintained or increased trade, improved ability to react in case of an outbreak of disease, maintaining a structured network of professionals able to react appropriately against a (future) threat, maintaining a critical level of infrastructure for disease control, increased understanding about a disease, and improved ability to react in case of an outbreak of disease.

understanding of the aim of the surveillance and its added value to the community are required. The composition of the focus groups should as much as possible represent providers and users of the system. For example, a focus group for a surveillance system for vesicular swine diseases should include representatives from swine industry, local swine farmers, private swine practitioners, and public animal health field officers. In addition to the questions, a relevant scenario to reflect collection of data and presentation of the findings can be used as a tool to obtain responses to determine the practicality of the system. Calba et al. [6] have developed a methodology based on participatory approaches to assess the acceptability of the system by its stakeholders looking at different aspects including their understanding and trust in the system organization (including its simplicity to operate) and objectives (cf. Sect. 3.4) [6, 14]. Using a community-based approach (CBA) and qualitative social science methods will aid in creating and ensuring a system that is understood, accepted, and practical to the community. Community members can be asked specific questions to determine their understanding of the specific surveillance system during the design and implementation of a project. CBAs have proven successful because the most appropriate solutions for problems that arise in communities are frequently best addressed by persons directly affected, who have intimate knowledge of the situation and involvement in decisions. A CBA is a cost-effective and efficient disease control method over the long term. There are two main parts to a CBA: situation analysis and community mobilization for empowerment. Situation analysis includes several parts: information analysis, stakeholder analysis, establishing contact with the community, participatory evaluation, and participatory planning. The United Nations High Commissioner for Refugees explained that information analysis is the phase in which is known information from existing documents and data. Community mobilization requires precise and accurate statements of the required actions from as well as the benefits to every entity of the stakeholders.

Stability, flexibility, and adaptability: Stability of the system in terms of its flexibility and adaptability related to unexpected health and/or political events should be assessed prior to and during the implementation of the program. Prior to implementation, the evaluators can provide a hypothetical scenario with a scoring sheet to determine the response and accommodation of the system to event such as emerging diseases or unexpected adverse health events. The scenario should be related to the specific aim of the surveillance system.

Cultural sensitivity: The system and its activities should be acceptable to the community in which it is applied. A social and cultural checklist that is used for assessing the evaluation of adaptability can be used both during the planning of the system and the evaluation as well. The Australian Institute of Health and Welfare has highlighted several great issues to be considered in the evaluation to account for those cultural aspects, for example, during the avian influenza outbreak in Indonesia in 2005–2006, leaders of mosques and villages were consulted on implementation of specific objectives of a surveillance system with the aim to enhance the reliability of the system [15]. Delabouglise et al. [4] have shown the importance of cultural and socioeconomic factors in the performances of avian influenza surveillance system performances in Thailand and Vietnam [4] (see Parts IV and VI).

Stakeholder communication: The method of communication of a surveillance evaluation will depend on the different stakeholders, their familiarity with the details of the surveillance system, and their anticipated or intended actions. How, when, and why stakeholders will be communicated with is an appropriate activity to undertake during the planning stages of the evaluation—so that the appropriate data is gathered at the outset and the appropriate method of distribution considered. The evaluation must be clear, action oriented, and easily distributed. It should also be geared to the particular stakeholder. Stakeholders who are directly involved in the surveillance, its design, and activities may require little need for interpretation of evaluation findings. Because they have significant knowledge of the system and underlying processes, details on the background, etc., will be less necessary. The evaluation report will be result oriented, allowing for interpretation. Evaluation reports intended for stakeholders who may not be as familiar with the surveillance system may require more information, including background, data collection methods, and analysis. Interpretation of the findings will need to be elaborated upon. Interpretive reports do not just provide the results of data collection, but put the results in context including, if appropriate, changes over time. When necessary, evaluation reports can also take the form of information sheets for lay audiences for those who may not have a high level of knowledge on the surveillance topic [1]. Depending on the surveillance system being evaluated, other means of communication of findings may be appropriate including peer reviewed journal articles, abstracts or posters given at professional meetings, lay press news items, books, book chapters, and web-based publications [1].

Overall sensitivity of system: Most systems require an overall high sensitivity particularly when their priority is for early detection of cases. Thus, the overall proportion of nondetected cases (i.e., the proportion of false negatives) of the system should be as low as possible. The evaluators should be able to estimate the overall sensitivity of the surveillance system by considering all the steps in the diagnosis of cases following either a conventional decision tree or the formula for estimating herd sensitivity with the adjustments for the various objectives in the final diagnosis and all the organizational and functional aspects of the system that are likely to influence its sensitivity.

Overall specificity of the final disease diagnosis: Similar to the above item of estimation of the overall sensitivity of the surveillance system, the overall specificity should be estimated using the same procedure. The overall proportion of false alarms (i.e., false positives) should be assessed with the aim to link it to the overall sensitivity. The implementers should be encouraged to have a reasonable proportion of false alarms; otherwise, the overall sensitivity will suffer and the resources will be poorly used.

Representativeness of the system: Complete documentation of the sampling design and its validation should be available for review by evaluators to ensure that the inclusion of animals and their premises are representative of the reference population and the functional and organizational aspects of the system that may influence its representativeness should be assessed. The plan should include the appropriate statistical adjustments so that inference to the reference population can be done.

Timeliness in measuring health events including the response time: The system should include a documented plan with various response options according to the expected outcomes from the system. The responses should be as much as possible comprehensive to include all the potential expected outcomes with scientific justifications and time periods. These responses are usually specific to the health events that are included in the system, but they are also linked to regulations and authorities. The evaluators should be able to review these responses with both scientific knowledge and regulations of the underlying the health events in the system. For instance, a surveillance stream for national brucellosis control program may include mitigation options when animals are serologically positive but with no history of clinical signs of the disease in contrast to a different mitigation option when the serologically positive animals are associated with farms that have a known history of events and/or clinical signs of the disease.

Usefulness of the system: The usefulness of the system will vary according the different stakeholders' needs but could be measured in terms of its impact and/or added value to reach its objectives and address those needs. The utility of the system could be measured by looking at its economic value and by considering all the organizational and functional aspects that will influence this aspect.

3.4.4 Implementation Phase

The second phase in the evaluation process concerns the implementation of the evaluation itself, including the assessment of evaluation attributes, analyzing the data with regard to addressing the evaluation question, and looking at strengths and weaknesses of the evaluation approach (Fig. 3.3). Parts III–V of this book cover these aspects in detail, providing relevant methodologies for the implementation phase.

3.4.5 Reporting Phase

During the synthesis step, the data are combined to form an overall assessment of the merit or worth of the surveillance program, or to summarize evidence across several evaluations. This can be done by using methods such as mult-criteria analysis or economic evaluation, looking at the cost-effectiveness, cost–benefit, or cost-utility of a surveillance program (see Sect. 3.3). At this stage, the evaluator can assess how can the findings from this evaluation be generalized to the future, to other sites, and to other strategies or if they are context-specific only. The reporting step is essential to ensure that the results will be taken over by the relevant stakeholders or the decision makers (Fig. 3.4). The initial requirements of the evaluation should be answered. Accessibility of the results to nonscientific audience can be ensured by following the 1:3:25 principle (1-page outlines, 3-page executive summary; 25-page findings and

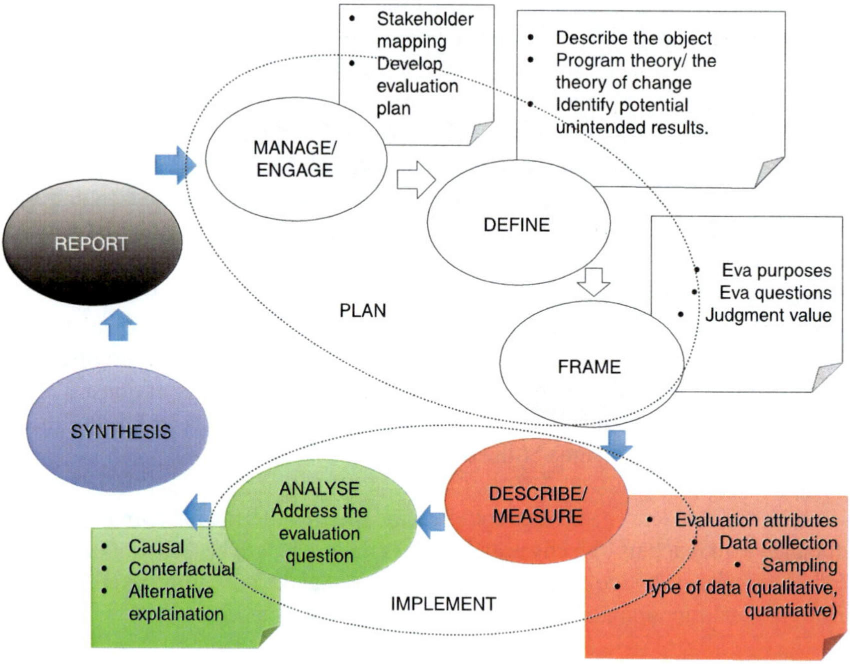

Fig. 3.3 Implementation phase of the evaluation process

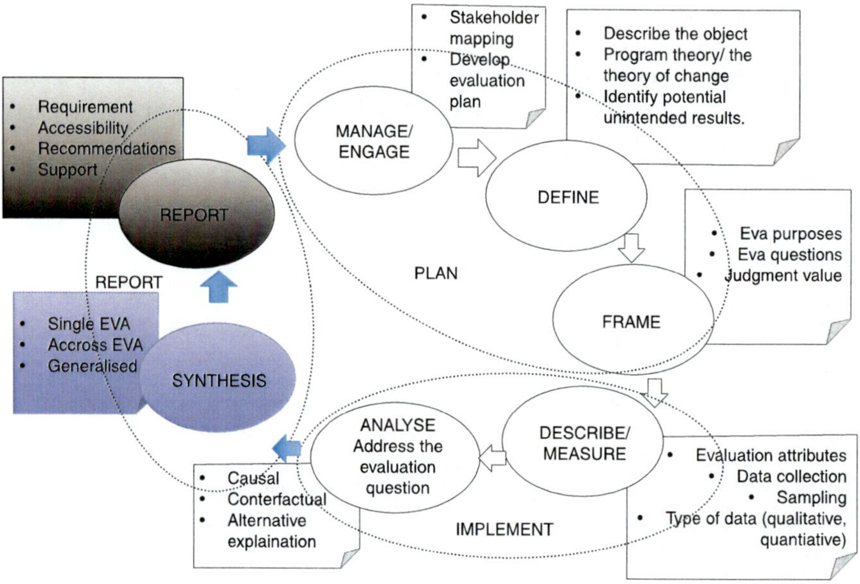

Fig. 3.4 The reporting phase of the evaluation process

methods) [16]. Recommendations should be defined with the decision makers and/or relevant stakeholders to be realistic and feasible; this could be done by actor consultation such as stakeholder workshops. To further support the use of the evaluation findings, the results can be translated into different target audience formats and communicated by mass media or publications in newsletters, scientific journals, etc. For more information on reporting the results of an evaluation, refer to the specific section (Reporting) in the RISKSUR Survtool (https://survtools.org) [8]. Part VI of this book provides critical elements on how to increase uptake of evaluation recommendations by decisions makers to ensure change.

3.5 Conclusion

We have seen and described in this chapter the important steps in the evaluation process: planning, implementing, reporting—highlighting the fact that defining the evaluation question(s) is a critical step as no evaluation should be performed without specific question(s) to be answered. We have seen that considering the organizational and functional aspects of the system is as important as its technical performances to ensure its good functioning. Taking such a comprehensive approach to evaluation (including economics) will ensure good performances and appropriate use of resources to health surveillance systems and will help to tackle issues linked to disease emergence and pandemic threat. The next chapter of this part will present the Survtool evaluation framework that promotes this integrated evaluation approach and its practical application in the field of animal and zoonotic disease surveillance.

References

1. Salman MD, Stark KDC, Zepeda C. Quality assurance applied to animal disease surveillance systems. Rev Sci Tech Off Int Epiz. 2003;22(2):689–96.
2. World Animal Healthe Organisation (OIE). Animal health surveillance. In: Terrestrial animal health code. OIE; 2019.
3. Antoine-Moussiaux N, Vandenberg O, Kozlakidis Z, Aenishaenslin C, Peyre M, Roche M, Bonnet P, Ravel A. Valuing health surveillance as an information system: interdisciplinary insights. Front Public Health. 2019;7:138. https://doi.org/10.3389/fpubh.2019.00138.
4. Delabouglise A, Antoine-Moussiaux N, Tatong D, Chumkaeo A, Binot A, Fournié G, Pilot E, Phimpraphi W, Kasemsuwan S, Paul MC, Duboz R, Salem G, Peyre M. Cultural practices shaping zoonotic diseases surveillance: the case of highly pathogenic avian influenza and Thailand native chicken farmers. Transbound Emerg Dis. 2017;64:1294–305. https://doi.org/10.1111/tbed.12506.
5. Delabouglise A, Dao TH, Truong DB, Nguyen TT, Nguyen NTX, Duboz R, Fournié G, Antoine-Moussiaux N, Grosbois V, Vu DT, Le TH, Nguyen VK, Salem G, Peyre M. When private actors matter: information-sharing network and surveillance of highly pathogenic avian influenza in Vietnam. Acta Trop. 2015;147:38–44. https://doi.org/10.1016/j.actatropica.2015.03.025.
6. Calba C, Antoine-Moussiaux N, Charrier F, Hendrikx P, Saegerman C, Peyre M, Goutard FL. Applying participatory approaches in the evaluation of surveillance systems: a pilot study

on African swine fever surveillance in Corsica. Prev Vet Med. 2015a;122:389–98. https://doi.org/10.1016/j.prevetmed.2015.10.001.

7. Calba C, Comin A, Conraths F, Drewe J, Goutard F, Grosbois V, Haesler B, Höreth D, Hoinville L, Lindberg A, Peyre M, Prieto VR, Rushton J, Staerk K, Schauer B, Traon D, Vergne T. WP1 - development of a conceptual evaluation framework 43; 2013.
8. Peyre M, Hoinville L, Njoroge J, Cameron A, Traon D, Goutard F, Calba C, Grosbois V, Delabouglise A, Varant V, Drewe J, Pfeiffer D, Häsler B. The RISKSUR EVA Tool (Survtool): a tool for the integrated evaluation of animal health surveillance systems. Prev Vet Med. 2019;104777 https://doi.org/10.1016/j.prevetmed.2019.104777.
9. Drewe JA, Hoinville LJ, Cook AJC, Floyd T, Stärk KDC. Evaluation of animal and public health surveillance systems: a systematic review. Epidemiol Infect. 2012;140:575–90. https://doi.org/10.1017/S0950268811002160.
10. Hoinville LJ, Alban L, Drewe JA, Gibbens JC, Gustafson L, Häsler B, Saegerman C, Salman M, Stärk KDC. Proposed terms and concepts for describing and evaluating animal-health surveillance systems. Prev Vet Med. 2013;112:1–12. https://doi.org/10.1016/j.prevetmed.2013.06.006.
11. Rushton J. The economics of animal health and production, first paperback edition. Wallingford, Oxfordshire, UK; Cambridge, MA: CABI; 2011.
12. CDC. Framework for evaluating public health surveillance systems for early detection of outbreaks recommendations from the CDC Working Group tment of health and human ser 53; 2004.
13. Hendrikx P, Gay E, Chazel M, Moutou F, Danan C, Richomme C, Boue F, Souillard R, Gauchard F, Dufour B. OASIS: an assessment tool of epidemiological surveillance systems in animal health and food safety. Epidemiol Infect. 2011;139:1486–96. https://doi.org/10.1017/S0950268811000161.
14. Schulz K, Calba C, Peyre M, Staubach C, Conraths FJ. Hunters' acceptability of the surveillance system and alternative surveillance strategies for classical swine fever in wild boar—a participatory approach. BMC Vet Res. 2016;12:187. https://doi.org/10.1186/s12917-016-0822-5.
15. Graham TW, Turk J, McDermot J, Brown C. Preparing veterinarians for work in resource-poor settings. J Am Veter Med Assoc. 2013;243(11):1523–8.
16. Canadian Health Services Research Foundation (CHSRF). Reader-friendly writing—1:3:25; 2001.

Check for updates

The EVA Survtool: An Integrated Framework to Plan Health Surveillance Evaluation

4

Marisa Peyre, Katja Schulz, Pham Thi Thanh Hoa, and Barbara Häsler

Abstract

Currently available frameworks for evaluation of surveillance systems in animal or human health often treat technical, process, and socioeconomic aspects separately instead of integrating them. The surveillance evaluation (EVA) Survtool, a support tool for the evaluation of animal health surveillance systems, was developed to provide guidance for integrated evaluation of animal health surveillance including economic evaluation. The tool was developed by international experts in surveillance and evaluation in an iterative process of development, testing, and revision; accounting for existing frameworks and guidance, scientific literature, and expert opinion elicitation. The EVA tool encompasses a web interface for users to develop an evaluation plan, a Wiki classroom to provide theoretical information on all required concepts, and a generic evaluation work plan to facilitate implementation and reporting of outputs to decision makers. The tool was used to plan and conduct epidemiological and economic evaluations of surveillance for classical and African swine fever, bovine virus diarrhea, avian influ-

M. Peyre (✉)
CIRAD, UMR ASTRE, Montpellier, France

ASTRE, CIRAD, INRAE, University of Montpellier, Montpellier, France
e-mail: marisa.peyre@cirad.fr

K. Schulz
Friedrich-Loeffler-Institut, Federal Research Institute for Animal Health, Institute of Epidemiology, Greifswald, Insel Riems, Germany

P. T. T. Hoa
CIRAD, UMR ASTRE, Hanoi, Vietnam

B. Häsler
Veterinary Epidemiology, Economics and Public Health Group and Leverhulme Centre for Integrative Research on Agriculture and Health, Department of Pathobiology and Population Sciences, Royal Veterinary College, Hatfield, UK

M. Peyre et al. (eds.), *Principles for Evaluation of One Health Surveillance: The EVA Book*, https://doi.org/10.1007/978-3-030-82727-4_4

enza, and Salmonella Dublin in five European countries. These practical applications highlighted the importance of a comprehensive evaluation approach to improve the quality of the evaluation outputs (economic evaluation; multiple attributes assessment) and demonstrated the usefulness of the guidance provided by the EVA tool. At the same time, they showed that comprehensive evaluations might be constrained by practical issues (e.g., confidentiality concerns, data availability) and resource scarcity. In the long term, the EVA tool is expected to increase professional evaluation capacity and help optimizing health surveillance system efficiency and resource allocation for both public and private actors of the surveillance systems.

The EVA Survtool is freely available online (https://survtools.org/user/login) and is shared under the principles of the noncommercial Creative Commons license 2017 (i.e., the tool can be freely used and shared for any noncommercial purposes but appropriate credit should be given, providing link to the license and changes made should be indicated). The tool is linked to the surveillance evaluation Wikispace (https://survtools.org/wiki/surveillance-evaluation/doku.php), which is also freely available.

Keywords

Health surveillance · Decision tool · Animal disease · Evaluation

4.1 Overview of the EVA Survtool

The tool has been organized into three main sections to capture all the elements critical to an evaluation process and highlighted by the experts during the iterative development process of the tool (Fig. 4.1) [1, 2]:

- Section (1): a general introduction to the tool and essential information on evaluation concepts, including evaluation attributes and economic methods to promote the understanding of the evaluation process and economic evaluation
- Section (2): guidance on how to define an evaluation plan based on steps 1 and 2 with data entry on the evaluation context and the evaluation question and steps 3 and 4 where the tool facilitates the selection of relevant evaluation attributes and assessment methods (including economic analysis)
- Section (3): guidance on how to perform the evaluation and how to report the outputs of the evaluation to decision makers

In the introduction section, the tool provides essential information on its organization and on how it was developed. A manual is also available for download to facilitate the use of the tool. This section further provides general information on

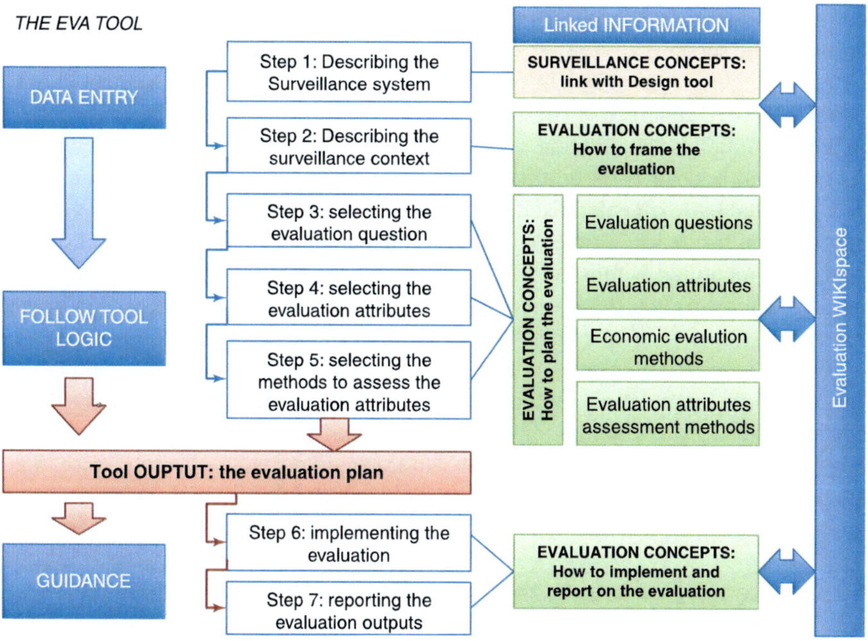

Fig. 4.1 General organization of the EVA tool. Section (1): general introduction to evaluation concepts and economic methods; Section (2): guidance on how to define an evaluation plan; and Section (3): guidance on how to perform the evaluation and how to report the outputs of the evaluation to decision makers. (From [3])

evaluation concepts, evaluation attributes, and economic evaluation methods to promote the understanding of the evaluation process and economic evaluation. An evaluation process should encompass three main aspects: planning, implementation, and reporting (Fig. 4.1). This should promote the implementation of "better" evaluation and therefore the quality of the data generated by those evaluations, along with the use of economic evaluation in the decision-making process.

4.1.1 Step 1: Describing the Surveillance System

Survtool takes the user step by step into describing the surveillance system and component under evaluation (https://survtools.org/wiki/surveillance-design-framework/doku.php?id=1-surveillance-system).

The first step in this process is the characterization of the surveillance system that you can do in the SURVEILLANCE SYSTEM tab. Here you can describe a NEW SURVEILLANCE SYSTEM or LIST EXISTING SYSTEMS that you have previously described. Within the tool, you need to either select a surveillance system from the drop-down list in the top right-hand corner of the screen or create a new surveillance system before you can use the design or evaluation tools. The name of the system that is currently active will be displayed in the top right-hand corner of the screen.

A surveillance system is defined here as a collection of various surveillance components that are all aimed at "describing health-hazard occurrence and contributing to the planning, implementation, and evaluation of risk-mitigation actions" [4] for a specific health hazard and in a defined region. A surveillance system is therefore characterized by (1) one defined hazard that is targeted by surveillance (a disease or another health threat); (2) the objective of the surveillance system (the following have been identified within the RISKSUR project: case detection, prevalence estimation, demonstrate disease freedom and early detection; see details below); and (3) the geographical area covered by the surveillance system.

These surveillance systems are designed within a context that includes (1) the specific animal population susceptible to the hazard in the region of interest; (2) characteristics of the distribution of the hazard (or hazard risk) at the population level, herd level, or animal level, which can impact the design of surveillance; and (4) political and economic context link to the surveillance system priorities.

4.1.2 Step 2: Describing the Surveillance Evaluation Context

The tool allows for a sound and standardized identification of the most relevant question adapted to the user and/or decision maker needs according to its specific surveillance context. The EVA decision tool provides this flexibility to adapt the evaluation protocol to the specific case study context including, for example, surveillance objective and decision maker needs.

The evaluation context provides the background information that will help to make choices about how the evaluation needs to be carried out (Why? What? How?). The tool then asks the user to enter information on the elements of the context (surveillance system and evaluation needs) that are essential to frame the evaluation and define the evaluation question and also to analyze and discuss the outputs of the evaluation by setting them back in their context (Table 4.1). Some of these context elements are being retrieved from the surveillance system description section.

4.1.3 Step 3: Selecting the Evaluation Question

The evaluation question is the most important aspect of the evaluation process. As evaluation is intrinsically linked to action, it makes little sense, and is of limited interest, to perform an evaluation without a specific objective for action. Indeed, an evaluation process with the aim to gather knowledge is qualified as a "quasi-evaluation" as it provides elements on how the system is working but no elements about why the system is performing this way and is therefore limited in terms of recommendation for corrective actions and improvement. This is especially important to consider in resource-scarce situation as evaluation has a cost, both in terms

Table 4.1 List of evaluation context elements included in the EVA tool and their relevance in the framing of the evaluation process (from [3])

Context elements	Relevance
Surveillance objective	Impacts on the selection of evaluation attributes
Hazard name	Provides information about the disease under evaluation that will impact the complexity of the evaluation (e.g., between animal disease and zoonotic diseases)
Geographical area	Provides information about the scale of the evaluation
Legal requirements	Provides information about the need to meet an effectiveness target or not
Strengths and weaknesses of the current approach	Provide summary information about the rationale behind the decision to evaluate - help the evaluator to frame the evaluation question
Stakeholder concerns about current approach	Provides information about the involvement and interest of decision makers in the evaluation process—help the evaluator to frame the evaluation question
Alternative strategies to consider	Provides information about the type of evaluation required (based on a counterfactual or not)
Do you want to evaluate or change the system or some components in the system?	Provides information about the level of evaluation
How many components will you include in this evaluation?	Provides information about the number of counterfactual considered
Are you considering risk-based options?	Relevant for the inclusion of the attribute risk-based criteria definition in the evaluation plan
Will you consider the costs of surveillance in your evaluation?	Provides information about the interest of economic evaluation
Do you know the current cost of your system and/or components?	Provides information about the data required
Do you have a budget constraint?	Provides information for the economic evaluation (meeting a budget target or not)

of human and financial resources, and should therefore provide meaningful and practical recommendations for improvement.

A list of 11 evaluation questions were defined within the EVA tool aiming to account for diverse evaluation needs including economics (Table 4.1). However, this list might not be exhaustive and could be reviewed based on feedback from users of the tool and/or comments made on the EVA wiki. A decision tree was also developed to assist the user with the choice of the evaluation question. In brief, the users are guided through a series of questions (11 in the longest pathway) to define their evaluation priorities (e.g., level of evaluation, system, or component; previous knowledge of effectiveness; need for economic analysis); and to identify the most relevant evaluation question. At the end of the pathway, the user is redirected to the evaluation question list and the tool will preselect the appropriate question.

In order to promote best practices in economic evaluation of surveillance, guidance and practical information on economic evaluation is provided both in the tool itself and the Wikispace. A series of relevant questions that allow defining an economic evaluation question has been developed to help frame the evaluation context and the evaluation questions according to this context. Out of the 11 evaluation questions defined in the tool, 5 are economic evaluation questions covering three common types of economic evaluation methods: least-cost assessment, cost-effectiveness, and cost–benefit analysis (Table 4.2).

Table 4.2 List of evaluation questions developed within the EVA tool and evaluation criteria and methods linked to each question (from [3])

Evaluation question	Evaluation criteria	Evaluation method
Evaluation at the component level		
Q1. Assess whether one or more surveillance component(s) is/are capable of meeting a specified technical effectiveness target	Effectiveness	Effectiveness attribute assessment
Q2. Assess the technical effectiveness of one or more surveillance components		
Q3. Assess the costs of surveillance components (out of two or more) that achieve a defined effectiveness target, where effectiveness is already known	Effectiveness Cost	Least-cost assessment
Q4. Assess the costs and effectiveness of surveillance components (out of two or more) to determine which achieves a defined effectiveness target at least cost, the effectiveness needs to be determined		
Q5–Q7. Assess whether a surveillance component generates a net benefit, the biggest net benefit or the biggest under a budget constraint for society, industry, or animal holder(s):		
Benefit to be measured in monetary terms	Effectiveness Monetary benefit Cost	Cost–benefit assessment
Benefit to be measured in nonmonetary terms or to be expressed as an effectiveness measure	Effectiveness Nonmonetary benefit Cost	Cost-effectiveness assessment
Benefit to be measured in both monetary and nonmonetary terms (or to be expressed as an effectiveness measure)	Monetary benefit Nonmonetary benefit/ effectiveness Cost	Cost–benefit and cost-effectiveness assessment
Evaluation at the system level		
Q8. Assess the functional aspects of surveillance that may influence effectiveness	Effectiveness	Functional attribute assessment
Q9. Assess the technical effectiveness of one or more surveillance components and the functional aspects of surveillance that may influence effectiveness		Effectiveness and functional attribute assessment
Q10. Assess the technical effectiveness of the surveillance system		Effectiveness attribute assessment
Q11. Assess the surveillance structure, function, and processes		Process assessment

4.1.4 Step 4: Selecting the Relevant Evaluation Attributes

The tool provides the full list of attributes organized by level of relevance according to the surveillance system under evaluation and the evaluation context and question. The user can then select the attribute(s) he wants to include in his evaluation. This selection could be done a priori, according to the data currently available on each attribute, or in a second step, by first selecting all the highly relevant ones and then reviewing the type of methods and data needed to assess each relevant attributes (see next step).

A total of 19 evaluation attributes were included in the final list consolidated within the RISKSUR project team (Table 4.3). The differences in relevance of evaluation attributes mainly depended on the surveillance objective (e.g., early detection, freedom from disease, case finding), the evaluation question (e.g., value attributes, organizational attributes), and in some situations on the surveillance design (e.g., risk-based surveillance).

4.1.5 Step 5: Selecting the Evaluation Attribute Assessment Methods Including Economic Analysis

A list of 70 different methods and/or specific applications of a method was retrieved from the scientific literature. Their characteristics including advantage, limits, and competences required to apply the methods were validated by the relevant experts and included in the EVA tool and the Wikispace (https://survtools.org/wiki/surveillance-evaluation/doku.php). The number of methods validated for each evaluation attribute is indicated in Table 4.3. The tool allows the user to select the most relevant method according to the list of attributes (selected in step 4) and the data availability.

Novel methods developed as part of the RISKSUR project were also included in the EVA tool including

- EVARisk to assess the risk-based definition criteria; EVARisk is a specific questionnaire developed to collect data on how risk criteria are defined when designing a risk-based surveillance approach. This questionnaire was developed based on a systematic literature review on risk assessment and risk-based sampling methods. A fact sheet document on the standard methods to define risk of risk-based surveillance was also produced based on the literature review to allow the user to qualitatively assess his/her risk selection approach compared to standard methodology available in the literature.
- AccePT to assess the acceptability, engagement, and benefits of a surveillance system [5] (see Part IV, Chap. 8); AccePT is based on participatory approaches and allows gathering semiquantitative information on the level of acceptability and/or benefits of the surveillance system by the actors [6]. The use of participatory approaches allows engaging the stakeholder in the evaluation process and in the definition of practical corrective actions to improve the system [6].

Table 4.3 Final list of evaluation attributes consolidated within RISKSUR project and number of related assessment methods

Category[a]	Attribute name	Attribute definition	Assessment methods[b]
Functional	Availability and sustainability	The ability to be operational when needed (availability) and the robustness and ability of system to be ongoing in the long term (sustainability).	2
Functional	Acceptability and engagement	Willingness of persons and organizations to participate in the surveillance system, the degree to which each of these users is involved in the surveillance. Could also assess their beliefs about the benefits or adverse consequences of their participation in the system including the provision of compensation for the consequence of disease detection.	4
Functional	Simplicity	Refers to the surveillance system structure, ease of operation, and flow of data through the system.	4
Functional	Flexibility, adaptability	The ability to adapt to changing information needs or operating conditions with little additional time, personnel, or allocated funds. The extent to which the system can accommodate collection of information about new health hazards or additional/alternative types of data; changes in case definitions or technology; and variations in funding sources or reporting methods should be assessed.	4
Functional	Compatibility	Compatibility with and ability to integrate data from other sources and surveillance components, e.g., one health surveillance (part of data collection and data management).	0
Functional	Multiple hazard	Whether the system captures information about more than one hazard.	1
Organizational	Risk-based criteria definition	Validity and relevance of the risk criteria selected and the approach/method used for their identification.	0

Organizational	Surveillance system organization	An assessment of the organizational structures and management of the surveillance system including the existence of clear, relevant objectives, the existence of steering and technical committees whose members have relevant expertise and clearly defined roles and responsibilities, stakeholder involvement, and the existence of effective processes for data management and dissemination of information.	6
Effectiveness	Coverage	The proportion of the population of interest (target population) that is included in the surveillance activity.	2
Effectiveness	Representativeness	The extent to which the features of the population of interest are reflected by the population included in the surveillance activity; these features may include herd size, production type, age, sex, or geographical location, or time of sampling (important for some systems, e.g., for vector-borne disease).	7
Effectiveness	False alarm rate (inverse of specificity)	Proportion of negative events (e.g., nonoutbreak periods) incorrectly classified as events (outbreaks). This is the inverse of the specificity but is more easily understood than specificity.	5
Effectiveness	Bias = accuracy	The extent to which a prevalence estimate produced by the surveillance system deviates from the true prevalence value. Bias is reduced as representativeness is increased.	7
Effectiveness	Precision	How closely defined a numerical estimate is. A precise estimate has a narrow confidence interval. Precision is influenced by prevalence, sample size, and surveillance approach used.	2

(continued)

Table 4.3 (continued)

Category[a]	Attribute name	Attribute definition	Assessment methods[b]
Effectiveness	Timeliness	Timeliness can be defined in various ways: • This is usually defined as the time between any two defined steps in a surveillance system; the time points chosen are likely to vary depending on the purpose of the surveillance activity. • For planning purposes, timeliness can also be defined as whether surveillance detects changes in time for risk mitigation measures to reduce the likelihood of further spread. The precise definition of timeliness chosen should be stated as part of the evaluation process. Some suggested definitions for the RISKSUR project are *For early detection and demonstrating freedom* • Measured using time—Time between introduction of infection and detection of outbreak or presence by surveillance system • Measured using case numbers—Number of animals/farms infected when outbreak or infection detected *For case detection to facilitate control* • Measured using time—Time between infection of animal (or farm) and their detection • Measured using case numbers—Number of other animals/farms infected before case detected *For detecting a change in prevalence* • Measured using time—Time between increase in prevalence and detection of increase • Measured using case numbers—Number of additional animals/farms infected when prevalence increase is identified	7

Effectiveness	Sensitivity (detection probability and detection fraction)	Sensitivity of a surveillance system can be considered on three levels. • *Surveillance sensitivity (case detection probability)* refers to the proportion of individual animals or herds in the population of interest that have the health-related condition of interest that the surveillance system is able to detect. Sensitivity could be measured in terms of *detection fraction* (number of cases detected divided by the coverage level) in a context of nonexhaustive coverage. • *Surveillance sensitivity (outbreak detection)* refers to the probability that the surveillance system will detect a significant increase (outbreak) of disease. This may be an increase in the level of a disease that is not currently present in the population or the occurrence of any cases of disease that is not currently present. • *Surveillance sensitivity (presence)* refers to the probability that disease will be detected if present at a certain level (prevalence) in the population.	13
Effectiveness	PPV	The probability that health event is present given that health event is detected.	2
Effectiveness	NPV	The probability that no health event is present given that no health event is detected.	1
Effectiveness	Robustness	The ability of the surveillance system to produce acceptable outcomes over a range of assumptions about uncertainty by maximizing the reliability of an adequate outcome. Robustness can be assessed using info-gap models.	0
Value	Cost	The concept of economic cost includes (1) the losses due to disease (e.g., reduced milk yield, mortality) and (2) the resources required to detect the disease by a system (e.g., time, services, consumables for surveillance). In economic evaluation, the resources used to detect disease are compared with the disease losses with the aim to identify an optimal balance where a higher economic efficiency is achieved. Estimation of the total economic cost stemming from losses and expenditures is called a disease impact assessment. Estimation of the resource expenditures only is called a cost analysis.	6 (including two nonpublished from RISKSUR members)

(continued)

Table 4.3 (continued)

Category[a]	Attribute name	Attribute definition	Assessment methods[b]
Value	Benefit	The benefit of surveillance quantifies the monetary and nonmonetary positive direct and indirect consequences produced by the surveillance system and assesses whether users are satisfied that their requirements have been met. This includes financial savings, better use of resources, and any losses avoided due to the existence of the system and the information it provides. These avoided losses may include the avoidance of • animal production losses • human mortality and morbidity • decrease in consumer confidence • threatened livelihoods • harmed ecosystems • utility loss Often, the benefit of surveillance estimated as losses avoided can only be realized by implementing an intervention. Hence, it is necessary to also assess the effect of the intervention and look at surveillance, intervention, and loss avoidance as a three-variable relationship. Further benefits of surveillance include maintained or increased trade, improved ability to react in case of an outbreak of disease, maintaining a structured network of professionals able to react appropriately against a (future) threat, maintaining a critical level of infrastructure for disease control, increased understanding about a disease, and improved ability to react in case of an outbreak of disease.	6

[a]Functional = attributes aimed to evaluate the system function; effectiveness = attributes aimed to evaluate the system performances; organizational = attributes aimed to evaluate the system management and process

[b]The assessment methods are available on the Wikispace online: https://survtools.org/wiki/surveillance-evaluation/doku.php

- A new approach to assess the effectiveness of the system [7] (see Part V); this new rationale to assess effectiveness consists in a generic rationale in which effectiveness of a surveillance system is expressed in terms of discrepancy between the modalities and intensity of ideal prevention and/or control measures (given a perfect knowledge of the true epidemiological status of a population and the modalities) and/or control measures that are likely to be actually implemented (often based on the analysis and interpretation of the data produced by a surveillance system).
- *A cost calculator tool*, which was developed by RVC, is provided to estimate the cost of health surveillance; the cost is essential to perform economic analysis. Economic analysis techniques encompassing least cost, cost-effectiveness, and cost–benefit assessments are listed and described in the tool and linked to the economic evaluation methods described in detail in the evaluation Wikispace. Further information on economic evaluation of surveillance system is presented in Part III of this book.

4.1.6 Steps 6 and 7: Implementing the Evaluation and Reporting on the Evaluation Outputs

The tool allows to produce a comprehensive evaluation plan that will support the evaluators in the implementation of the evaluation (see examples in case studies section below).

4.2 Practical Application of the EVA Survtool

4.2.1 Case Study 1. Evaluation of the Swine Disease Surveillance System in Vietnam

Information on swine disease srveillance in Vietnam was inputted in the EVA web tool in combination with information on the context of evaluation (e.g., decision maker, legal requirements). The tool generated an optimum selection of evaluation attributes and measurement methods to assess the efficiency, effectiveness (e.g., sensitivity), and also functional aspects influencing the overall performance of the surveillance system under evaluation. Then information on the evaluation protocol was exported from the EVA web tool into PDF file.

4.2.1.1 Evaluation Plan—Outputs of EVA Tool Steps 1–5

Evaluation name	Swine disease surveillance system in Vietnam
Evaluator name(s)	Thi Thanh Pham Hoa, Marisa Peyre

Selected Evaluation Question(S)

Evaluation question	EVA tool question number
Assess the costs and effectiveness of different surveillance scenarios to determine which achieves a defined effectiveness target at least cost, the effectiveness needs to be determined	Question 4
Assess whether a surveillance component generates a net benefit, the biggest net benefit or the biggest under a budget constraint for society, industry, or animal holder(s): Benefit to be measured in monetary terms	Question 5

Selected Evaluation Attributes

Evaluation attribute	Attribute assessed Yes/no	Justification on the choice/removal
Surveillance system organization	Yes	An assessment of the strengths and weaknesses of the surveillance system including the existence of clear, relevant objectives is an essential aspect of its evaluation to (1) identify the needs for improvement and aspects to be evaluated and (2) ensure meaningful recommendations.
Acceptability	Yes	Pig producers' acceptance to pig disease surveillance and control measures and qualitatively assessed based on DCE study results (qualified as either high, medium, or low).
Timeliness	Yes	Considered as highly relevant for early detection of cases (objective of swine disease surveillance in Vietnam) and has great influence on the effectiveness of interventions. Timeliness was defined here as the time between case detection and reporting by the farmer.
Sensitivity	Yes	Defined as the ability of the system to detect cases (the percentage of reported cases over the total number of cases occurring).
Economic efficiency (cost-effectiveness)	Yes	Among feasible (acceptable) options that comply with minimum legal requirements, the least-cost option should be chosen to use resources rationally.
Economic efficiency (cost–benefit)	Yes	Among feasible (acceptable) options that comply with minimum legal requirements, the option with the higher benefit/cost ratio should be chosen.

Assessment Methods

Attribute	Assessment method
Surveillance system organization	The system was mapped and qualitatively assessed using data on official veterinarian actions to animal disease reporting and management of disease outbreaks generated in the different studies performed under the framework of the same project and using social network analysis method [8] (see Part V).
Sensitivity	Quantitatively assessed using data generated in the discrete choice experiment (DCE) study previously performed [9] (see Part III).

Attribute	Assessment method
Timeliness	Assessed qualitatively as high, medium, or low according to the data generated in DCE study [9].
Acceptability and engagement	Quantitatively assessed using data generated in the DCE study [9].
Monetary benefits	Defined as the avoided losses (i.e., the monetary value of the number of pigs saved from infectious and/or culling). Assessed using an epidemiological simulation model (see Part V).
Costs	As the study compared different scenarios, only the variable costs were considered. The fixed costs such as veterinarian salaries were not included in the calculation as they would be the same for all scenarios. The costs considered were payment for veterinarians for movement control and daily disease reporting, costs of destroying pigs (disinfection, labors), and compensation payment for infected households (see Part III).

4.2.1.2 Implementation of the Evaluation: Step 6

Descriptive Analysis (Qualitative Assessment)

The objective of this task was to describe the surveillance system under evaluation and to build an action diagram (flow chart of the links and actins between actors of the system considered).

Animal disease information needs to be reported officially from pig farmers to commune para-veterinarians, then para-veterinarians report to commune people council and district veterinarians (Fig. 4.2). District veterinarians will report animal disease to district people's committee and province veterinarians. In case of emergency, animal disease can be reported by phone so that investigation of animal disease is performed at the same day or the day after disease reporting. Sampling for

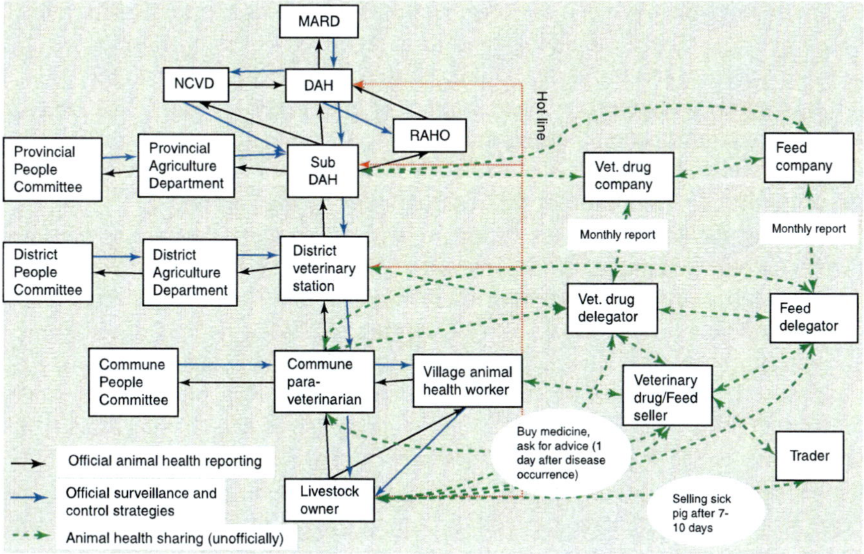

Fig. 4.2 Organization of the swine disease surveillance and control system in Vietnam. (From [8])

animal disease confirmation is often carried out by province veterinarians. Laboratory testing takes around 2 days for giving the results so the disease can be confirmed in 3–4 days. However, disease outbreak notification needs to be official and issued by provincial people committee before disease information is being sent to the national veterinary center (DAH). Process of official reporting of animal disease was considered by the farmers as complicated with several levels of veterinary services (commune, district, province, national center) (Fig. 4.2). The action of official veterinarians upon animal disease reporting was considered between medium to sufficient quality by pig farmers as veterinary officers often visit farm at the same day or the day after disease reporting and give advice on disease prevention and control. Control measures such as disinfection or destroying dead animals are applied to infected holdings even before disease confirmation by the laboratory. Pig farmers can report their swine disease to district/province/national level by the hotline. In each administrative veterinary service (i.e., district, province, or DAH), there are office staffs receiving animal health information through hotline and send to lower level (e.g., from DAH (national level) to sub DAH (province level), then to veterinary station (district level) for disease investigation. Disease progress is then reported daily to upper level. Control measures will be applied if necessary. Informal swine disease surveillance system also exists in parallel with formal surveillance system and is well developed with the involvement of private actors (Fig. 4.2). Feed/drug companies often provide free technical support for large pig farms or drug/feed shops as a market strategy. Drug/feed delegations from companies often visit farms and feed/drug shops to collect data on feed/drug sales as well as the swine disease information. When there are swine disease outbreaks at farm, they might give advice on diseases treatment or send technicians from the company to do disease investigation, take samples, and send to their laboratory for disease confirmation. Small pig holders often contact drug/feed shops to buy the drug and ask for advice of disease treatment when there is any disease problem at their holdings. They also get animal health information in surrounding areas from drug/feed sellers to consider the disease prevention measures at their holdings. According to pig farmers' perception, informal swine disease surveillance is effective in terms of timeliness and scale of animal health information transmission.

Acceptability of Surveillance and Control Policy by Pig Farmers

The willingness of pig farmers to report swine diseases at their farms depends largely on how veterinary officers interact and control the disease after reporting. Three scenarios of disease control measures were used to elicit farmers' preference to report swine diseases (Table 4.4) [9]. Scenario 2 (destroying only dead or unrecovered pigs in infected households with compensation of 70% market value of pig) was well accepted by most pig producers. Around 90% infected households would report pig diseases in their holding if they were certain of being compensated. Pig farmers mentioned that they can even accept the lower compensation level (50% market value of pig) for destroying only dead/unrecovered pig at their farm (scenario 3). However, scenario 1 (stamping out all pigs in infected households with compensation of 70% market value for culled pigs) was the least accepted by most

Table 4.4 Summary of the evaluation of swine disease surveillance in Vietnam

Surveillance and control scenarios	Description	Evaluation attributes			Total cost (USD)
		Acceptability	Timeliness	Sensitivity	
Scenario 0	Culling 100% pigs in holding, compensation 70% market value of pig, uncertainty of being compensated	Very low	10–12 weeks*	4%	37,070
Scenario 1	Culling 100% pigs in holding, compensation 70% market value of pig, certainty of being compensated	Low	> 4 weeks	52%	424,959
Scenario 2	Culling unrecovered pigs, compensation 70% market value of pig, certainty of being compensated	High	1–2 weeks	91%	241,548
Scenario 3	Culling unrecovered pigs, compensation 50% market value of pig, certainty of being compensated	Medium	2–3 weeks	84%	163,635

*Disease reporting at the end of disease outbreak (information derived from semistructured interview of pig farmers and local veterinarians)

pig farmers due to the unacceptability of mass culling of clinically healthy pigs and especially culling of healthy breeders. This low acceptability had a great impact on the reduction in the proportion of pig farmers willing to report swine diseases and therefore had significant influence on the performance of surveillance system.

Timelines of Swine Disease Reporting

Information on swine disease situation in the study area, swine disease ranking, and swine disease reporting was obtained from focus group discussions and key informant interviews [9]. Most pig holders mentioned that they will try to treat sick animals at least during 1 week before considering reporting; reporting will be based on the disease progress upon treatment. They will first contact the veterinary drug sellers or commune para-veterinarians who work as drug sellers or private veterinarians to buy drugs or ask for advice on disease treatment (Fig. 4.2). The commune para-veterinarian also waits one more week to see the result of the treatment and risk of disease spread. The quickest timing for reporting disease would therefore be at least 2 weeks even in case of high transmission rate between household. If the disease does not spread quickly, then the reporting would take even longer time as the veterinarians often give the advice for disease treatment first and assess the disease progress (i.e., the severity and/or spread rate) before reporting the disease to upper veterinary levels.

Compensation for culled pigs was considered as a good incentive for pig farmers to report swine disease early. However, if the farmers are not certain of being compensated for culled pigs, almost all of them will not report the disease. Some pig farmers would report the disease at the end of the outbreak when many infected pigs have died and management of dead pigs by the farmer is difficult (Table 4.4). Culling all pigs in the pig holding negatively affects early reporting even if the compensation is paid for culled pigs. Under this culling regulation, pig farmers consider to report only when infected pigs do not response to treatment and the disease spreads among most pigs in the pig holdings. Culling only unrecovered pigs and being compensated for culled pigs was perceived by farmers as a strong incentive to report early. Anyhow, pig farmers or commune veterinarians will still wait for the response of infected pigs to treatment, so the earliest reporting time will remain at 2 weeks.

Sensitivity of Swine Disease Surveillance System

As seen in the DCE study, under the current scenario (scenario 0) only 4% of the farmers actually report swine disease outbreak to the official surveillance system. Around half of pig farmers (50%) would report PRRS at their farms under scenario 1 (i.e., if they are certain to get compensated and if the compensation level is of 70% market value for culling all pigs in infected farms) [9]. However, nearly all pig farmers (90%) would report the disease if only dead/unrecovered pigs at their farms are destroyed and compensated with 70% market value (scenario 2). Most pig farmers (80%) even accepted a lower compensation level of 50% market value for destroying dead/unrecovered pig (scenario 3) [9].

4.2.1.3 Cost Analysis

The total surveillance and control costs for scenario 1 were nearly twice as high as scenario 2 costs and three times higher than scenario 3 costs [8]. This is due to the highest number of culled pigs in scenario 1 (culling of all pigs in infected holding). This led to the highest compensation payment and costs of pig destroying. Scenario 2 had higher costs than scenario 3 due to the higher compensation level and the higher number of culled pigs. The total cost of each scenario was mainly influenced by the amount of compensation payment for pig farmers and therefore by the number of culled and dead pigs compensated.

4.2.1.4 Cost-Effectiveness Analysis

Overall result: Scenario 2 was found to be the most effective in terms of acceptability, timelines, and sensitivity (Table 4.4). However, the total cost of scenario 2 was 1.5 times higher than scenario 3. Scenario 3 had a medium acceptability level, timeliness, and a 7% lower sensitivity level than scenario 2. In order to assess the added value of scenario 2 versus scenario 3 in terms of disease control, a cost–benefit analysis was performed.

4.2.1.5 Cost–Benefit Analysis

Benefit–cost ratio of scenario 0 could not be estimated as under this current scenario almost all pig farmers did not report the disease (Table 4.5). The disease spreads easily to surrounding areas without any control. A few farmers (4%) might report the disease when there are many dead pigs, but it is usually at the end of the outbreak. Thus, the benefit of control measures could not be estimated at the commune level using the simulation model developed in this study. Scenario 3 had the highest benefit–cost ratio (B/C = 5.2) compared to scenario 2 (B/C = 3.5) and scenario 1 (B/C = 1.1). The benefit–cost ratio of scenario 3 was higher than that of scenario 2 due to saved cost of compensation (i.e., lower compensation level and lower number of culled pigs).

4.2.1.6 Recommendations: Step 6 (Addressing the Evaluation Questions) and Step 7 (Reporting on the Evaluation Outputs)

The objectives of this task were to review the meaning of the results considering the surveillance system in its global aspects and provide recommendations for decision makers based on the economic evaluation results.

Quality of the Evaluation Performed

A comprehensive approach was used to perform economic evaluation of swine disease surveillance and control in Vietnam. Multiple attributes covering different aspects of surveillance system effectiveness and efficiency such as organization, function, and value of the system were considered. The effectiveness of surveillance system was assessed based on the cost-effectiveness analysis of different control options, which had a significant influence on the performance of surveillance system (i.e., proportion of farmer reporting). This economic analysis technique did not

Table 4.5 Cost–benefit analysis

	Control scenarios		
Items	Scenario1	Scenario 2	Scenario 3
Number of infected households	151	161	161
Number of uninfected households	10	0	0
Number of reported households	79	147	135
Number of culled pigs	5271	2945	2718
Number of dead pigs in infected farms (not reported)	1460	291	518
Number of saved pigs	4190	7685	7685
Total costs	424,959	241,548	163,635
Benefit of saved pigs	461,281	846,044	846,044
Benefit–cost (B/C) ratio	1.10	3.50	5.17

allow differentiating between the two most effective scenarios (2 and 3). A cost–benefit analysis was required to assess the added value of detecting 7% more cases (sensitivity) with a 50% increase in costs in terms of disease control. The results of the cost–benefit analysis highlighted the limited importance of an increase of 7% of surveillance sensitivity in terms of efficient disease control. This comprehensive evaluation provided meaningful recommendations; however, such evaluation could be time consuming and laborious and required simulation modeling and socioeconomic field studies (i.e., DCE) to provide information on farmer's decision-making useful for both quantitative evaluation (sensitivity) and qualitative evaluation (acceptability) of surveillance system. Other biases linked to the hypothesis used in the modeling study and the cost estimation have been identified and addressed to ensure validity of the recommendations and are described elsewhere [8].

Recommendations to Improve Surveillance Strategies

Control scenario involving destroying of only dead and unrecovered pigs and compensation of 70% of pig market value got the highest acceptability, but the scenario with compensation of 50% market value for unrecovered pigs gave the highest B/C ratio. Culling all pigs in infected households and compensation of 70% market value of pig were considered as limited effectiveness due to the low famers' acceptability even though the B/C ratio was 1.1. In case of endemic disease, this scenario was thought as wasted money as most farmers considered that they can treat sick animals and morbidity and mortality of the diseases depends much on the prevention of other diseases (e.g., classical swine fever, epizootic pneumonia, etc.). Keeping infected pigs at pig holdings in infection period showed the potential risk of disease spread to surrounding areas. However, improving biosecurity at pig holdings and ensuring proper outbreak management (i.e., disinfection, movement restriction, and vaccination) can help to prevent the disease spread. Indeed, previous study highlighted that emergency vaccination was a more effective strategy to control PRRS outbreaks rather than stamping out [10].

4.2.2 Case Study 2: Evaluation of Classical Swine Fever Surveillance System in Germany

The Federal State Rhineland-Palatinate in Germany comprises 24 districts and 12 municipalities, covering a total area of about 20,000 square kilometers. In this state, classical swine fever (CSF) infection in wild boars was detected in 1995 and between 1998 and 2009 with the two most recent outbreaks occurring in two separate parts in the beginning of 2009. Since 2002, infection in the wild boar population was controlled in some part by means of oral immunization with vaccination baits. In May 2012, the state was officially declared free from CSF. Since then, regular surveillance measures have to be applied to demonstrate freedom from the disease. In this case study, the current and alternative surveillance strategies to demonstrate were evaluated to demonstrate freedom from disease.

4.2.2.1 Evaluation Plan—Outputs of EVA Tool Steps 1–5

Evaluation name	Classical swine fever in Germany
Evaluator name(s)	Katja Schulz, Christoph Staubach, Marisa Peyre

Selected Evaluation Question(S)

Evaluation question	EVA tool question number
Assess the effectiveness of one or more surveillance component(s) or system(s) in relation to a surveillance objective and rank the options accordingly	Question 2
Assess the timeliness of different surveillance strategies and assess the acceptability in hunters of different surveillance strategies—These questions relate to the EVA tool question: "Assess the technical effectiveness of one or more surveillance components and the functional aspects of surveillance that may influence effectiveness"	Question 9
Assess the costs of surveillance component(s) or system(s) that achieve(s) a defined objective and rank them according to costs to identify the least-cost option	Question 3

Selected Evaluation Attributes

Evaluation attribute	Attribute assessed Yes/no	Justification on the choice/removal
Surveillance system organization	Yes	An assessment of the strengths and weaknesses of the surveillance system including the existence of clear, relevant objectives is an essential aspect of its evaluation to (1) identify the needs for improvement and aspects to be evaluated and (2) ensure meaningful recommendations.
Sensitivity	Yes	Sensitivity is a critical requirement to fulfill EU regulations for CSF. An improvement in timeliness is expected to lead to fewer outbreaks.
Timeliness	Yes	
Acceptability	Yes	Any change in a surveillance strategy for CSF is likely to be influenced by stakeholders.
Economic efficiency (cost-effectiveness)	Yes	Among feasible (acceptable) options that comply with minimum legal requirements, the least-cost option should be chosen to use resources rationally.

Assessment Methods

Attribute	Assessment method	
Surveillance system organization	Descriptive analysis (qualitative assessment)and SWOT analysis using OASIS trop tool (see Part IV)	
	Component 1	Component 2
Sensitivity and timeliness	Field data: Sensitivity of the whole surveillance system by using capture–recapture method (see Part V)	Simulation data (see Part V)
Acceptability and engagement	AccePT method (see Part IV)	

4.2.2.2 Implementation of the Evaluation: Step 6

Descriptive Analysis (Qualitative Assessment)

The objective of this task was to describe the surveillance system under evaluation and build an action diagram (flow chart of the links and actions between actors of the system considered).

Method: Application of the OASIS Trop protocol and collation of expert opinion.

System mapping examples (Fig. 4.3):

SWOT Analysis Report

The objective of this task was to gather information on the system performance process (strengths and weaknesses of the system). This was conducted using the OASIS Trop tool (accessible here: https://survtools.org/wiki/surveillance-evaluation/doku.php?id=surveillance-system-organisation).

The OASIS Trop tool results are presented in the following manner:

- Output 1 gives the satisfaction level of each criterion, which provides an indication of the functioning and the global situation of the surveillance system.
- Output 2 indicates the critical points of the surveillance system.
- Output 3 gives the scores of the quality indicators.

Output 1: Strengths and Weaknesses of the System: Fig. 4.4 demonstrates the strengths and weaknesses of the surveillance system process based on the application of the OASIS tool (described in Part IV) [11].

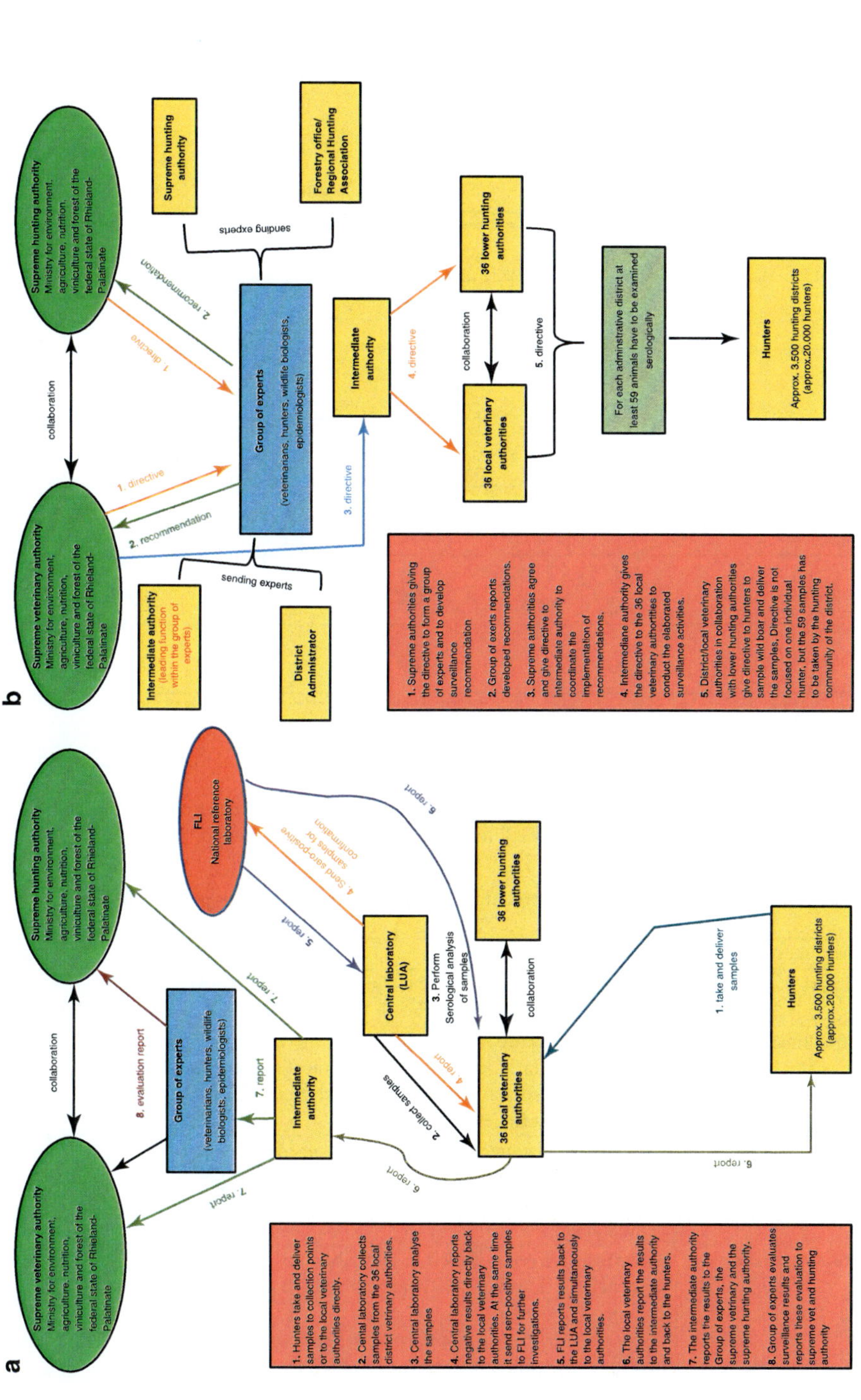

Fig. 4.3 Information flow (**a**: bottom-up; **b**: top-down) within the surveillance system of the currently implemented, active surveillance for classical swine fever in wild boar in times of disease freedom on the basis of the Federal State of Rhineland-Palatinate

Sections	Result of evaluation per each section	Percentage of satisfaction
Section 1: Objectives and context of surveillance		100%
Section 2: Central institutional organization		74%
Section 3: Field institutional organization		92%
Section 4: Laboratory		82%
Section 5: Surveillance tools		86%
Section 6: Surveillance procedures		86%
Section 7: Data management		90%
Section 8: Fromation		89%
Section 9: Communication		70%
Section 10: Evaluation		67%

Fig. 4.4 Strengths and weaknesses of the surveillance system process: level of compliance of each section of the system process according to an ideal system (OASIS Output 1)

Feedback on the results of the strengths and weaknesses of the system process (output 1)

Process section	Feedback/recommendations
Objectives (100%)	The objectives are clearly stated and documented and take into consideration all stakeholders.
Central unit (74%)	There is no specific steering committee but they are operational and they meet regularly (every day communication); their material and financial resources are not considered sufficient. However, the human resources are sufficient.
Field institutional organization (92%)	Only human resources in the field are considered as low sufficient (material and financial resources are very sufficient). Some limits in the representativeness as only some age groups are being hunted.
Laboratory (82%)	Some tests are not included in interlaboratory trials (pathology and sequencing); however, this is not considered as a limitation of the system. Laboratory has only a minor role in the surveillance system. Investigation team not assigned 100% on the task but could be mobilized upon request: Not considered as a limitation. Low specificity of the suspicion and confirmation tests. Delivery from laboratory to CU of results sometimes delayed but minor problem.

Process section	Feedback/recommendations
Surveillance tools (86%)	Limits in acceptability of the consequences of a suspicion or case for the source or collector data: Important constraints linked to control measures implemented. Specificity of the case definition is low, but this is not an issue as high sensitivity is preferred under freedom from disease objective. Some issue in the delay of sending samples to the laboratory. Not all but the majority >95% of the collection form and sample are correct.
Surveillance procedures (86%)	The surveillance is not exhaustive: No = caused by spatial aggregate + deficiencies minor (due to hunter engagement) + level of underreporting = between 15% and 30% (field agents); intermediary units <5% (assumed). No indemnities for hunters (data source); no awareness building. Limited representativeness: This bias justifies the need/will to change surveillance protocols in place. The samples obtained are based on the hunting bag and the hunting bag itself is already biased by several factors, e.g., hunting intensity, hunting ground, environmental conditions, season, hunting ethics, etc. Furthermore, randomly distributed over the hunting bag, e.g., no classification by age classes. Randomly distributed over the year following the hunting bag distribution, e.g., no classification by season.
Data management (90%)	A relational database exists and is considered adequate but does not hold all the data (only a majority). There is a delay in data input time, but this time lag is considered minor and does not affect the system efficacy.
Training (89%)	Some actors are not concerned by the initial training. There is no refresher training in place.
Communication (70%)	The frequency of report/publications is not planned by the network. There is a feedback of results to field actors but no means to control it. There is regular dissemination of reports, easy to control but no guarantee that it reaches all field actors. Communication system: Not all the actors use the communication means.
Evaluation (67%)	Performance indicators measured: Depending on the federal states sometimes major improvements are required. There is no external evaluation.

Output 2: Critical Points Analysis: The OASIS tool identifies seven critical points for the surveillance system using the hazard analysis critical control point (HACCP) method [12]:

- *Objectives:* This point assesses the capacity of the objectives to be coherent and consider the expectation of the different stakeholders and of the surveillance procedures to be appropriate with the surveillance objectives.
- *Sampling:* This point assesses the quality of the sampling.
- *Animation:* This point evaluates the quality of the trainings and the awareness of field agents and the organization of the surveillance system.

- *Tools:* This point assesses the quality of the collection, testing, analysis of the samples (i.e., the quality of the laboratory processes).
- *Collection and circulation of data:* This point assesses the quality of the samples and results collection and the system communication.
- *Processing and interpretation:* This point assesses the quality of the data management.
- *Dissemination and information:* This point assesses the quality of the communication of the results.

Figure 4.5 shows that the most critical point in the system in need of improvement is "dissemination and information." This has an impact on the level of acceptability and compliance with the system. Further, improvement could be made regarding sampling to improve representativeness. The points "tools and processing" and interpretation of data show smaller margins for improvement.

Output 3: Qualitative analysis of the evaluation attributes (how the system process affects the effectiveness and functional attributes of the system). The score of the performance and functional attributes results from a combination of scores of the different criteria from the OASIS Trop score grid. The size of the blue portion of each bar on the radar represents the level of the satisfaction for the performance attribute considered.

The freedom from disease surveillance system requires a higher sensitivity over specificity. However, the sensitivity of the system is not optimal (66%) as it is affected by the acceptability of the stakeholders (70%) and the representativeness (69%), which are two elements of the system to be improved (Fig. 4.6).

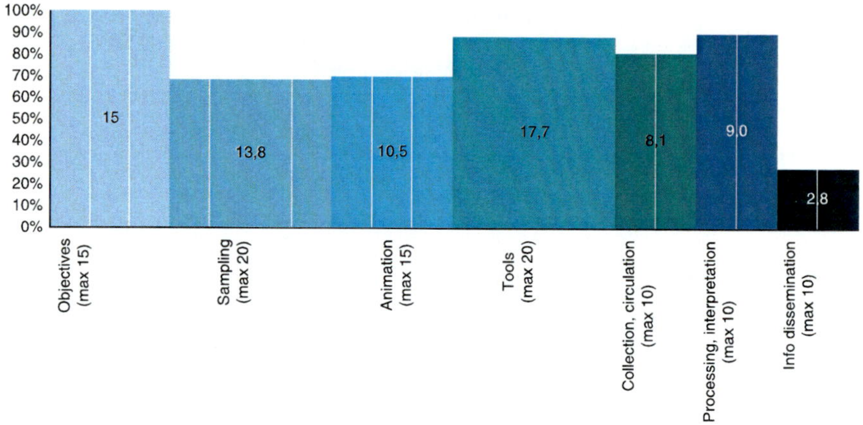

Fig. 4.5 Critical control point assessment of the classical swine fever system in Germany (OASIS Trop Output 2)

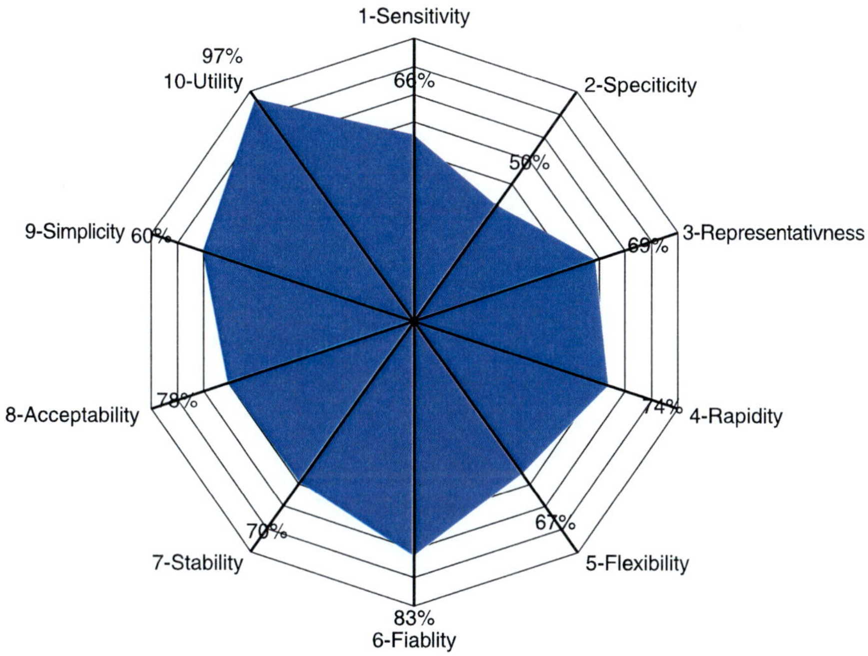

Fig. 4.6 Qualitative assessment of classical swine fever surveillance system performance and functional attributes (OASIS Trop Output 3)

Analysis of Changes in the System Process Incurred by the Change in Surveillance Design

A wide range of different active, passive, and combined surveillance scenarios were simulated as listed below varying the number of samples, targeted districts, frequency, types of samples, and age classes of animals. The strategies based on different age classes will only change the shooting behavior of the hunters, which means that they need to shoot more animals of a defined age group. The strategies based on defining districts will change the workload and reduce the cost for some veterinary authorities and some hunters (transport costs, sampling costs). The strategies based on season will change the workload and the cost within 1 year as the samples have to be delivered and picked up only in certain month, which impacts on transport and sampling costs. The strategies based on sample size will reduce or increase transport and sampling costs due to a lower or higher volume. Moreover, the costs are dependent on the examination of samples, that is, whether they were only serologically, virologically examined, or in both ways.

4.2.2.3 Cost Analysis

The aim was to assess the cost of the different options considered for the case study (current and novel design).

Method: A cost-effectiveness analysis was used to identify which strategies could achieve a defined target at the least cost [13]. First, all strategies that achieved

Table 4.6 Overall evaluation of all strategies, in which all three evaluation attributes and costs were investigated. S represents the score, whereby 1 constitutes the best result; sero = simulation of serological sample examination, vise = serological and virological sample examination (from [13])

Strategy	Sensitivity in %	S	Timeliness	S	Acceptability	S	Cost difference in Euro	S	Total score
S4 sero	99.76	1	0.129	2	1	1	0	3	1.8
S4 vise	99.82	1	0.133	1	1	1	14,018.4	5	2.0
S11 vise	99.47	1	0.124	3	−0.4	4	−27,146.4	2	2.5
S11 sero	99.27	1	0.12	5	−0.4	4	−28,800	1	2.8
S1 vise	99.99	1	0.122	4	0.9	2	14,018.4	5	3.0
S1 sero	99.95	1	0.117	6	0.9	2	0	3	3.0
S12 vise	99.91	1	0.12	5	−0.4	4	−27,146.4	2	3.0
S13 vise	99.82	1	0.117	6	−0.4	4	−27,146.4	2	3.3
S12 sero	99.82	1	0.115	8	−0.4	4	−28,800	1	3.5
S27 sero	99.96	1	0.116	7	−0.3	3	3,585.6	4	3.8
SI3 sero	99.72	1	0.113	9	−0.4	4	−28,800	1	3.8

a detection probability of at least 95% (i.e., an effectiveness of 100%) were identified. Second, the costs for each strategy were calculated using the cost calculation spreadsheet taking into account variable additional costs for labor, operations, and expenses associated with each strategy (https://survtools.org/wiki/surveillance-evaluation/doku.php?id=cost-analysis) (Table 4.6). The costs for each of the 100% effective scenarios were expressed as cost units (instead of euros) due to data confidentiality issues. To estimate these cost units, the costs of the reference strategy were estimated taking into account the variable costs for transport and analysis. The costs for the alternative surveillance strategies were then estimated and represented as a proportion relative to the estimated costs of the reference strategy.

Discussion: The cost assessment showed that—among all the scenarios that would comply with legislative requirements (i.e., 95% detection probability)—there would be 19 scenarios leading to lower surveillance costs when using serological testing and 11 scenarios when using serological and virological testing. Consequently, there are cost savings to be made in CSF surveillance in Germany.

4.2.2.4 Effectiveness Assessment

Sensitivity was assessed by measuring the detection probability. This was done using a simulation model [13]. The model was based on real data including population estimates, population structure, hunting data, and course of infection and used to determine the detection probability of infection within 1 year.

There were many scenarios that achieved the target effectiveness. The difference between random or real distributed sampling over the year was found to be very small. The sensitivity of serological examination was nearly as high as if performing both examinations. However, virological examination only was found to result in a lower sensitivity. When samples were examined serologically as well as virologically almost in all strategies, the detection probability was above 95% (in 21 from 24). When the samples were only examined virologically, the detection probability did not exceed 85%. The reference strategy was shown to have almost 100% detection probability. Most of the risk-based strategies showed a detection probability above 95% provided that the samples were not only examined virologically.

Timeliness was defined as the time between introduction and detection of a CSF virus infection. Using the model described above, for every repeated simulation with detection of the infection, timeliness was estimated as the number of months between introduction and detection of the infection. The results for the timeliness assessment were consistent with those found for sensitivity. The best timeliness could be seen in risk-based strategies that were taking into account the age of the animals. It was found that smaller sample sizes resulted in lower timeliness.

Acceptability, which provides evidence on the functional aspect of the surveillance strategies, was investigated using participatory methods as described previously [14]. Within the surveillance system for CSF in wild boar, hunters play a key role in sample collection. The acceptability by hunters and veterinarians of the current system as well as of some of the alternative strategies was examined [15] (Table 4.6) (see Part IV).

The trust in the system by the hunters was quite high (0.75). However, their acceptability of the objective of the system was moderate (0.4) and the acceptability of the operation even lower (0.1).

Their acceptability of the strategy in which only samples resulting from passive surveillance should be examined was very low (−1.3). This was mainly due to the fact that sampling dead, decomposing animals can be rather unpleasant. Interestingly, the hunters' acceptability of the strategy of taking 59 samples only quarterly was only moderate (0.4). The most accepted strategy was taking the 59 samples only within the age group of subadult animals (1). Remarkably, also the currently implemented active surveillance strategy was well accepted (0.9). It was not possible to present all scenarios to the hunters; therefore, only the results for a few scenarios are available. Because it was not straightforward to recruit hunters and they were mainly from one age group, there was a risk of bias and subjectivity.

4.2.2.5 Cost-Effectiveness Assessment

Overall Result: For each attribute, a rank was given to each attribute and the combined rank was determined weighing each attribute equally (Table 4.6). Doing this, it was possible to present an overall priority list of the potential scenarios.

4.2.2.6 Recommendations: Step 6 (Addressing the Evaluation Questions) and Step 7 (Reporting on the Evaluation Outputs)

The objectives of this task were to review the meaning of the results considering the surveillance system in its global aspects and provide recommendations for decision makers based on the economic evaluation results.

Quality of the Evaluation Performed

Because fewer data are commonly available on passive surveillance compared to active surveillance, the outcomes of the simulation model may not have full reliability. The differences in detection probabilities were found to be rather small (e.g., 99.9 vs. 99.5), which may be due to the simulation differences (1000 simulation runs). The combination of sensitivity analysis and timeliness analysis did produce important additional information. Even when strategies result in an equal detection probability, the timeliness can be the crucial factor for the final choice of a strategy.

The focus group discussion added value to the evaluation. It became obvious that some of the strategies, although they would be cheaper and more effective, would not be very well accepted by the hunters.

The final results of the analysis showed the benefit of combining different evaluation attributes and also performing an economic evaluation. Thereby, it was possible to identify the strategy resulting in the best overall performance, but it needs to be kept in mind that the attributes may need to be weighted differently, which would change the ranking of the combined performance assessment.

Recommendations for Surveillance Design Changes

While the current surveillance strategy has a good performance, it is worth considering to sample only in defined age groups. If a decision maker is interested in saving costs, it is advisable to discontinue the double serological and virological examination of the samples. The results suggest that the sample size could be decreased to 50 or even 40 samples per district as the 59 sample size calculation is based on the assumption of an infinite population and a homogenous distribution of infection with the population. Finally, the combination of different strategies (lower sample size within a defined age class) was found to be a feasible and cost-effective alternative.

4.3 Conclusion

The EVA tool provides a comprehensive framework for integrated evaluation of health surveillance, including a step-by-step guide on how to best perform the evaluation and providing a reference online platform for health surveillance evaluation methods. Its applications in the field highlighted the importance of such a comprehensive evaluation approach to improve the quality of the evaluation outputs (economic evaluation; multiple attributes assessment) and demonstrated the usefulness of the guidance provided by the tool itself. Comprehensive evaluations might be constrained by practical issues (e.g., confidentiality concerns, data availability) and resource scarcity. In the long term, the EVA tool is expected to increase professional evaluation capacity and help optimizing health surveillance system efficiency and resource allocation for both public and private actors of the surveillance systems.

References

1. Peyre M, Hoinville L, Njoroge J, Cameron A, Traon D, Goutard FL, Calba C, Grosbois V, Delabouglise A, Varant V, Drewe J, Pfeiffer DU, Haesler B. The RISKSUR EVA Tool: a tool for the integrated evaluation of animal health surveillance systems. Prevent Veter Med. 2018;173:104,777.
2. Peyre M-I, Dorea F, Haesler B, Comin A, Lindberg A, Schauer B, Staubach C, Schulz K, Goutard F, Van Schaik G, Staerk K, Hoinville L, Bisdorff B, Cameron A, Parry J, Brouwer A, Varant V, Traon D, Pinto J, Martinez Avilés M, Sanchez-Vizcaino JM, Ripperger J, Pfeiffer DU. RISKSUR decision support tools: towards improved design, evaluation and documentation of animal health surveillance [WWW Document]. Proc. ICAHS - 3rd Int. Conf. Anim. Health Surveill. Beyond Anim. Health Surveill. Rotorua New-Zealand 1–5 May 2017; 2017.
3. Peyre M, Hoinville L, Njoroge J, Cameron A, Traon D, Goutard F, Calba C, Grosbois V, Delabouglise A, Varant V, Drewe J, Pfeiffer D, Häsler B. The RISKSUR EVA Tool (Survtool): a tool for the integrated evaluation of animal health surveillance systems. Prev Vet Med. 2019:104777. https://doi.org/10.1016/j.prevetmed.2019.104777.
4. Hoinville LJ, Alban L, Drewe JA, Gibbens JC, Gustafson L, Häsler B, Saegerman C, Salman M, Stärk KDC. Proposed terms and concepts for describing and evaluating animal-health surveillance systems. Prev Vet Med. 2013;112:1–12. https://doi.org/10.1016/j.prevetmed.2013.06.006.
5. Calba C, Goutard FL, Vanholme L, Antoine-Moussiaux N, Hendrikx P, Saegerman C. The added-value of using participatory approaches to assess the acceptability of surveillance systems: the case of bovine tuberculosis in Belgium. PLoS One. 2016;11:e0159041. https://doi.org/10.1371/journal.pone.0159041.
6. Calba C, Antoine-Moussiaux N, Charrier F, Hendrikx P, Saegerman C, Peyre M, Goutard FL. Applying participatory approaches in the evaluation of surveillance systems: A pilot study on African swine fever surveillance in Corsica. Prev. Vet. Med. 2015;122:389–98. https://doi.org/10.1016/j.prevetmed.2015.10.001.
7. Grosbois V, Häsler B, Peyre M, Hiep DT, Vergne T. A rationale to unify measurements of effectiveness for animal health surveillance. Prev Vet Med. 2015;120:70–85. https://doi.org/10.1016/j.prevetmed.2014.12.014.
8. Pham TTH. Economic evaluation of swine disease surveillance system in Vietnam (PhD). Bangkok, Thailand: Kasetsart University; 2016.
9. Pham HTT, Peyre M, Trinh TQ, Nguyen OC, Vu TD, Rukkwamsuk T, Antoine-Moussiaux N. Application of discrete choice experiment to assess farmers' willingness to report swine diseases in the red River Delta region. Vietnam Prev Vet Med. 2017;138:28–36. https://doi.org/10.1016/j.prevetmed.2017.01.002.
10. Zhang H, Kono H, Kubota S. An integrated epidemiological and economic analysis of vaccination against highly pathogenic porcine reproductive and respiratory syndrome (PRRS) in Thua Thien Hue Province. Vietnam Asian-Australas J Anim Sci. 2014;27:1499–512. https://doi.org/10.5713/ajas.2014.14060.
11. Hendrikx P, Gay E, Chazel M, Moutou F, Danan C, Richomme C, Boue F, Souillard R, Gauchard F, Dufour B. OASIS: an assessment tool of epidemiological surveillance systems in animal health and food safety. Epidemiol Infect. 2011;139:1486–96. https://doi.org/10.1017/S0950268811000161.
12. Dufour B. Tehnical and economic evaluation method for use in improving infectious animal disease surveillance networks. Vet Res Inra/Elsevier. 1999:27–37.
13. Schulz K, Peyre M, Staubach C, Schauer B, Schulz J, Calba C, Häsler B, Conraths FJ. Surveillance strategies for classical swine fever in wild boar – a comprehensive evaluation study to ensure powerful surveillance. Sci Rep. 2017;7:43871. https://doi.org/10.1038/srep43871.

14. Calba C, Goutard FL, Hoinville L, Hendrikx P, Lindberg A, Saegerman C, Peyre M. Surveillance systems evaluation: a systematic review of the existing approaches. BMC Public Health 2015;15:448. https://doi.org/10.1186/s12889-015-1791-5.
15. Schulz K, Calba C, Peyre M, Staubach C, Conraths FJ. Hunters' acceptability of the surveillance system and alternative surveillance strategies for classical swine fever in wild boar - a participatory approach. BMC Vet Res. 2016;12:187. https://doi.org/10.1186/s12917-016-0822-5.

Part III

Methods for Economic Evaluation

The Economics of Surveillance

5

Keith Howe

Abstract

Surveillance is both a technical process and, because it uses scarce resources, an economic process. The product (or output) of surveillance is information. More precisely, surveillance is an intermediate product whose value derives from its role as an input to decisions about mitigating the effects of disease. Disease effects are twofold: lost benefits to people who could have consumed the goods and services disease-affected animals would have produced; the opportunity cost of resources allocated to disease mitigation which otherwise could have been allocated to other productive use. Production economics principles illuminate the key considerations. A surveillance information production function is a technical relationship showing how the quantity of information produced depends on the variable quantities of surveillance resources used. If scientific advance makes resources more productive, the production function shifts upwards to a new frontier of technical efficiency. But knowledge of technical efficiency is insufficient. For economic efficiency, information must be obtained at least cost. Furthermore, normally surveillance information is useful only when used in association with resources for intervention. Thus the relationship of most interest is a three-dimensional disease mitigation surface, illustrated here for avoided animal output losses as a function of variable combinations of surveillance and intervention resources. Surveillance and intervention are typically economic substitutes. The ratio in which they are combined depends on (a) the specific characteristics of the technical relationship between them and (b) their relative monetary costs of provision. Having also estimated the monetary value of output losses avoided for all combinations of surveillance and intervention, the maximum net benefits from mitigation, that is, overall economic optimum, can be obtained. No longer con-

K. Howe (✉)
Centre for Rural Policy Research, University of Exeter, Exeter, UK
e-mail: k.s.howe@exeter.ac.uk

M. Peyre et al. (eds.), *Principles for Evaluation of One Health Surveillance: The EVA Book*, https://doi.org/10.1007/978-3-030-82727-4_5

strained to specify *ex ante* a functional form for econometric estimation, modern computers potentially facilitate simulation of mitigation surfaces and the derivation of economic efficiency measures as never before.

Keywords

Health economics · Surveillance · Evaluation

5.1 Introduction

Definitions of surveillance naturally tend to focus on its technical aspects. Thus Häsler [1] describes surveillance as being for early warning when disease (re-) occurs, to detect infection or disease, to measure prevalence of incidence of pathogens or hazards found in animal populations or along the food chain, to inform intervention activities to reduce or eradicate disease, and to document freedom from disease, infection, or the level of chemical contaminants in food products. In summary, core surveillance activities are data collection, measurement, documentation, and communication.

Central to the present context is that all those activities depend on use of real resources for their implementation—animal owners, field workers, scientists, test equipment, laboratories, data recording and reporting facilities, and so on. In that sense, Thacker's [2] more general definition of surveillance as a scientific, factual tool that informs policy decisions and the allocation of resources for disease control is more comprehensive for its explicit recognition that surveillance is also part of an economic process, that is, it affects resource allocation decisions. But still the definition is deficient. The missing element is reference to the economic product of surveillance, the purpose it serves by producing something people value, and so want the benefits it provides. From an economics perspective, disease control is not an end in itself. Rather, the objective is to diminish the negative consequences of disease, better described as mitigating disease effects, thus reducing value losses for people's benefit and hence enhancing their sense of well-being.

5.2 Surveillance Information Is an Economic Product

In brief summary, the purpose of surveillance is to produce information to assist decision-makers in responding to disease, whether it is actual or in prospect. Importantly, information is the result, or product (synonym output), of processing data; data and information are different conceptually, and must not to be confused [3, 4]. Moreover, in economic terms surveillance information is typically an intermediate, not final, product; surveillance information is an input to another process, that of decision-making about actions to be taken for disease mitigation. Specifically, the information acquired from surveillance helps decision-makers make choices about what interventions, if any, should be made to mitigate negative disease effects.

However, surveillance information could be regarded as a final product if its purpose is the accumulation of scientific knowledge about, say, an emerging disease currently not considered to be of actual economic consequence, although potentially it may become so in future. In that context, information represents a stock of knowledge that can be drawn on at some future date, if required. It is closer to the end product of an epidemiological survey explicitly designed to obtain knowledge, not surveillance in its full sense, even though provided by a surveillance system.

Although simple in concept, surveillance information as a product is multidimensional. It is a flow variable, its purpose to report the outcomes of actual or expected consequences of disease (e.g. incidence, geographical dispersion, rates of change over calendar time) as a basis for decisions about what to do. The process is dynamic in the sense that surveillance is about documenting and promoting actions when facing changes, whether from a state of disease absence which switches to disease present, or then mapping (often literally) the progress of disease over real time as its consequences are experienced throughout an animal population. It follows that assuring the quality or, in other words, the technical efficiency of surveillance is of major importance, typically under conditions of uncertainty, reflecting the current state of disease science, analytical capacity including human skills and knowhow, and capacity of decision-makers to take the correct action. Such quality conditions must obtain for all quantities and combinations of resources committed to surveillance.

5.3 Surveillance Is a Production Process

In the following explanation, it is assumed that the surveillance system is optimally efficient in a technical sense. In other words, at any given time the technical information obtained from any level and configuration of specific surveillance resources is always the maximum (or 'best') possible. Moreover, it helps to think of surveillance information as a single homogeneous product. Similarly, surveillance resources can be conceptualised as homogeneous units of aggregated individual elements. It follows that a technically optimal surveillance system is one for which the information produced is the best possible for any given level of resource use. Implicitly, it follows that the individual elements which comprise aggregate units of resource correspondingly must be optimally combined in technical sense; if suboptimal at any level, so will be the surveillance information produced.

The above interpretation facilitates explanation of important relationships by use of simple production economics principles. A basic introduction for animal health economics and production is found in Rushton [5], and a more advanced and general treatment in Beattie et al. [6]. The ultimate objective for applied economists is to quantify relationships as an aid to policymakers in the process of decision-making. But it cannot be stressed too strongly that even without quantification anyone concerned with policymaking needs to understand the fundamental logic of the economic principles when taking decisions about committing resources to surveillance. Economics really is too important to be left to the experts [7].

In general terms, the resource–product relationships described recall other applications in animal health. The generic term for any relationship involving the transformation of resources into products is a production function. Here, the product is surveillance information, and so Fig. 5.1 shows two stylised examples of surveillance information production functions (SIPFs). Consistent with the discussion above, these describe optimally efficient relationships or 'best-practice frontiers'. By assumption, the curves display diminishing returns, indicating that adding more resources to generate more surveillance information (variable resources) does so at a diminishing rate when other resources are in fixed supply, at least in the short term. Specifically which resources are considered fixed will depend on actual circumstances in any given case. But personnel equipped with the necessary analytical skills is a candidate if, for instance, coping with a burgeoning accumulation of data in a fast developing disease outbreak stretches capacity to its limit; indeed, capacity constraints similarly may apply when conditions are not extreme. The assumption is defensible because it reflects experience of similar relationships found widely in the real world. In brief, it means that the technical efficiency with which variable resources are used in production when others are fixed eventually declines.

However, while the overall shape of any SIPF is unlikely to be linear (no diminishing returns), it is conceivable that diminishing returns set in slowly. It means that successive increments of variable surveillance resources add to information by increments that decline progressively in very small amounts. In mathematical

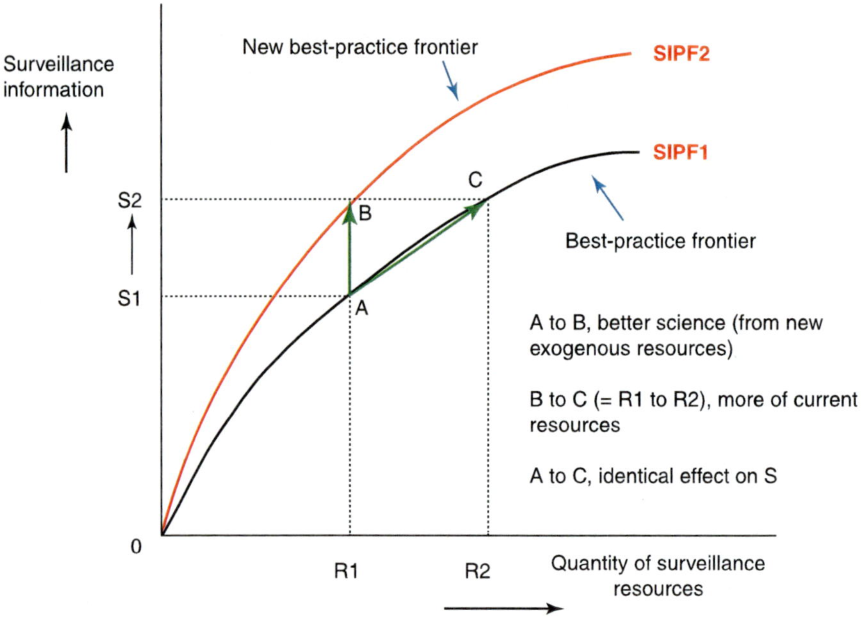

Fig. 5.1 Surveillance information production functions (SIPFs) and technical efficiency

economics terms, the marginal productivity of surveillance resources tends to zero over a large quantitative range of resource use. This could occur as a result of 'learning by doing'; personnel become more experienced and adept at data collection, interpretation, and analysis as the scale of other surveillance resources provided in support of activities increases.[1] Whether in fact this is so is a question for investigation in specific cases. Certainly, it is expected that the marginal product[2] of variable surveillance resources approaches zero at some level of their use.

5.4 Choice of Surveillance Approach

Figure 5.1 draws attention to an important consideration for decision-makers concerned with policies aimed at improving surveillance information. Suppose that currently OS1 information product is obtained for a given disease from OR1 resources on SIPF1, and animal health policymakers consider that OS2 information product is desirable. This objective may result from evidence that a particular disease threat is imminent or an exotic disease is now considered of sufficient concern to merit greater surveillance attention than hitherto.

There is more than one way to approach finding a solution, of which Fig. 5.1 illustrates the two extremes. Vertical AB indicates increased productivity of existing quantities of surveillance resources; in other words, improve the quality of resources currently in use. For example, scientists advance understanding of the disease and its behaviour in the susceptible animal population, personnel are brought up to date in all relevant respects (animal owners and veterinarians skilled in observation, diagnosis, ability to use test equipment, analytical techniques for interpretation of test results, institutional structures fully equipped to facilitate rapid communication to those responsible for consequent interventions), and so on.

Given sufficient time, this first solution implies providing significant new resources for scientific research aimed at understanding a specific disease or diseases in general, and improving practical capacities for surveillance. Collectively, these are exogenous resources (thus excluded from the Fig. 5.1 model) injected to achieve technical progress, a generic term for enhanced productivity. A successful outcome has the effect of rendering SIPF1 apparently redundant as SIPF2 replaces it as the new best-practice frontier. But Fig. 5.1 also suggests that even with SIPF1 and current knowledge OS2 is achievable by increasing OR1 quantity of resources to OR2 (from A to C), say by employing more veterinarians and associated personnel in surveillance, providing them with necessary equipment, and supplementing

[1] Indeed, increasing returns might occur at very low levels of variable resource use. Consider the example of a new surveillance facility being established, a laboratory fully equipped except for its complement of scientists. As staff with different skills are appointed and begin to interact productively, the overall efficiency of resource use may well increase, at least over a range of numbers employed.

[2] Marginal product is the increment of product (here, surveillance information) that results from an increment of (surveillance) resources.

existing resources for disseminating information to animal owners about how to minimise, or preferably avoid, disease spread. In cases of highly infective diseases, for example, foot and mouth disease, sometimes this latter requirement applies also to the general public.

According to the model, adding (OR2 – OR1) resources with respect to SIPF1 has the same effect on surveillance information as OS2 – OS1, the effect of introducing new resources to shift SIPF1 upwards to SIPF2. But SIPF2 and SIPF1 are presented as extremes, and so AB and AC similarly locate extreme possibilities. In practice, there is an array of different combinations of scientific advance and additional resources which also satisfy the policy objective of raising OS1 to OS2 surveillance information output. SIPF1 is technically inferior to SIPF2 and so becomes the now second-best-practice efficiency frontier to the latter's best practice. But implicitly between the two is an array of surveillance information production functions, SIPFi for $i = 1, 2, 3, \ldots\ldots n$, offering different combinations of efficiency improvement both from adding new resources and adding currently available resources to those already in use.

Given scope for planning ahead before making a choice, the crucial economic question is which of all feasible options achieves the policy objective, that of more surveillance information at least cost. The caveat is that choice may be constrained by practical circumstances. It is one thing having sufficient time to conduct surveillance ahead of a disease outbreak, or to monitor prevalence changes for endemic disease of low infectivity and scope for spread throughout an animal population, and quite another when a sudden unforeseen outbreak of a highly infective disease demands immediate action—the so-called 'fire brigade' approach. In those circumstances, in effect there is no decision to make; it is made already in the light of prior information about the expected consequences of not intervening to mitigate outbreak effects, both technical and economic. The important issue of intervention is considered below.

If resources are to be committed for a long period ahead, their opportunity cost that explicitly accounts for time must be taken into account, that is, the net present value of benefits forgone as a result of not allocating resources to their alternative use expected to yield highest net benefits. In the simplest case, a choice may need to be made between allocating surveillance resources to disease X rather than disease Y (a competitive relationship); in other circumstances, allocating resources to disease X may contribute positively to disease Y surveillance (a complementary relationship). The same criterion applies to investment in surveillance in general, such as whether society benefits more from animal health surveillance than from human health surveillance, given that the two categories overlap for zoonoses. Taking into account the specific technical characteristics of relationships in actual cases is fundamental to economic choices in resource allocation decisions. Multiple disease surveillance systems and One Health perspectives (see Case Study 2) are extensions of these considerations.

5.5 The Value of Surveillance

Surveillance information is commonly defined exclusively according to its technical specifications, but increasingly it is recognised that economics must be taken into account [8–11]. As noted above, the resources committed to surveillance have an opportunity cost, not only in terms of trade-offs between different diseases, or categories of disease, but overall for society as a whole. However, translating the technical production function relationships into value terms presents problems. On the one hand, the monetary value of surveillance resources (financial costs of employing scientists and veterinarians, maintaining laboratories, purchasing test equipment, transport provision, paying for dissemination activities, etc.) normally can be estimated with acceptable accuracy; on the other hand, valuing surveillance information is problematical.

5.5.1 Cost-Effectiveness Criteria

Owing to its multifaceted technical aspects, it is unsurprising that economic evaluation tends to focus on cost-effectiveness criteria, that is, how cheaply specified technical requirements for surveillance can be satisfied. In relation to Fig. 5.1, this is equivalent to technical specification of, say, OS2 surveillance information, and then calculating which of OR1 and OR2 quantities of resources—or some intermediate quantity supplemented by exogenous resources to raise productivity—achieves OS2 at least financial cost. In this simple theoretical model, units of surveillance resource give rise to units of surveillance information assuming homogeneous quality for each of the variables. Relaxing that restrictive assumption, and reinterpreting the surveillance resources horizontal axis as measuring equal increments in financial expenditure instead of equal units of aggregate physical resources, we can think of unpacking those units into their component parts. That way, the composition of OS1 financial expenditure in terms of its separate technical elements identifies the most cost-effective system for conducting surveillance consistent with production of OS2 information.

Note that cost–benefit analysis is presented later, when dealing with the link between surveillance and intervention.

5.5.2 Willingness-to-Pay Approaches

In the absence of valuations directly observable from market prices, as necessarily they are, approximations to non-monetary values for stakeholders' willingness to pay for surveillance are derived by indirect methods. Other approaches to surveillance valuation are by discrete choice experiments [12] and contingent valuation

[13, 14]. Inevitably, answers may vary according to who is asked—individual livestock farmers directly affected in the event of disease outbreak, epidemiologists aware of effects at population level, and so on. Certainly these procedures are a step in the right economic direction when other data are unavailable.

In interim conclusion, surveillance system design is both a technical and an economic matter. Choices made about the design and resourcing of surveillance systems affect the flow of information in quantity and quality. Thus the level of financial provision for surveillance, and implicitly the availability of real resources for it, is a consideration that justifies close scrutiny (see, e.g., [15]). The key question to be answered in making all resource allocation decisions is, 'is it worth it?' The question is only partly answered by the cost-effectiveness criterion because it requires consideration of not only the costs of resources but also surveillance benefits. Often the focus may be on particular interest groups, livestock farmers for instance, but ultimately it is an issue for society at large.

5.6 Surveillance and Intervention Are Interdependent

Economic evaluation is *always* about relationships between variables. Consequently, full economic evaluation of any production process cannot be made without reference to both costs and benefits. These are measured using money as the unit of account because it is the only feasible way to compare real resources and products which are technically dissimilar and to aggregate them if required, as is frequently so.

The task of measuring the benefits of surveillance is anyway complicated because its value is not independent of decisions made to make interventions, and therefore use additional resources with the purpose of mitigating disease effects, on the basis of the information acquired. As previously noted, surveillance is not an end in itself, not even, say, if its purpose initially is to acquire a better understanding of disease aetiology ostensibly for its own sake.

Figure 5.2 summarises the relationship between surveillance, intervention, and their common purpose, which is to avoid benefits lost to people as a result of animal disease. The origin of benefit losses is reductions in production of all the goods and services animals provide for people's consumption that are caused by animal disease [an example of the wider range of animal (or zoonotic) disease impacts has been described in [17]—Box 5.1]. Without disease, more animal products would be available to people, enabling them to enhance their well-being. Also, resources

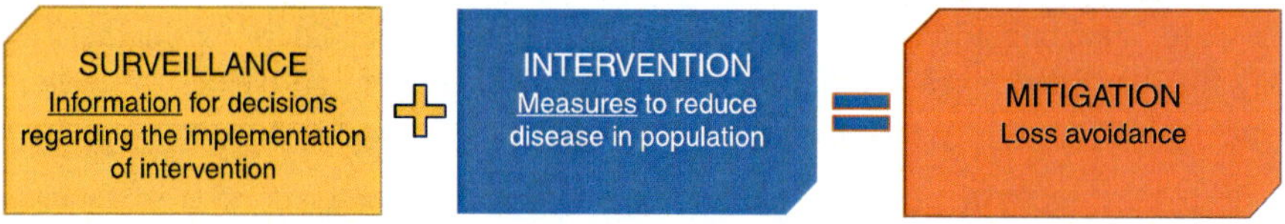

Fig. 5.2 The relationship between surveillance, intervention, and loss avoidance. (Source: [16])

Box 5.1 The Wider Range of Disease Impacts

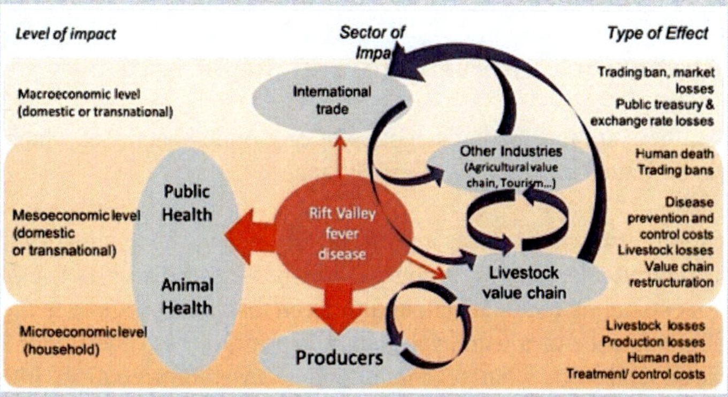

Socio-economic impacts of Rift Valley fever per sector, level, and type of effects induced. The links between the disease and the different sectors and level impacted (health-related costs) are represented by straight (red) arrows; the links between the different sectors and level impacted (non-health-related costs) are represented by the curved (blue) arrows. (Adapted from [17])

Regarding resources, although different according to their particular characteristics, both surveillance and intervention employ an array of resources including scientists, field workers, administrators, test and treatment equipment, laboratories, data processing facilities, means of transport, and more, all variously combined. Some resources (e.g. laboratories, full-time personnel, in institutions such as the UK's Animal and Plant Health Agency) are fixed in the short term, and others variable according to the particular disease, or diseases, to be addressed at any given time.

As also previously noted, monetary costs of resources are relatively straightforward to identify and calculate, amounting to the sum of expenditures on wages and salaries, equipment, rents and depreciation on buildings, etc., incurred over a given time period. Moreover, surveillance and intervention resources can be separately identified, if imperfectly, and costs allocated accordingly. But the benefits from disease mitigation are attributable to both surveillance and intervention. Even if the objective for surveillance is initially viewed as to provide information as the final product, putative future benefits still cannot be categorically attributed to surveillance alone. Account must be taken of the possibility that interventions will be

[3]At risk of stating the obvious, that is not to say existing surveillance and associated resources suddenly are able to metamorphose seamlessly into something quite different. Some are transferable to other uses (e.g. scientists) while even they, along with highly specialised resources, will be differently employed from the outset if there is reduced need over the long term to mitigate negative effects of animal disease.

necessary, even if only on a very limited scale. The reason lies in the specific characteristics of benefits, which need careful definition.

5.7 Surveillance, Intervention, and the Benefits

In summary, there are four main categories of economic benefits of which only the first may be attributed exclusively to surveillance.

1. Intervention resources saved as a result of surveillance enabling advance preparation and rapid intervention response if or when disease occurs. Thus a precondition for estimating monetary expenditures on resources incurred in the event of disease is existence of a technical plan, blueprint, or best guestimate outlining what to do and with what resources under different scenarios. Intervention resources have an opportunity cost. So, to the extent that effective surveillance facilitates saving intervention resources, the benefits from reallocating unneeded intervention resources to alternative uses are attributable to surveillance [18].
2. Losses avoided in animal production, and therefore resource productivity, as a result of interventions informed by surveillance helping to reduce animal morbidity and mortality. Most easily understood in relation to farm livestock production, reduced milk yields, higher abortions and calf mortality, premature death of adult animals and so higher herd replacement rates, are all examples of disease-induced physical output losses. So are the benefits people feel from avoided suffering or death of their companion animals, and avoided loss of transport and traction services provided by equine and bovine animals on which people rely, and so on. All such losses avoided represent economic benefits, sources of people's well-being which encompass products both tangible (e.g. goods, such as farm livestock products) and intangible (e.g. services, such as pet companionship, traction and transport, recreation, assistance). Losses may be avoided either by taking preventive measures in anticipation of disease occurring (prophylaxis) or by cure, which prevents the further accumulation of losses additional to those already incurred into the future.
3. In cases of zoonoses, human losses experienced as morbidity and mortality affecting people in their role as factors of production (diminished efficiency and availability for productive economic activity) and in itself (dissatisfaction with quality of life) should also be added [19], additional costs incurred by health services. Avoided fear of the potential impacts of zoonoses on people, of which bovine spongiform encephalopathy is a classic example, is also a benefit.
4. Avoided negative externalities, the wider societal value losses incurred because of disease, for example, national or international trade disruption because of movement constraints placed on animals and related goods to limit or prevent infectious disease spread, reduced tourism, and associated loss of net incomes.

Category 2 is central to explanation of how surveillance contributes to economic benefits in general, and so the following section sets out the detailed analytical framework in relation to loss avoidance in animal production. Categories 3 and 4 are essentially extensions of that framework, for reasons explained.

5.8 Relationship Between Surveillance, Intervention, and Disease Mitigation[4]

Surveillance and intervention are conceptually distinct and contribute together to mitigate the adverse effects of animal disease. To recall, a reduced quantity (and/or quality) of animal products people want is a disbenefit because people are denied the possibility of consuming as much as would be available to them in the absence of disease. It follows that only when surveillance and intervention are considered simultaneously is it possible to consider the value of disease mitigation, the avoidance of benefit losses that would occur in its absence. In other words, the value of surveillance can only be meaningfully interpreted taking intervention into account.

In principle, the focus may be on value to livestock farmers, pet owners, the thoroughbred racehorse industry, or any other group in society to whom animals matter. However, society as a whole is commonly the unit of most concern, not least because the ultimate purpose of economic analysis is to illuminate the implications for people's well-being of choices made in resource allocation that affect us all.

Nevertheless, it simplifies explanation to confine definition of benefits to the following avoided losses: raw material animal products intended for human food consumption, for example, litres of milk, kilogrammes of beef, pig meat, or sheep meat, poultry meat, and eggs; lost companionship from pets and people's concern for animals' welfare, also representing benefit losses to the people affected, whether to owners or anyone who cares about the well-being of animals; and reduced availability of animals as means of transport or traction. Collectively, these avoided losses of goods and services provided by animals are summarised as variable A.

By definition, zoonotic disease, Z, affects people's own health, while epidemics such as of foot and mouth disease cause still wider 'negative externalities', E, the full range of costs that are indirect spin-off effects of animal disease into other spheres of the economy. Disruption to everyday life occasioned by movement restrictions on both animals and people, including loss of tourism, are prime examples. These pose different kinds of measurement problems beyond the scope of the present discussion, but do not invalidate the essential principles. So, remembering that total economic losses, L, caused by animal disease are $L = A + Z + E$, the magnitude of each variable contribution depending on the precise circumstances and disease, here attention is confined to

$$A = f(S,I) \tag{5.1}$$

[4]This section is based on Howe et al. [20] 'Economic principles for resource allocation decisions at national level to mitigate the effects of disease in farm animal populations'. Epidemiology and Infection, 2013; 141 (1): 91–101, http://journals.cambridge.org/repo_A856SFJs

where A = animal product losses avoided, S = surveillance resources, and I = intervention resources.

Also as before in relation to surveillance resources, we reasonably hypothesise diminishing returns to variable intervention resources that also contribute to disease mitigation. Plotting the three-variable relationship in eq. (1) gives Fig. 5.3, a stylised hypothetical example of a disease mitigation surface for epidemic disease. Particular features of the surface are as follows.

Along axis *OH*, allocating more resources to intervention with no surveillance at all nevertheless enables production losses to be avoided. But if any given level of I is supplemented by surveillance (all curves in the direction *OJ*), more losses are avoided. The interpretation along axis *OJ*, increasing surveillance with no intervention, is less straightforward.

With respect to surveillance resources, the relevant lower boundary of the production surface is *OK*, a curvilinear relationship on the horizontal plane tracing out the path of increasing avoided production losses vertically above, *OL*, for the lowest feasible levels of intervention consistent with any loss avoidance. In other words, however small scale in practice, there must be some provision made for intervention for surveillance to have any practical purpose at all. Also along curve *OL*, intervention resources are shown as limiting the ability of more surveillance to reduce losses above the level corresponding to point *L*′, where curve *OL* flattens, indicating that thereafter the marginal product of surveillance resources, dA/dS is zero. In simple

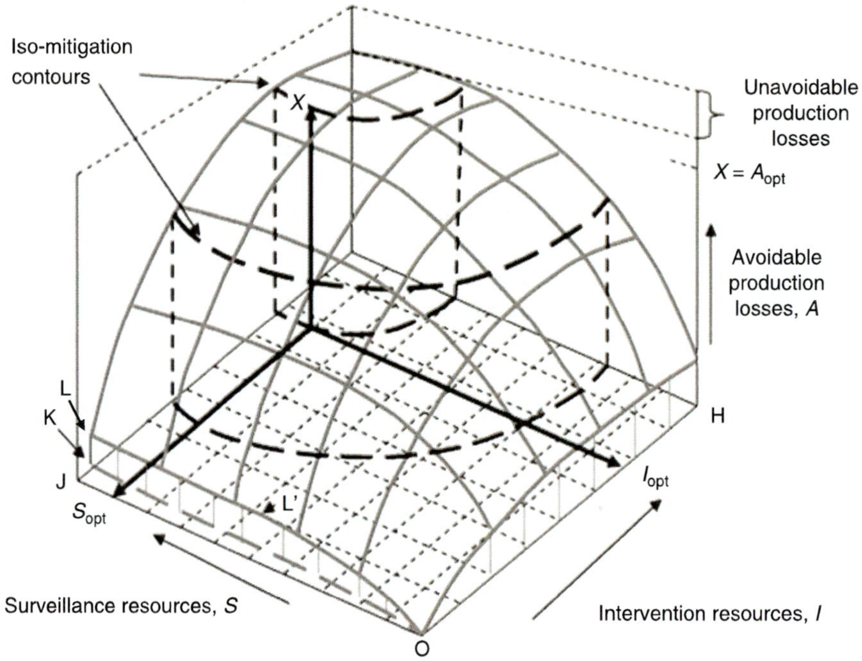

Fig. 5.3 Hypothetical epidemic disease mitigation surface, diminishing returns to S and I

terms, the scale of all resources devoted to disease mitigation is too small to have a significant beneficial effect.

At the opposite extreme, a feature of the mitigation surface is flattening towards its apex, indicating the assumed impossibility of eliminating all production losses. At high levels of resource use both surveillance and intervention have zero marginal products (i.e. $dA/dS = dA/dL = 0$, no more losses avoided). In some cases eradication of a disease is feasible, and so with no possibility of future losses the unavoidable losses are zero.

5.8.1 Iso-Mitigation Maps and Technical Relationships Between Surveillance and Intervention

Figure 5.3 also shows three out of a theoretically infinite number of contour lines that can be drawn around the mitigation surface. Translated to the horizontal plane, the contour lines become an iso-mitigation map plotting variable combinations of S and I that give rise to different fixed levels of A. Their particular characteristics in the case of a given disease or class of diseases depend exclusively on the technical relationship between *S*, *I*, and *A*. Thus a starting point for analysing the role of surveillance in loss mitigation is to establish the precise characteristics of that technical relationship, and then to examine the economic implications of what is found.

To generalise, it is instructive to begin by describing the technical relationship between *S* and *I* in terms of a single parameter, the Hicks elasticity of substitution, σ, a measure of the ease with which surveillance and intervention resources can be substituted for one other.

Mathematically,

$$\sigma = \left[\mathrm{d}(S/I)(S/I) \right]\left[(\mathrm{d}S/\mathrm{d}I)\mathrm{d}(\mathrm{d}S/\mathrm{d}I) \right]$$

In words, σ is the proportional change in the ratio of *S* to *I* resource use relative to the proportional change in rate of technical substitution of *I*, intervention resources, for *S*, surveillance resources.[5]

Constructed independently of Fig. 5.3, Fig. 5.4 shows the implications for the shape of iso-mitigation curves, and hence substitutability between *S* and *I*, of three values for σ; the limits infinity and zero, and unity. The values for σ are shown for increasing magnitudes of *A* and incorporate a curve for *A2*, where $\sigma = 1$ which more closely approximates to the implications of a mitigation surface such as Fig. 5.3.

[5] This is more complex than the more usual definitions of elasticities in economics, having the useful property of expressing substitution possibilities as a single value. Also, d*S*/d*I* strictly defined in mathematics measures the variable effect on *S* for a unit increase in *I*, whereas in the present context its inverse, d*I*/d*S*, that is, how many intervention resources can be saved by a unit increase in surveillance resources, intuitively may seem of greater interest. The mathematical refinement makes no substantive difference to the arguments.

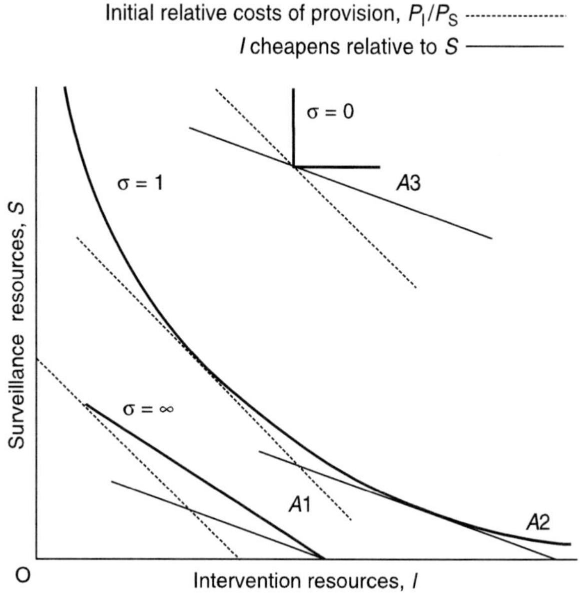

Fig. 5.4 Implications of the Hicks elasticity of substitution, σ, for mitigation resource allocation under two sets of relative costs of providing surveillance, S, and Intervention, I; iso-mitigation curves for losses avoided, $A3 > A2 > A1$

5.8.2 Budget Constraints and Monetary Costs of Loss Avoidance

Reference to the Hicks elasticity of substitution, σ, has the important function of reminding anyone concerned with the evaluation of surveillance in particular, or disease mitigation in general, that constantly the initial focus must be on assessing the technical characteristics of surveillance and intervention with regard to scope for their substitution. Once that is established, the relative costs of their provision come into play.

Economic efficiency and technical efficiency are different. Economic efficiency requires identification of the combination of S and I that minimises the cost of achieving a given level of avoided losses, A, having taken into account their relative costs of provision. The reason is that in any real-world context there is normally a financial limit, a budget constraint, on the expenditures that can be made on real resources for surveillance and intervention.

Thus,

$$B = P_S.S + P_I.I \tag{5.2}$$

where B = total budget available, P_S = monetary outlay (price, or cost of provision) per unit of surveillance resources, S = quantity of surveillance real resources, P_I = monetary outlay (price, or cost of provision) per unit of intervention resources, and I = quantity of intervention real resources.

The least-cost combination of S and I is found uniquely where $P_S \cdot dS = P_I \cdot dI$. Any other outcome costs more, inequality indicating that the cheaper of S and I should be substituted for the more expensive.

Rearranging terms,

$$dS / dI = P_I / P_S \tag{5.3}$$

where dS/dI = rate of technical substitution of I for S, and P_I/P_S = monetary cost of providing I relative to S.

Figure 5.4 illustrates the implications of different values of σ for least-cost mitigation for two ratios of the monetary cost of providing S relative to I. The total budget available to finance both surveillance and intervention resources increases with distance from the origin.

A straight line iso-mitigation contour such as $A1$ has the property that $\sigma = \infty$, making S and I perfect technical substitutes; a unit change in S, say, always has the same (i.e. constant) effect in terms of how much of I resources will substitute for no change in losses A. The consequence for resource allocation is that the cheaper of S and I per unit of their provision will account for all loss avoidance activities. But as already noted from Fig. 5.3, should the relative monetary costs favour surveillance S, there must be at least some provision for intervention, however small, because the immediate response to any disease incidence identified by surveillance must be to trigger activities aimed at inhibiting its progress. There is no point in conducting surveillance if there is no intention or possibility of intervening to do something about it, however limited the intervention resources employed.

For $\sigma = 1$, the less expensive resource substitutes for the relatively more expensive, both S and I making a contribution to loss avoidance. In general, the greater the magnitude of σ the more sensitive is the least-cost solution for budget allocation between S and I for changes in their relative costs of provision. Each of the three iso-mitigation contours in Fig. 5.3 are drawn to be broadly in the vicinity of $\sigma = 1$ to draw attention to the real-world observation that both S and I typically contribute to loss avoidance. In practice, depending on the particular disease or class of diseases, $\infty > \sigma > 0$ is normally expected to be the case.

Where $\sigma = 0$, S and I must be used in fixed proportions; substitution is impossible irrespective of changes in their relative costs of provision, and S and I are described as perfect complements. In effect, they are to be treated as a single resource, say M. Arguably, disease mitigation policies in practice are typically designed as if $\sigma = 0$, if only because few discrete options for combining S and I are ever considered. Clearly, a comprehensive assessment of the options is likely to be demanding on research time and other resources. Not only is resource allocation between surveillance and intervention subject to budget constraints, so is scope for financing research to ascertain the technical feasibility and economic efficiency of different approaches to loss avoidance. But relative to the value of the information acquired, the effort nevertheless may prove worthwhile.

5.8.2.1 The Overall Economic Optimum for Combining Surveillance and Intervention

Should there be no budget constraint on resources allocated or, more realistically, a case is to be made for investing funds in disease mitigation, the following optimising criteria apply.

First, treat S and I as an aggregate resource, M. Then $\mathrm{d}A/\mathrm{d}M = P_M/P_A$ which, rearranged, is

$$P_A\left(\mathrm{d}A/\mathrm{d}M\right) = P_M \tag{5.4}$$

That is, the value of the marginal product of all mitigation resources, M (aggregate of surveillance and intervention resources) in terms of losses avoided equals the cost per additional unit of mitigation resources provided. Should the left-hand side exceed the right-hand side, total net benefits from mitigation can be increased by using more resources; if the converse, reduce mitigation resources to increase net benefits.

But since M comprises S and I,

$$\mathrm{d}A/\mathrm{d}M = \left(\partial A/\partial S\right)\mathrm{d}S + \left(\partial A/\partial I\right)\mathrm{d}I \tag{5.5}$$

In words, the overall marginal effect of adding units of mitigation resources can be decomposed into two parts, the addition to avoided losses contributed by a unit increase in surveillance resources and the addition to avoided losses contributed by a unit increase in intervention resources.

Following the logic of (5.4), we require that

$$P_A\left(\partial A/\partial S\right) = P_S \text{ and } P_A\left(\partial A/\partial I\right) = P_I$$

are solved simultaneously for S, I, and A. The result amounts to the consequence of searching across an iso-mitigation map until the level of A is reached at which both S and I are in least-cost combination and the total monetary value of losses avoided (total benefits) minus the monetary cost of surveillance and intervention (total costs) is maximised. Point '*x*' in Fig. 5.3 associated with *S opt* and *I opt* illustrates the idea.

5.9 Further Considerations in Economic Evaluation

The above discussion has outlined and elaborated standard production economics principles to the evaluation of animal disease surveillance. The single most important conclusion is that to proceed beyond cost-effectiveness analysis, which provides information about the implications for monetary expenditure on resources aimed at achieving a technical objective, two conditions must be fulfilled. First, the benefits accruing to surveillance must be defined in economic, not technical, terms and measured in equivalent monetary units; second, recognition that benefits do not accrue exclusively to surveillance but also to interventions made in the light of surveillance information. Thus any standard social cost–benefit approach to evaluation, should it be contemplated, must incorporate both surveillance and intervention resources, and address the challenging task of expressing the benefits of mitigating disease effects in monetary units.

As previously explained, to keep the exposition simple the discussion largely overlooked the fact that in many cases of animal disease the benefits of total losses avoided, L, extend beyond variable A to $L = A + Z + E$, where Z is zoonotic and E is wider externality effects. Intuitively, if the $A = f(S, I)$ evaluation indicates efficient resource allocation by showing that net benefits are increased by mitigation, society must be better off because both Z and E similarly will be reduced. Two caveats apply.

First, the evaluation framework outlined here implicitly assumes that all measured benefits are private, that is, they accrue directly only to livestock farmers, pet owners, or users of animals as other forms of personal resource; so secondly, no account is taken of any negative externalities, Z, associated with zoonotic disease on people's health, the implications for demands on human health service resources, and the potential loss of productivity by workers to the detriment of gross domestic product. Therefore, Z negative externalities are indeed expected to fall. Evaluation needs recourse to human health economics, a distinct area of enquiry complementary to animal health in specific contexts. Foundation texts include McGuire et al. [21], McPake et al. [22], and Drummond et al. [23]. One Health has emerged (or perhaps re-emerged, [24]) as an integrating framework for all such dimensions.

Second, in cases of major public disruption caused by the steps taken to curtail epidemic disease such as foot-and-mouth, still more externalities must be taken into account. But these are not always wholly detrimental. For example, a farmer's failure to report signs of foot-and-mouth disease in a north of England pig herd in 2001 led to a national epidemic [25]. Its costs extended far beyond the farm sector. The National Audit Office [26] estimated that compensation and other payments to farmers (i.e. money transfers from taxpayers to farmers) were expected to total nearly £1.4 billion; direct costs of measures to deal with the epidemic, including the purchase of goods and services to eradicate the disease, were nearly £1.3 billion; other public sector costs were £0.3 billion. In the private sector, the areas most affected by the epidemic were agriculture, the food chain and supporting services, incurring net costs of £0.6 billion; tourism and supporting industries lost revenues of between £4.5 billion and £5.4 billion. However, the UK Treasury estimated that the net overall economic effect of the epidemic amounted to less than £2 billion, or just 0.2% of Gross Domestic Product (GDP), because many of the losses suffered by individuals and firms in agriculture and tourism led to equivalent amounts of money being spent in other sectors of the economy. The nature of economic activity is such that costs incurred by one sector may be offset to a greater or lesser extent by benefits to another.

Kompas et al. [27] developed a stochastic optimal control model consistent with the simplified framework outlined here which they applied to surveillance activities to guard against a potential entry of FMD in the United States. Having taken border quarantine expenditures as given, the optimal level of surveillance activity against a disease incursion and spread was estimated by minimising the present value of the major direct and indirect costs of the disease, as well as the costs of the surveillance and disease management and eradication programmes.

5.10 New Directions for Surveillance Evaluation

This Chapter has concentrated on the microeconomic principles that underpin the practice and appraisal of surveillance evaluation. For economists, they are the core of a framework that should underpin quantitative evaluations. Equally, veterinary scientists engaged in surveillance policymaking or guiding evaluation undertaken by economists need to understand the broad principles outlined; for instance, they do not need to know how to estimate an elasticity of substitution, but understanding the principle and knowing why it matters is indispensable for making efficient resource allocation decisions.

Direct estimation of production functions from empirical data has a long history in economics, but presents two main challenges to analysts. First, the initial requirement is to identify and obtain quantitative estimates for resource and product data as inputs to econometric estimation of the equations. Attention has been drawn to problems arising, such as the fact that although market price data for farm livestock production frequently is available, indirect methods have to be used to estimate people's willingness to pay for, say, animal companionship or welfare. Should production function estimation be an option, Beattie et al. [6] usefully summarise the properties of different functional forms[6]; Heathfield and Wibe [28] and Chambers [29] are earlier foundation texts, while Hackman [30] is mathematically challenging and revives attempts made long ago to integrate engineering and economics [31, 32]. In all cases, not least the present context, the foundation of all production function analysis is knowledge of technical relationships.

The widespread availability of computers and spreadsheets potentially has revolutionised scope for analysing the implications of technical relationships between surveillance and intervention in mitigating disease effects. No longer is it necessary to experiment with different predetermined functional forms in parameter estimation or necessarily have recourse to complex mathematics. In principle, identifying the technical resource requirements for different specifications of surveillance methods and related interventions, acquiring data and making monetary estimates for losses avoided, can all be brought together to simulate outcomes of different potential choices to be made.

As yet, the principle has not been translated into standard practice. If relationships are expressed in condensed three-dimensional form consistent with Fig. 5.3, outcomes for different disease mitigation surfaces might well turn out to exhibit topographical variations and irregularities unconstrained by the smoothing effects of preselected mathematical models. Häsler's practical tool designed initially for the Swiss Federal Veterinary Service (2011) and RISKSUR [34] with its EVA component (2013), which both incorporate cost-effective and cost–benefit approaches, are steps in that direction (see Chap. 4) (https://survtools.org/) [33].

Finally, a novel dimension yet to be thoroughly explored is the concept and measurement of social capital [35, 36]. People's personal relationships, social network support, civic engagement and trust, and cooperative norms are all factors critical to

[6] Pages 71–81, including Tables 2.1 and 2.2.

ensuring that the technical efficiency frontier (Fig. 5.1) and mitigation surface (Fig. 5.3) can be reached (see Part V—Methods to evaluate health information sharing networks). Important questions are: is the underlying science of surveillance reliable and the outcome of research conducted with integrity; can experts and animal owners conducting surveillance be relied upon to report the truth; are the institutions responsible for surveillance, intervention, and decision-making efficiently structured to operate on the basis of trust and ease of cooperation; are data on monetary values for resources and products (hence avoided losses) reliable? Gilbert et al. [37] is relevant in this context, as is Rich et al. [38], who consider system-wide effects throughout the livestock supply chain (see Part IV—Qualitative evaluation approaches) [39–42].

In conclusion, there remains ample scope to apply novel approaches to economic evaluation of animal disease surveillance, all founded on a sound theoretical basis that acknowledges its role in providing information for decisions about interventions aimed at mitigating the detrimental effects of animal disease for people's well-being.

References

1. Häsler BN, Howe KS, Stärk KDC. Conceptualising the technical relationship of animal disease surveillance to intervention and mitigation as a basis for economic analysis. BMC Health Services Res. 2011;11:225. http://www.biomedcentral.com/1472-6963/11/225
2. Thacker SB. Surveillance. In: Gregg MB, Dicker RC, Goodman RA, editors. Field epidemiology. New York: Oxford University Press; 1996. p. 16–32.
3. Blackie MJ, Dent JB, editors. Information systems for agriculture, Applied Science Publishers; 1979.
4. Dunn ES. Social information processing and statistical systems—change and reform. New York: Wiley-Interscience; 1974.
5. Rushton J, editor. The economics of animal health and production. Washington, DC: CABI; 2009. 364 pp.
6. Beattie BR, Taylor CR, Watts MJ. The economics of production. 2nd ed. Malabar, Florida: Krieger Publishing Company; 2009. 299 pp.
7. Howe KS. The allocation of resources for animal health. In: 'The economics of animal health', revue scientifique et technique, World Organisation for Animal Health (OIE), 36:1; 2017, pp. 35–48.
8. Drewe JA, Hoinville LJ, Cook AJ, Floyd T, Stärk KD. Evaluation of animal and public health surveillance systems: a systematic review. Epidemiol Infect. 2012;140:575–90.
9. Drewe JA, Hoinville LJ, Cook AJ, Floyd T, Gunn G, Stärk KD. SERVAL: a new framework for the evaluation of animal health surveillance. Transbound Emerg Dis. 2015;62:33–45.
10. Klinkenberg D, Nielenb M, de Mourits MCM, Jong MCM. The effectiveness of classical swine fever surveillance programmes in The Netherlands. Prev Vet Med. 2005;67:19–37.
11. Stärk KDC, Häsler B. The value of information: current challenges in surveillance implementation. Prev Vet Med. 2015;122:229–34.
12. Phama HTT, Peyre M, Trinhc TQ, Nguyend OC, Vud TD, Rukkwamsuke T, Antoine-Moussiauxf N. Application of discrete choice experiment to assess farmers' willingness to report swine diseases in the red River Delta region, Vietnam. Prev Vet Med. 2017;138:28–36.
13. Calba C, Antoine-Moussiauxc N, Charrierd F, Hendrikxe P, Saegerman C, Peyre M, Goutard FL. Applying participatory approaches in the evaluation of surveillance systems: a pilot study on African swine fever surveillance in Corsica. Prev Vet Med. 2015a;122:389–98.

14. Mitchell RC, Carson RT. Using surveys to value public goods: the contingent valuation method. Resources for the Future, Washington D.C.; 1989, 463 pp.
15. Keusch GT, Pappaioanou M, González MC, Scott KA, Tsai P. Sustainable financing for global disease surveillance and response. In: Keusch GT, editor. Sustaining global surveillance and response to emerging zoonotic diseases, Chapter 6. Washington, DC: National Academies Press; 2009. p. 187–204.
16. Häsler B, Rushton J, Stärk KDC, Howe KS. Surveillance and intervention expenditure: substitution or complementarity between different types of policy. In: Livestock disease policies: building bridges between science and economics. Paris: OECD; 2013. p. 89–108.
17. Peyre M, Chevalier V, Abdo-Salem S, Velthuis A, Antoine-Moussiaux N, Thiry E, Roger F. A systematic scoping study of the socio-economic impact of Rift Valley fever: research gaps and needs. Zoonoses Public Health. 2015;62:309–25. https://doi.org/10.1111/zph.12153.
18. Stärk KDC, Babo Martins S, Häsler B. Surveillance without intervention: is there a value? Proceedings of the Conference of the International Society for Veterinary Epidemiology and Economics, November; 2018, 16 pp.
19. Narrod C, Zinsstag J, Tiongco M. A one health framework for estimating the economics costs of zoonotic diseases on society. EcoHealth. 2012;9:150–62. https://doi.org/10.1007/s10393-012-0747-9.
20. Howe KS, Häsler BN, Stärk KDC. Economic principles for resource allocation decisions at national level to mitigate the effects of disease in farm animal populations. Epidemiol Infect. 2013;141(1):91–101. http://journals.cambridge.org/repo_A856SFJs
21. McGuire A, Henderson J, Mooney G. The economics of health care. London and New York: Routledge; 1988, 260 pages.
22. McPake B, Kumaranatake L, ansd Normand, C. Health economics: an international perspective. London and New York: Routledge; 2002. 286 pp.
23. Drummond MF, Sculpher MJ, Torrance GW, Stoddart GL. Methods for the economic evaluation of health care programmes. 3rd ed. Oxford: Oxford University Press; 2005, 379 pp.
24. Bresalier M, Cassidy A, Woods A. One health in history. In: Zinsstag J, Schelling E, Whittaker M, Tanner M, Waltner-Toews D, editors. One health: the theory and practice of integrated health approaches. Wallingford, Oxfordshire, 480 pp.: CABI International; 2015. https://doi.org/10.1079/9781780643410.0001.
25. Mansley LM, Dunlop PJ, Whiteside SM, Smith RGH. Early dissemination of foot-and-mouth disease virus through sheep marketing in February 2001. Vet Rec. 2003;153:45–50.
26. National Audit Office. The 2001 outbreak of foot and mouth disease. Report by the comptroller and auditor general. HC 939 Session 2001-2002: 21 June 2002. The Stationery Office, London; 2002.
27. Kompas T, Che TN, Van Ha P. An optimal surveillance measure against foot and mouth disease in the United States. Crawford School of Economics and Government, The Australian National University. Working papers in International and Development Economics. November; 2006, 23 pp.
28. Heathfield DF, Wibe S. An introduction to cost and production functions. London: Macmillan Education; 1987, 193 pp.
29. Chambers RG. Applied production analysis—a dual approach. Cambridge: Cambridge University Press; 1988. 331 pp.
30. Hackman ST. Production economics—integrating the microeconomic and engineering perspectives. Berlin: Springer; 2008, 520 pp.
31. Chenery HB. Engineering production functions. Q J Econ. 1949;63(4):507–31.
32. Chenery HB. Process and production functions from engineering data. In: Leontief W, et al., editors. Studies in the structure of the American economy. New York: Oxford University Press; 1953.
33. Peyre M, Hoinville L, Njoroge J, Cameron A, Traon D, Goutard F, Calba C, Grosbois V, Delabouglise A, Varant V, Drewe J, Pfeiffer D, Häsler B. The RISKSUR EVA Tool (Survtool): a tool for the integrated evaluation of animal health surveillance systems. Prev. Vet. Med. 104777; 2019. https://doi.org/10.1016/j.prevetmed.2019.104777.

34. RISKSUR. Development of an integrated evaluation matrix. Providing a new generation of methodologies and tools for cost-effective risk-based animal health surveillance systems for the benefit of livestock producers, decision makers and consumers. Project no. 310806, EU seventh Framework programme; n.d.
35. Scrivens K, Smith C. Four interpretations of social capital: an agenda for measurement. Working Paper No. 55, OECD Statistics Directorate; 2013.
36. Siegler V Measuring social capital. Office for National Statistics; 2014.
37. Gilbert WH, Häsler N, Rushton J. Influences of farmer and veterinarian behaviour on emerging disease surveillance in England and Wales. Epidemiol Infect. 2014;142:172–86. https://doi.org/10.1017/S0950268813000484.
38. Rich KM, Denwood MJ, Stott AW, Mellor DJ, Reid SWJ, Gunn GJ. Systems approaches to animal disease surveillance and resource allocation: methodological frameworks for behavioral analysis. PLoS One. 2013;8(11):e82019. www.plosone.org
39. Calba C, Cameron A, Goutard F, Grosbois V, Haesler B, Hoinville L, Lindberg A, Pinto J, Peyre M, Pfeiffer D, Traon D, Vergne T. The EVA tool: an integrated approach for evaluation of animal health surveillance systems. Report for the deliverable No. 1.4; 2013.
40. Calba C, Goutard FL, Hoinville L, Hendrikx P, Lindberg A, Saegerman C, Peyre M. Surveillance systems evaluation: a systematic review of the existing approaches. BMC Public Health. 2015b;15:448. https://doi.org/10.1186/s12889-015-1791-5.
41. Claridge T. Social capital research; 2004. https://www.socialcapitalresearch.com/.
42. Häsler BN. A practical guide for the economic assessment of veterinary surveillance at national level. In: Economic assessment of veterinary surveillance programmes that are part of the National Control Programme for Switzerland, PhD monograph, chapter 5. London: Royal Veterinary College, University of London; 2011. p. 127–47.

6 Applications of Principles to Case Studies Focusing on Non-Monetary Surveillance Values

Barbara Häsler, Alexis Delabouglise, Nicolas Antoine-Moussiaux, Thang D. Phan, Duan C. Dao, Thanh T. Nguyen, Hoa T. T. Pham, Bao D. Truong, Xuan N. T. Nguyen, Ton D. Vu, Khong V. Nguyen, Hien T. Le, D. Tatong, W. Phimpraphi, S. Kasemsuwan, Marisa Peyre, and Sara Babo Martins

B. Häsler (✉)
Royal Veterinary College, London, UK
e-mail: bhaesler@rvc.ac.uk

A. Delabouglise · H. T. T. Pham
ASTRE, CIRAD-International Centre of Agricultural Research for Development, Montpellier, France

N. Antoine-Moussiaux
FARAH-Fundamental and Applied Research for Animals & Health, University of Liège, Liège, Belgium

T. D. Phan · T. D. Vu
Center for Interdisciplinary Research on Rural Development, Vietnam National University of Agriculture, Hanoi, Vietnam

D. C. Dao
Faculty of Veterinary Medicine, Vietnam National University of Agriculture, Hanoi, Vietnam

T. T. Nguyen · K. V. Nguyen
National Institute of Veterinary Research, Hanoi, Vietnam

B. D. Truong · X. N. T. Nguyen · H. T. Le
Faculty of Animal Science and Veterinary Medicine, Nong Lam University, Ho Chi Minh City, Vietnam

D. Tatong
The 6th Regional Livestock Office, Phitsanulok, Thailand

W. Phimpraphi · S. Kasemsuwan
Faculty of Veterinary Medicine, Kasetsart University, Nakorn-Pathom, Thailand

M. Peyre
CIRAD, UMR ASTRE, Montpellier, France

ASTRE, CIRAD, INRAE, University of Montpellier, Montpellier, France

S. B. Martins
Institute of Global Health, Faculty of Medicine, University of Geneva, Geneva, Switzerland

M. Peyre et al. (eds.), *Principles for Evaluation of One Health Surveillance: The EVA Book*, https://doi.org/10.1007/978-3-030-82727-4_6

Abstract

A central aspect of economic evaluations of surveillance components or systems is to estimate the value of the information that is being generated by surveillance. Importantly, the value of information is determined by the user of the information. This value is often realised through decisions on interventions that are implemented to manage disease in populations with the associated reduction of disease costs in human and animal populations including effects on the wider society. The economic efficiency of such processes can be measured within a single sector or across sectors (e.g. animal health surveillance creating benefits streams in human populations) applying standard economic evaluation techniques. Depending on the context, people may have different demands and uses for information expressed in distinct information-seeking behaviour and willingness to pay for information or knowledge. Hence, private and public stakeholders may attribute different values to surveillance depending on their decision needs. Moreover, cultural and socio-economic factors shape not only the value of surveillance, but also people's decisions around their livelihoods, income generation, prevention, and disease management strategies. Therefore it is important to understand behaviours, processes, motives, and justifications around health management and surveillance. A range of case studies are presented that describe wider benefits of surveillance and illustrate how non-monetary benefits can be assessed using stated preference elicitation methods, such as discrete choice experiment. Moreover, they demonstrate how understanding of local value systems and contexts allows appraising wider surveillance attributes that ultimately affect the performance and economic efficiency of surveillance.

Keywords

Health economics · Surveillance · Evaluation · Case studies

6.1 Introduction

6.1.1 Overview

This chapter starts with examples of economic efficiency[1] studies conducted in surveillance and then explores in more detail the challenge of capturing non-market values of surveillance using four case studies. Each case study is self-contained and includes a description of the context, rationale, and research question; an explanation of the methods used; a summary of the key findings; and a short discussion.

[1] Economic efficiency is interested in using resources in a way that maximises a defined objective relevant to the economic unit under consideration, such as farm, sector, or national level. For example, if national welfare is to be maximised, economic efficiency aims at combining resources in a way to achieve this objective.

6.1.2 Examples of Economic Efficiency Studies

The theoretical framework outlined in Chapter 5 provides the foundation for the economic evaluation of surveillance. Several published studies provide evidence of its validity. These studies assess the economic efficiency of surveillance with different methodologies taking into account the relationship of surveillance with intervention and mitigation.

Three levels of criteria for economic efficiency can be described: (1) the leading criterion is optimisation, which defines how the net benefit accruing to society from allocating scarce resources to disease mitigation is maximised; (2) the acceptability criterion concerns whether the benefits stemming from a mitigation policy at least cover its costs, thus making a strategy justifiable from an economic point of view; and (3) the cost-minimisation criterion applies when achieving a technical target for mitigation without quantification of the benefit is the policy objective [1].

In studies striving for *optimal economic efficiency*, the net benefit is maximised or, in other words, resources for surveillance are used in an optimal combination that balances the losses caused by the disease and the expenditures needed for its mitigation [2]. This approach was, for example, used by Kompas *et al.* [3], who identified the optimal level of surveillance activity against a disease incursion and spread by minimising the present value of the major direct and indirect costs of the disease, as well as the costs of the surveillance and disease management and eradication programmes. A similar approach was chosen by Guo *et al.* [4], who kept the intervention fixed (based on the assumption that the intervention and its implementation would be perfect) and used combined simulation and multi-criteria decision models to identify technically and economically efficient surveillance set-ups. However, optimisation approaches for surveillance evaluation are still scarce; more often found are cost–benefit, and cost-effectiveness analyses [5].

In cost–benefit analysis, the *economic acceptability* is assessed by estimating whether the benefits outweigh the costs of a new strategy or policy compared to the status quo (i.e. the baseline). All surveillance and intervention resources and all benefits of mitigating disease effects must be expressed in monetary units (see Howe, Chap. 5). These costs and benefits of surveillance and intervention, direct and indirect, including market and nonmarket values, are then compared in order to find out if a strategy generates a positive net value (i.e. whether the benefits are larger than the costs). Because the impact of surveillance cannot be measured directly as a mitigation outcome, it is only possible to quantify the loss avoidance resulting from the combination of surveillance and intervention, and to compare it to the expenditure for surveillance and intervention. An illustration of this concept can be found, for example, in Häsler *et al.* [6], where the elimination programme for bovine virus diarrhoea in Switzerland is used to estimate a residual margin over the intervention cost, which constitutes the maximum additional expenditure potentially available for surveillance without the net overall benefit from mitigation becoming zero. This margin can then be compared to the expenditures of various surveillance options. Other cost–benefit analyses of surveillance have, for example, used combined economic–epidemiological simulation models to estimate the positive and negative monetary effects of distinct combinations of surveillance and intervention actions. An application of this concept with explicit costing of zoonotic effects in the human population was presented by Babo Martins [7] for the case of West-Nile virus in Italy where the benefits of the programme were calculated as the avoided costs of hospitalisation and avoided compensation for transfusion-associated disease of human cases. Another example is Tambi et al [8], who used combined epidemiological and economic modelling of rinderpest in Ethiopia to compare the likely costs and benefits of an epidemio-surveillance system with those of other options (including no intervention) in an *ex ante* (i.e. prospective) analysis. The epidemiological part focused on a state-transition SEIR ('susceptible', 'exposed', 'infectious', 'recovered') disease transmission model. The economic part was a social cost–benefit analysis model that focused on welfare changes to consumers and producers in an economic surplus analysis assuming productivity gains related to disease eradication. In studies focusing on cost-effectiveness, the aim is also to assess *economic acceptability* by comparing the costs of surveillance resources with performance (effectiveness) targets, which may be considered a proxy for an outcome of benefit (e.g. timeliness or sensitivity). However, a cost-effectiveness analysis can inform resource allocation meaningfully only if its effectiveness measure has an interpretable value [5]. For example, it should be known what the economic value is (expressed in monetary terms) of a higher probability of disease detection to be able to make a decision on expenditures for surveillance. It is not uncommon for cost-effectiveness studies of surveillance to report the costs of surveillance options in comparison to performance targets and report, for example, results such as the 'costs per percentage increase in probability of detection' or the 'costs per day of earlier detection' without providing an estimate of the economic value of these outcomes. In these cases, it is left to the decision-makers to interpret the effectiveness measure and consider its (economic) consequences or in other words to address the question whether the investment needed for the change in effectiveness is economically worthwhile (i.e. is it worth it?).

When a specified surveillance target (and its value) is accepted as a given, often a *least-cost analysis* is used to identify the cheapest option among different possible options that produce the same outcome. In this type of analysis, the financial cost of the option is the dominant determining factor; the outcome or value of the outcome is fixed. This is, for example, the case for surveillance where the design including species, sample type, and sampling frequency is stipulated by national or international legislation. In these cases, the surveillance planner does not have flexibility with the design, but can only think about ways of implementing the required plan in the cheapest way possible.

Box 6.1 Economic Analysis (SurvTools— Peyre et al. [9]—https://survtools.org/)
Economic analysis of surveillance components or systems is an aid to decision-making as it informs the allocation of resources to surveillance. It shows the consequences of resource use for different surveillance options and helps to identify which of these is to be preferred from an economic point of view. A unifying underlying principle is to provide a measure of the relative value attached to competing alternative strategies and thereby make judgements on the economic efficiency. Various economic analysis methods are available with corresponding criteria for decision-making (e.g. least-cost analysis; cost-effectiveness; cost–benefit). They all depend on valuation of the inputs and consequences or effects, both of monetary and non-monetary nature. A breadth of valuation techniques exist; some of them are illustrated in this chapter.

6.1.3 The Challenge of Capturing Non-Market Values

It is widely acknowledged that surveillance produces values that go beyond tangible loss avoidance in animal and human populations or wider tangible effects on society, such as loss of tourism in the case of a disease outbreak (see Text Box Chap. 5). These zoonotic and wider externality effects are included in the extended loss function $L = A + Z + E$ (see Howe, Chap. 5).

There are dimensions to the value of surveillance that so far have been explored only marginally. Surveillance has been described to generate intellectual and social capital, technical reassurance and feelings of safety, capacity, contentment, and 'peace of mind' [5, 7]. As mentioned above 'People's personal relationships, social network support, civic engagement and trust, and co-operative norms, are all factors critical to ensuring the technical efficiency frontier and disease mitigation surface can be reached'. In other words, the information generated by surveillance can be heavily influenced by the context within which it occurs and the private actors in the system who make decisions on surveillance activities (e.g. disease reporting) and the use of the surveillance information for disease prevention practices and production strategies. For example, Figuié et al [10] documented informal animal health surveillance networks in Thailand and Vietnam that operate outside conventional surveillance systems as collective action groups that are united by shared values and interests. Depending on the context, the need for public authority-driven surveillance may be an abstract notion to the private actor with limited usefulness and consequently variable compliance. Moreover, there are costs and benefits that are not immediately obvious and consequently difficult to capture (e.g. the social and cultural importance attributed to cockfighting, see below).

Over the past years, progress has been made to identify and measure non-market values of surveillance using either surveys or qualitative approaches (see Part IV – Qualitative

Evaluation Approaches). Babo Martins [7] used qualitative interviews with animal and public health policymakers, advisors, and scientists involved in policy design and implementation of zoonoses surveillance to explore the benefits of One Health surveillance. Examples in animal health include choice experiments in the UK to assess the UK farmers' willingness to pay for bovine tuberculosis vaccines [11], consumers' willingness to pay for different *Salmonella* infection control methods in pork [12], farmers' willingness to pay for sanitary information at different geographical levels in Corsica [13], and farmers' willingness to report swine diseases in Vietnam [14]. In this chapter, the use of qualitative research methods and stated preference methods is presented to illustrate the potential of their use in surveillance and capture wider perceived benefits that, on the one hand, provide important information for decisions on investments into surveillance and, on the other hand, allow gaining insights into perceptions that influence the behaviour of private actors and consequently the success or failure of mitigation programmes.

6.2 Case Study 1: Evaluation of Costs and Benefits of Passive Surveillance Through Qualitative Surveys: Results of Surveys Conducted in Vietnam and Thailand

6.2.1 Introduction

Surveillance systems are implemented to produce epidemiological information aimed at informing the planning and implementation of appropriate disease control measures [15]. In the case of passive surveillance, the supply of epidemiological information to government stakeholders is under the control of primary information holders, that is, livestock producers or other actors of animal production systems. It makes the economic evaluation of passive surveillance systems particularly complicated as the expected upward flow of epidemiological information is the result of decentralised choices operated by private actors.

Evaluators of passive surveillance need to identify the costs and benefits perceived by primary information holders as they can substantially depart from societal costs and benefits considered by government planners. Surveys implemented to collect such data are faced with three major issues. First, compliance of private actors to government rules is, by nature, a sensitive issue involving a moral judgement (reporting disease suspicions might be perceived as the right attitude from the society's standpoint) and, as such, questions on disease reporting are vulnerable to obsequiousness bias: interviewees are likely to tell the answer which they feel is expected by the interviewer rather than the truth. Second, passive surveillance can be an abstract notion that does not necessarily make sense as a whole to the viewpoint of private actors: they may be aware of the legal obligation of reporting some specific health events to authorities, but they might not perceive the purpose of the surveillance system and its practical effects (better knowledge of the epidemiological situation of the disease and more efficient implementation of control measures). Finally, perceived costs and benefits are potentially diverse and complex and may vary according to the socio-economic context and the livestock production systems. Standardised data collection (e.g. through questionnaire surveys) are difficult to implement without preliminary knowledge of the nature costs and benefits under study.

In consequence, perceived costs and benefits are best addressed through qualitative surveys based on semi-structured interview techniques [16]. Investigators use a checklist of themes to address during interviews but they conduct it like a discussion, using open questions and letting participants talk as much as possible about their opinions, perceptions, and daily practices related to livestock diseases and sanitary information management (see Part IV—Qualitative Evaluation Approaches). Interviewers can use probing questions or interactive tools to encourage participants to think deeper on some aspects of the discussion. They also can use interactive tools like ranking, proportional piling, or matrix scoring to build lists of items (e.g. disease names, list of actors with whom information is exchanged) and rank them according to specific criteria [16]. If necessary, interviews may need to be repeated in order to enhance progressively the confidence of participants. Primary information holders are livestock farmers, but other types of information holders (e.g. slaughterers, feed sellers) can be identified during surveys. Therefore, an adapted snowball sampling method is most appropriate [17].

The interest of these methods is illustrated by a case study on the passive surveillance of Highly Pathogenic Avian Influenza (HPAI) Surveillance in Vietnam [18] and Thailand [19]. Vietnam and Thailand have very different poultry production industries. Poultry products in Thailand are mostly supplied by a limited number of integrated settings of high biosecurity standards managed by private agro-industrial companies [20]. Nevertheless, backyard chicken farming, specialised in native chicken breeds, is still widely practised by rural households for home consumption of chickens, sale of chicken meat, and cockfighting. The survey focused on these backyard native chicken farmers. In Vietnam, on the other hand, most poultry are produced in backyard or small-scale commercial farms with limited investments in biosecurity. The survey focused on households keeping backyard poultry as well as commercial poultry farms of varying size (from 100 to 10,000 birds per production cycle).

6.2.2 Materials and Methods

The data collection method is explained in details in [18, 19]; a summary is provided here.

Study areas were subdistricts of Hải Dương (HD) province (North Vietnam), Đồng Nai (DN) and Long An (LA) province (South Vietnam), and Sukhothai (SK) province (North Thailand).

6.2.2.1 Participatory Approaches and Snowball Sampling Method

The sampling strategy followed a snowball sampling pattern. First, several group interviews of poultry farmers were performed in each study area. Participants were contacted with the help of local authorities. Five to twenty poultry farmers were interviewed at once. Each group interview gathered farmers from the same production system and production scale, and one or several group interviews were conducted for each production system. Poultry farmers who displayed willingness to participate in the study were then asked for individual interviews. The number of these individual interviews was determined by adapting the concept of saturation to the objective of the study [21]: saturation was considered to be reached when 10 additional interviews did not provide any new information on costs and benefits compared with all previous interviews. During this first phase of interviews, other categories of actors were identified as being targets of information exchanges on HPAI suspicions. Individuals belonging to those additional categories of actors and in contact with individuals from the initial sampling frame were then asked to participate in the study. Those who accepted were interviewed individually. Additionally, group and individual interviews of government veterinarians were conducted.

Topics of focus group interviews were as follows:

i. Actors involved in the poultry value chains (sources of funding and credit, suppliers of feed, breeds and medicines, buyers of farm products) were listed.
ii. Relative importance of general problems affecting poultry farmers and origins of these problems were assessed using simple ranking.
iii. Names used locally for poultry diseases occurring in the area were scored according to their impact on income, rates of mortality and duration using proportional piling (PP) [16]. Reported names of diseases characterised by both high mortality rate (>50% in one poultry flock) and short duration (<5 days in one flock) were used to define HPAI suspicions which were referred to in subsequent interviews.
iv. Farmers were then asked which actions were taken when facing a disease suspicion, and these actions were scored according to their relative likelihood using PP.

Individually interviewed poultry farmers, government veterinarians, and other actors identified by snowball sampling were asked more in-depth and sensitive questions using qualitative semi-structured interviews.

i. They were asked to provide information on the different ways of managing disease suspicion cases when it appeared in poultry farms.
ii. They were asked about the positive and negative consequences of reporting a disease suspicion to authorities.
iii. Impact flow charts were used to identify the negative and positive consequences of disease suspicion reporting for different types of actors. Participants first identified the list of actors impacted by disease suspicion reporting. Then, they assigned different signs and colours to each type of actors to indicate whether the effect was positive or negative.

6.2.2.2 Analysis of Qualitative Data

Qualitative data were analysed using thematic analysis [22]. Meaning units, that is, information or judgements expressed in interviews, were attributed specific codes. Codes were then grouped into subthemes and themes. Identified themes corresponded to specific factors influencing the perception of the HPAI passive surveillance system by participants, either positively or negatively. Each subtheme and theme was linked to the number of interviews it was extracted from. Moreover, to be considered as relevant, themes and subthemes that concerned several categories of actors had to be mentioned by participants from all the concerned categories. All statistical analyses were made using R.2.15.3 software [23]. Degree of agreement between interviewees and groups of interviewees' rankings and scores obtained by PP was assessed by non-parametric Kendall test of concordance [24], using the kendall.global function of the vegan package [25]. Statistical significance of the Kendall coefficient was shown by permutation test.

6.2.3 Results

6.2.3.1 Choices Operated by the Different Stakeholders Facing HPAI Suspicion

Among names of poultry diseases mentioned in focus group interviews with farmers, several ones matched the HPAI suspicion definition (i.e. caused more than 50% mortality in poultry flocks in less than 5 days), including Newcastle Disease, fowl cholera, Gumboro disease, and duck plague. In the Thailand study area, Newcastle Disease, 'Diarrhoea' (interpreted as 'Fowl cholera'), and 'Plague' (a general word used to qualify a rapid and massive mortality) also matched this definition.

Scores of the different options considered by poultry farmers in response to HPAI suspicion according to their likelihood differed between focus groups and, above all, between study areas. There was a higher agreement (measured through Kendall test of concordance) between groups of interviewees of similar study areas than between groups of similar farming scales. In the Vietnam study areas the main mentioned options were asking support from a private actor (feed seller, veterinary shop, and feed company), rapid sale of the poultry, warning of other farmers, and self-reliance (Fig. 6.1). Reporting of the event to veterinary authorities was never mentioned. In the Thailand study area, the main priority of farmers was to warn other poultry farmers of the disease occurrence, mainly cockfighting practitioners, but reporting to veterinary authorities and village heads was considered as an option in some group discussions.

6.2.3.2 Perceived Cost and Benefits of Sharing Health Information

In the Vietnam study areas, six themes related to perceived costs and benefits of HPAI passive surveillance were identified from individual interviews.

Theme 1. Benefits associated with government intervention in disease management: Clearance of the poultry farms from the disease, avoidance of disease spread to other farms, avoidance of environmental pollution (due to the release of dead

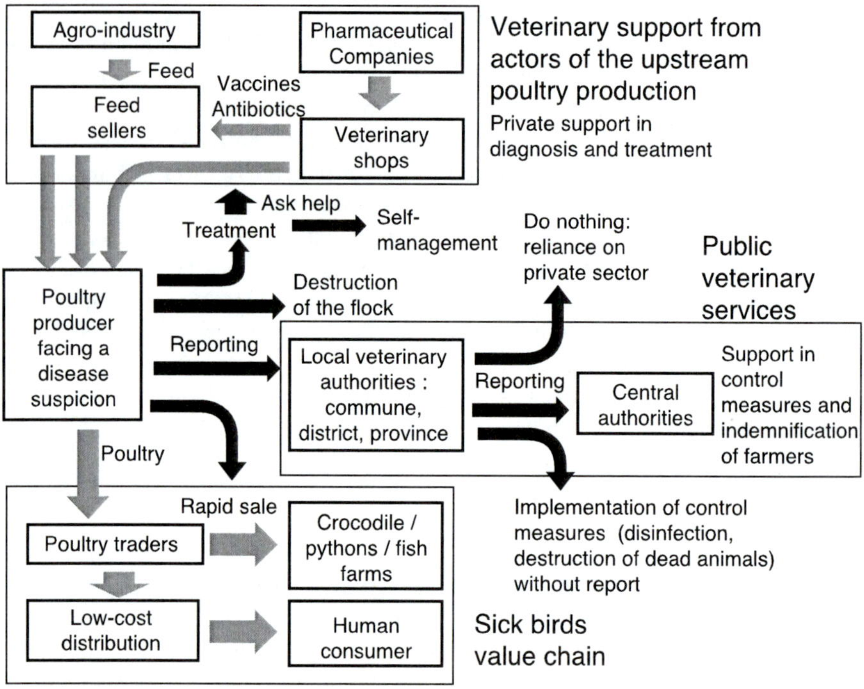

Fig. 6.1 Choices operated by poultry farmers and government veterinarians interviewed in Vietnam when facing avian influenza suspicion (grey arrow: commercial linkage; black arrow: decision). [18]

birds in the rice fields, water ponds, and rivers), protection of public health, and financial indemnities given in compensation of the destruction of affected poultry flocks.

Theme 2. Benefits from the reception of information on HPAI suspicions: Farmers used such information to adapt their prevention measures (biosecurity, vaccination) and anticipate variation in poultry market prices.

Theme 3. Uncertainty about the outcome of HPAI suspicion reporting: From private actors' viewpoint, veterinary authorities were, in most cases, taking no action in response to HPAI suspicions reports and, for this reason, were not trusted as source of help in disease management.

Theme 4. Transaction costs related to HPAI suspicion reports: Farmers reported long waiting times before obtaining support from authorities, including financial indemnities, while they were faced with short delays to refund their credit on feed purchase to feed sellers. Administrative procedures and fees were also reported.

Theme 5. Limits of local authorities' resources: The local government veterinary staffs reported having limited financial and technical resources available to control the disease in case of HPAI confirmation, which limited their willingness to notify the suspicion to the higher administrative level.

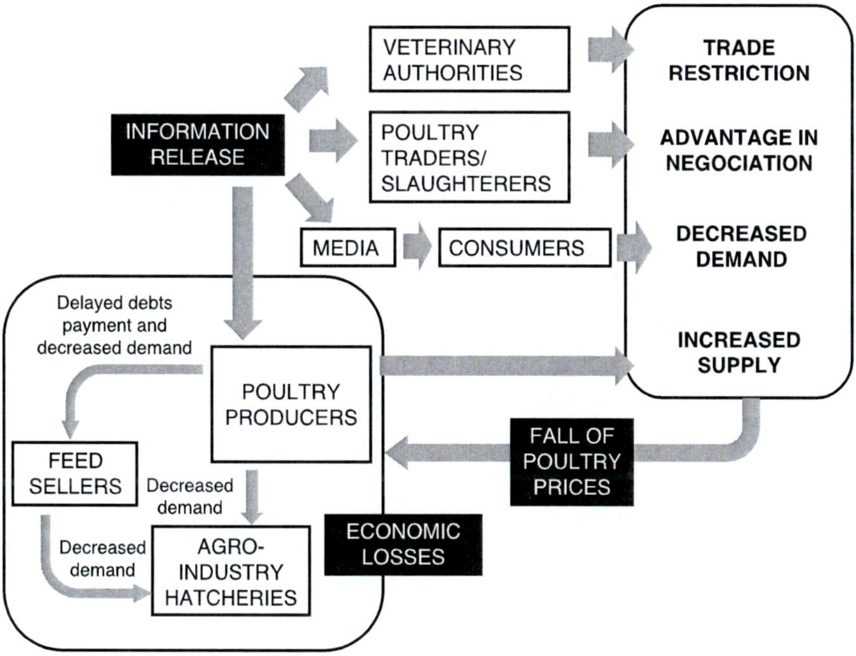

Fig. 6.2 Market effects of the release of information on avian influenza suspicions perceived by survey participants in Vietnam. [18]

Theme 6. Anticipation of market impacts: Poultry sale prices were anticipated to successively drop and increase following poultry disease outbreaks notifications and, therefore, HPAI surveillance was perceived as a factor of market instability. The price drop was due to early sale of poultry by farmers afraid of the disease, reluctance of consumers to purchase poultry, implemented movement restriction, and advantage of poultry traders in price negotiation (Fig. 6.2).

In the Thailand study area, six themes were identified:

Theme 1. Benefits associated with government intervention in disease management: Veterinary services provided veterinary products for free to farmers in response to a report of HPAI suspicion, even if HPAI was not confirmed, and financial indemnities were given in compensation of the destruction of affected poultry flocks.

Theme 2. Financial losses associated with the culling of cocks used for cockfighting: The value of these cocks specially trained for cockfighting competitions was reportedly much higher than the market price of standard birds sold for meat and financial compensations provided by veterinary authorities.

Theme 3. Loss of selected breeds of cocks aimed at fighting due to mass culling in affected farms.

Theme 4. The emotional link between farmers and their cocks that was disrupted by the mass culling policy.

Theme 5. The perceived moral fault of culling healthy animals out of purpose of consumption.

Theme 6. The fear of causing a conflict with cockfighting practitioners by reporting HPAI suspicions.

6.2.4 Discussion

The study illustrates how the perception of passive surveillance by its local stakeholders is affected by the socio-economic context in which it operates and, in particular, the type of livestock farming systems it targets. This is demonstrated by the qualitative differences between observation made in Vietnam and Thailand.

Benefits and costs of passive HPAI surveillance identified in Vietnam were strongly linked with the commercial nature of the poultry farming activity practised in the study areas. Large-scale as well as small-scale farmers were mostly concerned by the financial income generated from poultry flocks. Risk aversion, time preference, lack of trust in veterinary services, and compensation policy were key components of their decision-making process. Although the level of compensation might be close to the poultry market price, rapid sale of affected flocks was still perceived as a quicker and safer alternative to reduce income losses. Besides, the potential impact of the spread of disease information on the poultry market also was a major concern for farmers as well as veterinary government staff. Such market disturbances have been well characterised and quantified for avian influenza in several countries by multi-market or even computable general equilibrium models [26]. These impacts are complex and entail many distributional effects, besides the overall loss for society. Some examples may be extracted from the present study. First, consumers may transfer their demand for meat from poultry to swine products, the latter sector then generating more profit. Second, from their use of health information, traders also generate more profit during epizootics at the expense of poultry producers. Third, some poultry farmers adopt alternative strategies such as timing the sale of their flocks in the period of high deficit of poultry supply that just follows the epizootics to generate higher profits.

In the Thailand study area, poultry farming was mainly practised for the purpose of cockfighting. The social, cultural, and political importance of this activity [27] and the perceived brutality of the mass culling policy implemented in the past by the government of Thailand in response to HPAI outbreaks were a major explanation to the defiance of native breed chicken farmers towards the passive surveillance system. Even actors not involved in cockfighting activities were reluctant to report HPAI suspicions out of fear of causing conflicts with cockfighting practitioners. However, no possibility of sale of sick poultry was mentioned, contrary to Vietnam.

Native chickens sold for consumption were considered as quality products, and buyers were reported to check the health status of birds before purchase.

The results highlight the link between implemented disease control measures and effectiveness of passive surveillance. Control actions, being anticipated by actors, influence their decision-making. Farm disinfection, management of dead birds, and supply of veterinary products appear in the same way as compensation scheme as an incentive element of the control policy resulting from reporting.

Private actors of the poultry production expressed a need for early information on occurrences of poultry diseases. A major part of the Vietnamese poultry production is concentrated in small-scale farming systems and most farmers cannot afford constant investments in biosecurity and prevention measures. Information on disease occurrences is especially useful for such farmers who can adapt their choices (preventive measures or early sale of animals) according to the obtained information on disease threats.

Finally, it is notable that some of the perceived costs and benefits of the HPAI surveillance system do not have a market value, such as the social and cultural importance attributed to cockfighting, ethical concerns associated with mass culling, or the effect of price drop on other poultry farmers. But the effects of those costs and benefits on the decision-making to report or not a health event should be taken into consideration when defining disease management policies

6.2.5 Implication in Terms of Disease Management Policy

The effectiveness of passive surveillance systems depends on the decentralised decision-making of actors of livestock value chains who are the primary holders of animal health information. In consequence disease management policies need to be adapted to the specific needs and constraints of the private and local actors they rely upon. This study identifies some ways for improvement such as reducing the administrative burden associated with disease reporting and tailoring disease management intervention to answer farmers' needs. For instance, it appears that farmers would greatly benefit from a rapid support in cleaning and disinfection of farms upon reporting suspicions and without waiting for HPAI confirmation. In general, co-construction of surveillance and disease control strategies with local actors and end-users of health information should be an objective of surveillance systems development programmes, through the use of participatory approaches or specific methods like companion modelling (see Part IV).

6.3 Case Study 2: The Economic Value of One Health Surveillance—An Assessment of the One Health Approach to *Campylobacter* Surveillance in Switzerland

6.3.1 Introduction

In Switzerland, and in response to the observed increasing trend in human campylobacteriosis cases, the animal and the human health authorities enhanced collaborative disease surveillance and intervention efforts for *Campylobacter* with the intention of improving the disease management. For this, the *Campylobacter* platform, a stakeholder group composed by the poultry industry, researchers, and public health and animal health national and cantonal authorities, was formed [28]. A regular surveillance system in broiler chicken was also implemented.

The *Campylobacter* platform and the increased surveillance efforts constituted a shift from the previously instituted system, which was essentially based on the monitoring of human cases. In such One Health approach to surveillance [29, 30] it is of interest to explore whether overall resources are used more efficiently by collaborative or integrated approaches to surveillance than by a surveillance system with disconnected, sector-specific components. Using a previously developed framework to guide the assessment [31], this study investigated how surveillance activities across the two sectors linked to public health and animal health decision-making and triggered activities and interventions, and explored costs and benefits of the two approaches to surveillance and disease mitigation. More details on the study can be found in Babo Martins et al. [32].

6.3.2 Methods

The data collection method is explained in details in Babo Martins et al. [32]; a summary is provided in the following paragraphs.

Figure 6.3 summarises the conceptual framework of the links between surveillance of zoonoses in the animal population, the wider public health disease mitigation system, and benefit components associated, used as a basis for this study.

In this study, the One Health approach to *Campylobacter* mitigation was considered as the system in place since 2009 and up to 2013, where information generated by surveillance efforts in the poultry population and in the human population was integrated in the *Campylobacter* platform.

The steps proposed in the above-mentioned framework were as follows: an initial conceptualisation of the links between surveillance and triggered interventions, the identification of costs and benefits, and a final step of valuation of costs and of potential benefits. Based on discussion with experts involved in the activities and literature review [28], information on the type of surveillance activities, integration mechanisms and activities, and interventions prompted by the information generated in both the animal and the human health sectors was identified. A cost estimation model was developed and populated with data provided by the Swiss Federal

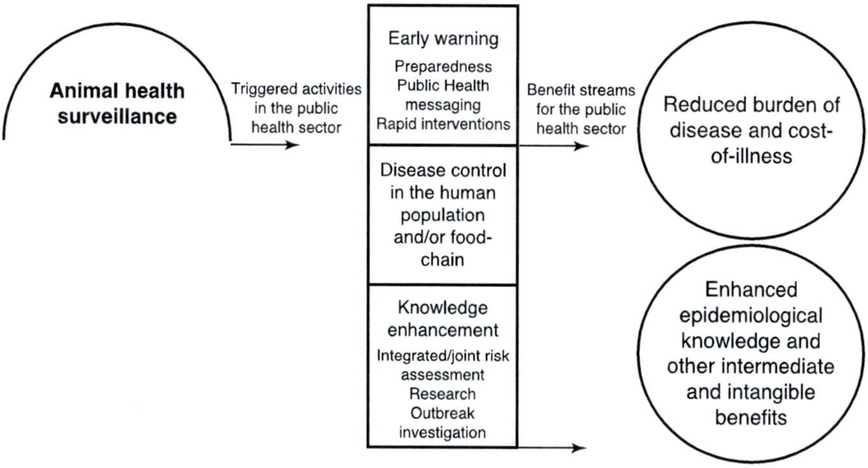

Fig. 6.3 Conceptual framework of the links between surveillance of zoonoses in the animal population, the wider public health disease mitigation system, and associated benefit components

Food Safety and Veterinary Office (FVO) and Federal Office of Public Health (FOPH). The cost model included all relevant labour costs and expenses accrued by surveillance activities, running costs of the *Campylobacter* platform, and costs of interventions and activities triggered by surveillance information across both sectors in the timeline of the analysis. From the benefit streams identified, potential changes in the impact of disease in the human population were explored by calculating disability-adjusted life-years (DALYs) [33] for 2008 and 2013, building upon the stochastic model used in Denmark for the estimation of the burden of foodborne disease [34].

6.3.3 Results

In the One Health approach, the information generated by surveillance in the animal population and by human cases monitoring shared in the *Campylobacter* platform triggered activities concerning biosecurity messaging in poultry farms and public health messaging on hygienic measures for chicken meat handling and prevention of cross-contamination. Integration of surveillance information was also used to perform cross-sectorial risk assessments and identify gaps in the knowledge base for *Campylobacter* infection in the country and research needs. Three main benefit streams were identified. A first benefit stream linked to the potential to generate a reduction in the direct and indirect impacts of the disease in the human population, namely on the burden of disease or cost of illness. This potential benefit stream was further explored in the study. The potential to reduce the direct and indirect impacts of disease in the animal population, ultimately contributing to a reduction in human infection, was identified but not assessed. The final benefit stream related to a set of intermediate or intangible benefits, connected to enhanced knowledge, performance of risk assessments and triggering of research, such as intellectual capital, and to social capital, generated through the intrinsic value of multi-sectorial collaboration and networking.

The One Health approach represented a marginal cost when compared to the uni-sectorial system, with almost half (48%) of the total expenses in 2009–2013 being absorbed by commissioned research on *Campylobacter* in Switzerland, followed by the surveillance and monitoring activities in poultry and humans, respectively. In the same timeline, a 3.4–8.8% increase in the average total burden of disease of campylobacteriosis was estimated, from 1609 (95% CI: 1330, 1947) to 2756 (95% CI: 2412, 3140) DALYs in 2008 to 1751 (95% confidence interval (CI): 1478, 2069) to 2852 (95% CI: 2520, 3227) DALYs in 2013, in the best- and worst-case scenarios considered, respectively.

6.3.4 Discussion

This study provides an example of how costs and benefits of surveillance conducted in a One Health approach can be identified. The framework used as the basis for economic assessment allowed the identification of cross-sectorial cost items and benefits streams, associated to *Campylobacter* in Switzerland in the period in analysis, through the conceptualisation of its links to activities and intervention. The study also demonstrates the challenges surrounding the valuation of costs and benefits of One Health surveillance approaches, particularly those generated in system at an early stage of implementation such as the One Health approach to *Campylobacter* mitigation in the time frame of this analysis.

In the first five years of the system, the level of the expenditure increased with a cross-sectorial approach to surveillance and intervention for *Campylobacter* in the country, particularly in research funding and surveillance activities in poultry. In line with the nature of these activities, information generated contributed mainly to the assessment of trends, to perform risk assessments, and to shape research efforts. Accordingly, in these initial 5 years, the nature of benefits was intangible, including the generation of intellectual capital. Such intellectual capital created by surveillance can later generate monetary value when it is used to inform control measures that mitigate the impact of the disease and generate a measurable health effect. Cost-effectiveness or cost–benefit tools can, at that stage, be used to estimate how One Health approaches to surveillance and mitigation compare in economic terms with uni-sectorial approaches.

6.3.5 Implication in Terms of Disease Management Policy

Gains in information and knowledge have been recognised as benefits from wider One Health approaches [35, 36]. However, for surveillance activities, such benefits are rarely incorporated into economic assessments [37]. To understand the overall added value of One Health surveillance, the assessment of these assets should be an integral part of the analysis, particularly in surveillance systems that are mainly informing assessments and producing knowledge. Stated preference elicitation methods, such as conjoint analysis, presented and further explored in other case studies in this chapter, could be a useful tool to gain further insight into this set of benefits of One Health surveillance approaches.

6.4 Case Study 3: Quantifying the Perceived Benefits and Costs of Surveillance Through Discrete Choice Experiments: A Pilot Study in North Vietnam

6.4.1 Introduction

The method explained in Chap. 5 is useful for identifying and understanding the costs and benefits associated with passive surveillance from the viewpoint of its primary information holders. However, it does not allow to quantify the effect of each factor on the actor's decision-making, and so, does not allow to measure the relative effect of each of the identified attributes on the effectiveness of surveillance.

To answer this gap, a quantification method based on stated preferences was built and tested, using the example of reporting of Highly Pathogenic Avian Influenza (HPAI) suspicions by poultry farmers to veterinary authorities in Vietnam. The method was composed of two phases with distinct objectives: first, quantifying the value attributed by survey participants to the reception of information on poultry diseases occurring in their area, using contingent valuation; second, quantifying the value of attributes of passive surveillance (anticipated costs and benefits of HPAI suspicion reporting) based on their relative effect on the reporting likelihood of survey participants, using choice-based conjoint analysis.

This section introduces the method of data collection and data analysis as well as preliminary results of the pilot study implemented in Hải Dương province (North Vietnam). A more detailed description of the method can be found in [18, 19]).

6.4.2 Materials and Methods

6.4.2.1 Contingent Valuation to Estimate the Benefits of Health Information Sharing

The benefits considered by the individuals from receiving information on poultry disease outbreaks were estimated by contingent valuation [38]. All types of poultry diseases were included, not only HPAI, in order to match actors' interest for epidemiological information on poultry diseases in general. Semi-structured interviews were performed to list the benefits of early information about the sanitary situation of poultry flocks in the region. The participants had to think of how they could use such information and what could be the expected gains or avoided losses from the anticipated actions. Then, contingent valuation was applied. It consisted in offering a virtual contract from a company providing information to the participant at a certain cost. Two factors were considered: the price the participant was willing to pay to receive information in an appropriate timing (i.e. to allow enough time for implementation of prevention and control measures) and the price the participant was willing to accept as a compensation to deliver information himself within an appropriate timing.

6.4.2.2 Discrete Choice Experiment to Value the Non-Monetary Costs and Benefits

Second, a modified protocol of discrete choice experiment was applied to value the non-monetary costs and benefits linked to the HPAI suspicion reporting process [39]. The participant had to list and explain the different options he/she was willing to consider when confronted to a hypothetical scenario of disease suspicion (50% mortality in less than 2 days) in his/her chicken flock, and the relative consequences (financial and non-financial) upon reporting or not reporting the disease suspicion to the authorities. Then the farmer was asked to estimate a relative likelihood to the three possible actions: (i) reporting the HPAI suspicion to authorities, (ii) not reporting the HPAI suspicion to authorities, and (iii) discuss with other people in the community about the need to report or not (Fig. 6.4). The objective of the third option was to give a possibility for the participant to opt out, as well as a possibility for the respondent to give a more detailed explanation of the social interactions

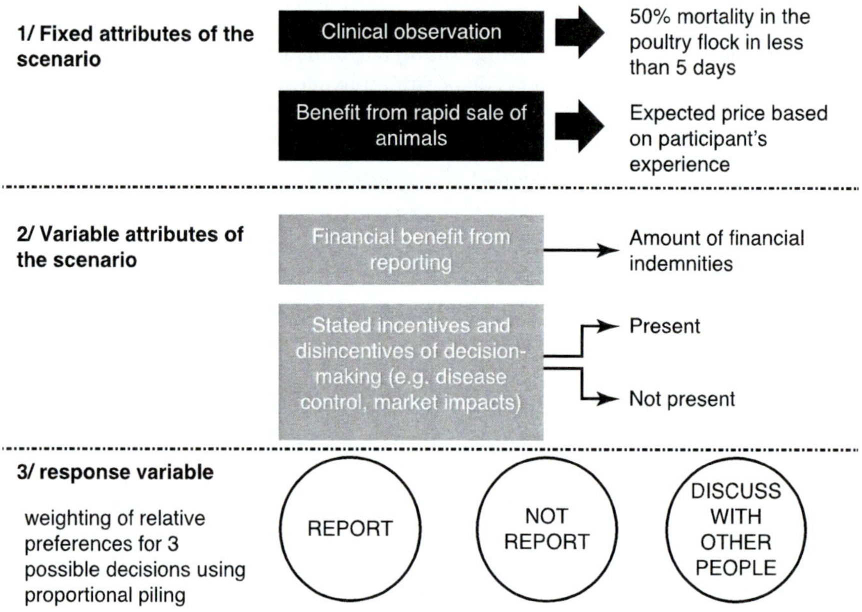

Fig. 6.4 Structure of the adapted discrete choice experiment tool. Scenarios are composed of fixed attributes and variable attributes. Responses of participants were a scoring of relative preference for three types of decisions using proportional piling. [18, 19]

conditioning the decision-making process. The likelihood of each option was quantified using proportional piling [16]: a set of 100 counters was divided and ascribed to each above-mentioned option by participants, in quantity proportional to the relative likelihood of choosing this option. Different scenarios were then tested by varying the levels of indemnities provided by the government upon report. The motives for the stated likelihoods were assessed at each step and considered as incentives or disincentives of the decision-making. The participant was then asked to assign likelihoods to each action in situations where the incentives and disincentives considered were not applicable (e.g. assign likelihood of each action when considering that authorities provide or do not provide help in disease management following a disease suspicion report). The presence/absence of these incentives and disincentives were considered as the qualitative attributes to be valued through the different choice scenarios (Fig. 6.4).

All statistical analyses were made using R.2.15 [23]. Results from contingent valuations were analysed through descriptive statistics. Results from the adapted discrete choice experiment were analysed considering the stated likelihoods of action as probabilities of choice. Being collected following distinct interview processes according to each individual case, data were analysed individually. To allow for the statistical estimation of utility coefficients of the different scenario attributes with standard statistical package, each individual probability gathered through proportional piling was simulated as resulting from a mock sample (n = 100 for the each scenario). A multinomial logistic regression model was applied to derive the monetary values of attributes [39] from data collected for each individual, using the 'mlogit' package [40]:

$$P = \frac{e^{b_r X_r}}{\sum_j e^{b_j X_j}}$$

with X being the vector of the attributes of the scenario (non-monetary and monetary incentives and disincentives), b being a vector of utility coefficients of the scenario attributes to be estimated, r being the report option, and j the choice set.

6.4.3 Results

The contingent valuation tool and the adapted discrete choice experiment were tested, with 21 and 17 poultry producers, respectively, of Hải Dương province (North Vietnam), of which 4 were female and the rest male. They were all small-scale farmers producing between 100 and 1000 broiler chickens per cycle.

The anticipated costs of poultry farmers for reporting HPAI suspicions were the fear of being responsible for the losses incurred by other producers and feed sellers, due to the drop of poultry prices in case of notification, and the transaction costs (administrative procedures and delays before receiving financial indemnities, as compared with the immediate payoff obtained by selling the affected flock). From the 17 interviews performed in HD with broiler chicken producers, 11 results were interpretable. Failures to obtain interpretable results arose from inability or unwillingness of participants to envisage hypothetic scenarios. For five farmers the effect on prices and resulting losses for other farms did not affect their decision (null cost). For five other farmers this cost had an impact that could be quantified at a median value of 442 USD (range: 108–2979 USD) (exchange rate: 1 USD = 21,000 Vietnam Dong). One farmer considered the impact of notifications on the income of other farmers was priceless (absolutely intolerable). Five farmers did not mention the transaction costs of reporting. For six other farmers these transaction costs could be estimated as a median value of 694 USD (range: 236–1081 USD). Seven farmers did not mention the benefit of help in disease management. For four other farmers this benefit could be estimated as a median value of 292 USD (range: 248–829 USD).

A quantified value of acceptable price for getting disease outbreak information (willingness to pay) could be obtained from 13 out of the 21 interviews performed in HD with broiler chicken producers. The median value was 0.04 USD (range: 0.005–0.05 USD) per chicken per cycle, which corresponds to about 1% of the chicken sale price.

6.4.4 Discussion

Stated preferences method is based on the elicitation of specific choices of participants under hypothetic scenarios with specific attributes. It is usually applied to assign a value to goods or attributes of goods which do not have a market [39]. In animal health, stated preferences were used, for example, to evaluate the willingness of farmers to pay for the extension of local veterinary services [41] or for vaccination programmes against livestock diseases, based on their attributes [11, 42]. Classically, stated preferences require data collection using standardised questionnaire-based approaches. Survey interviewees are required to make discrete choices in response to several sets of scenario attributes and model coefficients are estimated on the overall sample of participants (see Sect. 6.5).

The data collection protocol presented here was adapted to allow flexibility in conducting interviews with survey participants and defining scenario attributes. This flexibility was essential, given the complex and sensitive nature of the topic. It enabled to ascertain that participants had a good understanding of the proposed scenarios, the different choices they were faced with and their potential consequences, and to explore thoroughly the different incentives and disincentives conditioning their decision process. The method was well adapted to identify scenarios and relevant attributes that matched participants' specific perceptions. Proportional piling was used in conjoint analysis as a way to capture relative probabilities of decisions in response to change in scenarios attributes. These attributes were progressively adapted by the interviewer all along the exercise until capturing changes in probability that were precisely linked with the factor of interest.

A substantial proportion of the pilot interviews failed to produce relevant data. Indeed, the applicability of the tool proved to depend on the knowledge and experience of participants with the topic of the evaluation (poultry diseases and suspicion reporting) and their ability or willingness to consider hypothetic scenarios that could significantly diverge from their personal experience.

6.4.5 Implication in Terms of Disease Management Policy

The willingness of farmers to contribute financially and informationally to the suggested 'service of health information' highlights their interest in a well-functioning surveillance system and a direct illustration of the public value that such systems are creating. However, the fact that farmers did not consider this service to be synonymous of the actual surveillance system points to a lack of return of information to these users, hence pointing to the foregone creation of value. A flowing back of information to end-users is thus needed to realise the full social potential of surveillance. This case study illustrates how stated preference methods may be used at the individual level as a tool for in-depth qualitative investigation of actors' decision-making and attitude towards implemented or envisioned policies. The present results point particularly to the importance of disease management interventions and market impacts on the decision to report or not to report cases, which also appeared as resulting from social interactions, beyond the sole individual weighing of costs and benefits.

6.5 Case Study 4: The Willingness to Forego Compensation: Application of the Discrete Choice Experiment to Evaluate Swine Disease Surveillance in Vietnam

6.5.1 Introduction

Farmers' decision to report cases, and therefore the effectiveness of passive surveillance, crucially depends on the institutional framing of animal disease surveillance and control. Indeed, farmers' anticipation of consequences shapes their final decision to report [43, 44], which implies that passive surveillance cannot be considered separately from the planned control actions. Applying to swine diseases in two provinces of the Red River Delta, in the North of Vietnam, this case study applied discrete choice experiment (DCE) to evaluate passive surveillance as an institutional object, characterised by policy options as perceived by field actors. More details on the study can be found in Pham et al. [14].

6.5.2 Materials and Methods

6.5.2.1 Discrete Choice Experiment Applied to Passive Surveillance

As mentioned in the previous case study, discrete choice experiment (DCE) is part of the so-called stated preference method. It aims at estimating the value of goods or their characteristics (also called attributes) based on the analysis of choices made by individuals facing virtual alternatives between different kinds of the good to be evaluated. Such virtual choices are needed in cases in which real transactions on markets cannot be observed to obtain these estimations. Similar approaches were adopted by other authors to identify and evaluate farmers' reporting decisions [45] and animal disease control measures [42, 46].

By analysing the trade-off that the interviewees make between the policy options and compensation throughout their virtual choices, the DCE protocol allows for an estimation of the willingness of farmers to accept or to forego compensation facing different policy arrangements. This willingness may also be directly understood as a willingness to report, as the survey includes the possible choice of not reporting. Finally, this willingness to report may also be expressed as probabilities of reporting decisions, hence as an evaluation of the foreseen effect of different policy options on passive surveillance.

6.5.2.2 Definition of Policy Options To Be Tested

A DCE protocol needs to elaborate different profiles of the good to evaluate, to be proposed as alternatives. These profiles represent different combinations of characteristics, here policy options, relevant to the actors' decision-making. Those were identified through a participatory survey consisting of 18 focus groups with farmers and key informant interviews. The policy options included were as follows: (1) uncertainty of being compensated in case of animal disease reporting; (2) delivery time of compensation payment; (3) pig culling in case of disease reporting; (4) burden of administrative procedures for disease notification and getting compensation payment; (5) movement control in case of disease notification; and (6) compensation levels in case of animal culling. Each option was then assigned different modalities (attributes' levels) on the basis of the survey results and from a literature review on veterinary regulations in Vietnam [47, 48], as detailed in Table 6.1. Compensation level was expressed as a percentage of the market price for the live body weight (LBW) of a fattening pig, considering a fixed market price of Vietnam Dong (VND) 48,000 per kg LBW. Compensation levels were set at 50%, 70%, and 80% of market price.

6.5.2.3 Study Location and Participants

The DCE survey was conducted in eight communes of four districts of two provinces, based on pig density, extent of pig production, diversity of pig farming systems, and occurrence of notified swine infectious diseases (PRRS, FMD, and CSF). Stratified random sampling was carried out based on production types (mixed vs. fattening farm) and production systems (small vs. large farm, based on a threshold of 20 sows and/or 200 fattening pigs). Target sample size was 120 pig farms in each province (30 large farms and 90 smallholders). According to the WHO guideline on discrete choice experiments in public health research, a minimum sample size of 30 is required for each sub-group of the main sample to perform econometric analysis [49]. Each farmer was asked to make 12 virtual choices. Each choice consisted of two unlabelled disease-reporting alternatives and one opt-out alternative (non-reporting alternative).

Table 6.1 Policy options used in the discrete choice experiment to estimate farmers' willingness to report swine disease in two provinces of Northern Vietnam

Attribute	Levels
Probability of being compensated	Uncertain
	Certain
Compensation level (Vietnam Dong per kilogram live body weight)	24,000
	33,600
	38,400
Animal culling policy	Dead/unrecovered pigs
	All pigs at farm
Administrative procedures of disease reporting and compensation payment	Simple
	Complicated
Movement control in outbreak area	No movement ban
	Movement ban
Delivery time of compensation payment	3 months
	6 months
	1 years

From March to July 2015, face-to-face interviews in Vietnamese were conducted, resulting in 196 completed questionnaires in total (out of 240 pig holders contacted for interview). Mixed pig farms represented 81% of sample (keeping sows, growers, and fattening pigs), while 19% kept fattening pigs only. Small pig farms with 6 sows and 100 fattening pigs on average were dominant in both provinces (79% and 88%, respectively).

6.5.3 Results

From the selected policy options, all showed a statistically significant influence ($p < 0.01$) on farmers' decision-making, except the administrative procedures burden. No significant difference was observed between provinces. As expected, higher compensations increased the likelihood of reporting, allowing for the calculation of the so-called 'willingness to accept compensation' for negatively perceived policy options or 'willingness to forego compensation' for positively perceived policy options. The strongest influence on decision-making was obtained for the certainty of receiving compensation and for culling policy, the preferred option being to restrict it to not-recovering pigs only. Movement restriction and delayed compensation payment also reduced the probability of farmers' disease reporting but showed a lesser weight in decision-making. Regarding the desired policy changes, the highest willingness to forego compensation is obtained for restricting the culling policy to non-recovering pigs only and for shortening the compensation delivery time from 1 year to 3 months, amounting to 71% and 25% of the market price, respectively (Fig. 6.5).

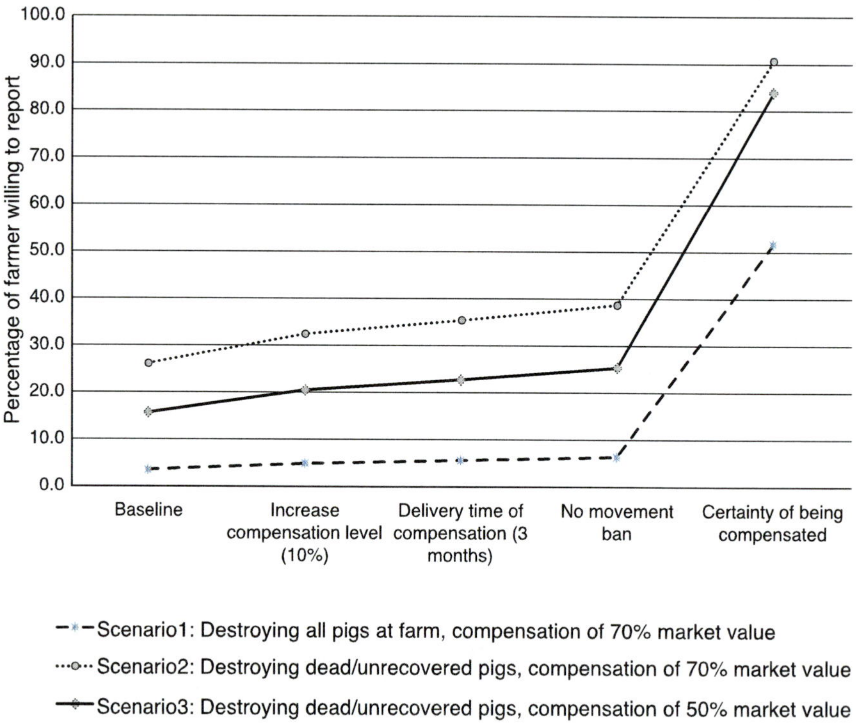

Fig. 6.5 Probability of swine disease reporting by farmers under different scenarios of control policy. (From Pham et al. [14])

With regard to the policy options that were considered, the current situation in Vietnam is defined as follows: uncertainty of being compensated, movement restriction, total culling in affected farms, complicated administrative procedures, compensation level equal to 70% of market price, and compensation delay of six months. Based on scenarios simulation, under this policy setting, the probability of case reporting was estimated at only 4% (95% CI: 0.9–14.3%). A change in the culling policy to restrict it to unrecovered pigs in affected farms brings this reporting probability up to 26% (95% CI: 6.2–65.4%). If farmers were certain of being compensated, probability of disease reporting would rise up to 52% in case of total culling in affected farms (95% CI: 16.8–85.3%) and up to 91% (95% CI: 59.7–98.5%) in case of targeted culling. Making administrative procedures less cumbersome, allowing free movements of uninfected pigs in the area, and increasing the compensation payment to 80% of market value do not significantly increase the proportion of farmers willing to report. In accordance with the calculated willingness to forego compensation, under the favourable options of a targeted culling policy and certainty of compensation, the scenario testing a lower compensation level (50% market value) could deliver an estimated probability of reporting as high as 84% (95% CI: 47.9–96.8%).

6.5.4 The Burden of Distrust, the Unbearable Cost of Massive Culling Outweighs Compensation Levels

The willingness to forego compensation highlights the true barriers opposed to disease notification from the perspective of Vietnamese pig holders' decision-making. Indeed, compensation is classically considered critical in disease control policies as an incentive to case reporting and compliance with culling actions [50]. Hence, policies often focus on this rate, with recommendations, for healthy and diseased animals, ranging from 75 to 90% of the reference price [50]. Yet, this case study brings a quantitative illustration of the secondary importance of compensation level in farmers' decision-making. Two policy elements are pointed as more relevant to this decision: *the certainty of compensation payment and the culling strategy*. As the present method mobilises stated preference, it is primarily handling perceptions of a policy by stakeholders rather than policy itself. Therefore, it is useful to translate these results into their perceptual equivalent, meaning that policy efforts have to increase the confidence in compensation payment and the acceptability of stamping out strategies. Clearly, in the present situation, the effort made to ensure a compensation level as high as 70% of the market price is totally overweighed by a lack in these two components coming up to massive underreporting behaviour. On the contrary, lower compensation rates may allow for an effective passive surveillance provided that confidence and acceptability are fostered. Similarly to compensation level, movement restriction and delivery time of compensation are minor although significant decision factors.

The lack of acceptability of stamping out strategies may be understood from qualitative in-depth interviews having accompanied the present DCE protocol. First, the destruction of clinically healthy pigs is perceived as a waste of resources and food, which is deemed unacceptable. Second, compensation rates based on fattened pig prices is considered as not relevant to compensate the culling of clinically healthy breeding stock that present a higher value as a built capital. Third, notifiable swine diseases such as PRRS and FMD are endemic in Vietnam, which leads farmers to perceive these diseases as a usual burden that does not call for stamping out strategies, then perceived as 'over-reaction'. According to Vietnamese disease control policy ([47, 48], culling upon disease confirmation applies for all pigs in the farm in case of a new outbreak or if the outbreak occurs in a limited area (few households in the village/commune). Targeted culling of non-recovering pigs already applies for wider outbreaks or in recurrently affected zones. Thus, the Vietnamese policy is not totally at odds with farmers' wishes but the wider acceptability of restricted culling invites to apply this strategy in a maximum of relevant cases. A true stamping out should be decided under very strict conditions, with both a profound work to promote its acceptability *ex ante* and a follow-up of farmers upon implementation.

The lack of confidence in compensation payment is the other main barrier for disease reporting identified through this case study. This relates to a more profound distrust in veterinary authorities and control measures, which is, indeed, known as an important barrier to disease reporting [43, 44, 51]. The timeliness and reliability of compensation delivery are critical elements in building this missing trust [50]. Finally, we could understand from open interviews that the flexibility of procedure, as mentioned here above, makes things unclear for farmers. These results suggest the importance of clarifying culling rules with adequate communication strategy.

6.5.5 Implication in Terms of Disease Management Policy

Delay in detecting and culling infected animals has been found as key factors of diseases spread, undermining the efficacy of control programmes [52, 53]. Conversely, the efficacy of control programmes, the acceptability, and the clarity of their procedures appear as feedback drivers of surveillance efficacy. This case study illustrates how discrete choice experiment can be mobilised to investigate the barriers to a timely disease reporting by farmers. Combined with qualitative interviews to grasp profound motives and justifications of farmers' choices, it proved useful to inform the needs for policy framing of communicable disease management. The present case particularly highlights the need for renewed communication strategies around animal disease control policy, to clarify the latter and build trust with farmers. Stamping out proved a critical factor in their decision-making. Therefore, there is a need to mobilise this measure with scrutiny in accordance with the epidemiological situation of the region, and to communicate duly about its need, legitimacy, and modalities in order to increase its acceptability.

6.6 General Discussion

This chapter has focused on practical applications used to describe and estimate wider surveillance values as well as factors that influence them.

Some aspects of the value of surveillance are quantifiable using market values, in particular the monetary losses avoided in animal populations (e.g. reduction in yield, loss of animals) and human populations (e.g. losses due to absence from work). In addition, some of the wider externality effects, such as the losses caused by a reduction of tourism due to disease outbreaks, can be measured in monetary terms. The comparison of the loss avoidance achieved through disease surveillance and control with the resource costs accrued for these activities allows determining the economic efficiency of surveillance, as described in Chap. 5 and illustrated in various studies (see, e.g., examples mentioned in this chapter or the RISKSUR outputs: http://www.fp7-risksur.eu/progress/publications-presentations).

While several studies focused on the value of surveillance for animal diseases, recent work has elaborated the theoretical foundations to extend the existing concepts to One Health or integrated health surveillance [7]. Benefit streams in the human health sector resulting from information generation in the animal health sector are expected to be generated from disease reduction in human populations that can be attributed to earlier or better knowledge produced by animal health surveillance—conceptually similar to considerations in the animal health sector. However, Babo Martins [7] found that there is a considerable time lag from the generation of information in animal health to interventions in the public health sector. In other words, the information is more often used to assess trends and trigger research, all of which can be used at a later point in time to inform the design of interventions. Consequently, the quantification of benefit streams in a One Health surveillance setting requires a long-term time frame to be able to estimate their economic value. This leads to situations where intangible benefits to surveillance are identified, such as intellectual property, experience, knowledge, which in the future may be used to realise a tangible value as explained in Case Study 2. In other contexts, the measurement of intellectual capital, knowledge, or research information is a question of interest to research institutions, governments, or funding bodies.

Importantly, the concept of value is not static, but varies with time, geographic setting, culture, etc. Thus, the value of surveillance is strongly determined by the context, as illustrated in Case Study 1 where qualitative studies on avian influenza surveillance identified clear differences in the perception of the usefulness of surveillance information in Vietnam and Thailand. Large-scale poultry farmers were mainly interested in financial income resulting from poultry flocks and used the surveillance information received to make decisions to sell their poultry (a risky practice in terms of disease spread) and maximise their income. This example clearly shows that the intended use (and consequently potential benefits) of surveillance information as conceptualised by public authorities (protection of animal and human populations by enabling interventions) may differ from private stakeholder interests and use. Consequently, any study aiming to estimate the value of a surveillance policy should take care to define clearly the viewpoints of the analysis and to reflect on different stakeholder perceptions and how these could be integrated in the study. This was highlighted by the results from Thailand, where the social, cultural, and political importance of cockfighting determined the value of poultry and was consequently the major driver of producers' perception of surveillance and disease reporting behaviour.

To understand the full value of surveillance, the assessment of non-monetary benefits should be an integral part of the analysis. Stated preference elicitation methods, such as conjoint analysis, have been presented in this chapter to explore their usefulness in generating new insights into surveillance values. They are based on the elicitation of specific choices of participants under hypothetic scenarios with specified attributes. They are commonly used to assign a value to goods or attributes of goods which do not have a market [39]. Case Studies 3 and 4 are examples of applications of these methods in an animal health context. From a methodological perspective, they showed the importance of having flexibility in interviewing people and defining scenario attributes to make sure that people were able to understand in detail the choices and consequences to gain robust insights into their decision process. In combination with qualitative interviews, profound motives and justifications of farmers' choices may be understood. In Case Study 4, information was gained on the two policy elements relevant for farmers' disease reporting behaviour, namely, the certainty of compensation payment and the culling strategy. This knowledge is useful for policymakers to be able to generate surveillance systems that are functional, accepted, and effective. In this case, contextual factors and local value systems influenced important signals in the surveillance pathway and therefore directly affected the value of surveillance that could be realised.

In conclusion, the case studies presented are examples of approaches that do not only help to identify perceived values of surveillance that may not be immediately obvious to the analyst, but they also allow describing, conceptualising, and quantifying non-monetary surveillance benefits. Finally, they are also helpful to characterise contextual factors, which directly affect functional and performance attributes of surveillance and in consequence its economic value. Together with the theory outlined in Chap. 5 and techniques to assess economic efficiency, they allow conducting robust and effective economic evaluation of animal health surveillance.

References

1. Häsler BN. A practical guide for the economic assessment of veterinary surveillance at national level, in economic assessment of veterinary surveillance programmes that are part of the national control programme for switzerland, PhD Monograph, Chapter 5, Royal Veterinary College, University of London; 2011;127–47.
2. Howe KS, Häsler B, Stärk KDC. Economic principles for resource allocation decisions at national level to mitigate the effects of disease in farm animal populations. Epidemiol Infect. 2013;141:91–101. https://doi.org/10.1017/S095026881200060X.
3. Kompas T, Nhu Che T, Van Ha P. An optimal surveillance measure against foot-and mouth disease in the United States. Australia: Crawford; 2006.
4. Guo X, Claassen GDH, Oude Lansink AGJM, Saatkamp HW. A conceptual framework for economic optimization of an animal health surveillance portfolio. Epidemiol Infect. 2016;144:1084–95. https://doi.org/10.1017/S0950268815002022.
5. Häsler B, Delabouglise A, Martins BS. Achieving an optimal allocation of resources for animal health surveillance, intervention and disease mitigation. Rev Sci Tech OIE. 2017;36:57–66. https://doi.org/10.20506/rst.36.1.2609.
6. Häsler B, Howe KS, Presi P, Stärk KDC. An economic model to evaluate the mitigation programme for bovine viral diarrhoea in Switzerland. Prev Vet Med. 2012;106:162–73. https://doi.org/10.1016/j.prevetmed.2012.01.022.
7. Babo Martins S. Economic assessment of surveillance in a "One Health" context. University of London; 2017.
8. Tambi EN, Maina OW, Mariner JC. Ex-ante economic analysis of animal disease surveillance. Revue Scientifique et Technique (International Office of Epizootics). 2004;23(3):737–52. https://doi.org/10.20506/rst.23.3.1517. PMID: 15861869.
9. Peyre M, Hoinville L, Njoroge J, Cameron A, Traon D, Goutard F, Calba C, Grosbois V, Delabouglise A, Varant V, Drewe J, Pfeiffer D, Häsler B. The RISKSUR EVA Tool (Survtool): a tool for the integrated evaluation of animal health surveillance systems. Prev Vet Med. 2019:104777. https://doi.org/10.1016/j.prevetmed.2019.104777.
10. Figuié M, Peyre M-I, Binot A. Surveillance of infectious animal diseases in southeast asia. Promoting the multiplicity of information networks. Perspect. - Cirad 1–4. 2013. https://doi.org/10.19182/agritrop/00040.
11. Bennett R, Balcombe K. Farmers' willingness to pay for a tuberculosis cattle vaccine. J Agric Econ. 2012;63(2):408–24. https://doi.org/10.1111/j.1477-9552.2011.00330.x.
12. Mørkbak MR, Christensen T, Gyrd-Hansen D. Consumers' willingness to pay for safer meat depends on the risk reduction methods—a Danish case study on Salmonella risk in minced pork. Food Control. 2011;22:445–51. https://doi.org/10.1016/j.foodcont.2010.09.024.

13. Calba C, Antoine-Moussiaux N, Charrier F, Hendrikx P, Saegerman C, Peyre M, Goutard FL, Applying participatory approaches in the evaluation of surveillance systems: A pilot study on African swine fever surveillance in Corsica, Preventive Veterinary Medicine, 2015;122(4):389–98. https://doi.org/10.1016/j.prevetmed.2015.10.001.
14. Pham HTT, Peyre M, Trinh TQ, Nguyen OC, Vu TD, Rukkwamsuk T, Antoine-Moussiaux N. "Application of discrete choice experiment to assess farmers' willingness to report swine diseases in the Red River Delta region, Vietnam." Preventive Veterinary Medicine. 2017;138:28–36.
15. Hoinville L. Animal health surveillance terminology. Final report from Pre-ICAHS workshop; 2011. http://www.fp7-risksur.eu/sites/fp7-risksur.eu/files/partner_logos/icahs-workshop-2011_surveillance_tewrminology_report_V1.2.pdf. Accessed 23/1/2014.
16. Catley A, Alders RG, Wood JL. Participatory epidemiology: approaches, methods, experiences. Vet J. 2012;191(2):151–60. https://doi.org/10.1016/j.tvjl.2011.03.010.
17. Sadler GR, Lee HC, Lim RS, Fullerton J. Recruitment of hard-to-reach population subgroups via adaptations of the snowball sampling strategy. Nurs Health Sci. 2010;12(3):369–74. https://doi.org/10.1111/j.1442-2018.2010.00541.x.
18. Delabouglise A, Antoine-Moussiaux N, Phan TD, Dao DC, Nguyen TT, Truong BD, Nguyen XN, Vu TD, Nguyen KV, Le HT, Salem G, Peyre M. The perceived value of passive animal health surveillance: the case of highly pathogenic avian influenza in Vietnam. Zoonoses Public Health. 2016a;63(2):112–28. https://doi.org/10.1111/zph.12212.
19. Delabouglise A, Antoine-Moussiaux N, Tatong D, Chumkaeo A, Binot A, Fournie G, Pilot E, Phimpraphi W, Kasemsuwan S, Paul MC, Duboz R, Salem G, Peyre M. Cultural practices shaping zoonotic diseases surveillance: the case of highly pathogenic avian influenza and Thailand native chicken farmers. Transbound Emerg Dis. 2016b; https://doi.org/10.1111/tbed.12506.
20. Heft-Neal S, Otte J, Pupphavessa W, Roland-Holst D, Sudsawasd S, Zilberman D. Supply Chain auditing for poultry production in Thailand. Rural Development Reasearch Consortium; 2008. http://www.fao.org/ag/againfo/programmes/en/pplpi/docarc/rep-0809_thaipoultrychain.pdf. Accessed 11/1/2013.
21. Bowen GA. Naturalistic inquiry and the saturation concept: a research note. Qualitat Res. 2008;8(1):137–52. https://doi.org/10.1177/1468794107085301.
22. Graneheim UH, Lundman B. Qualitative content analysis in nursing research: concepts, procedures and measures to achieve trustworthiness. Nurse Educ Today. 2004;24(2):105–12. https://doi.org/10.1016/j.nedt.2003.10.001.
23. R Core Team (2014) R: a language and environment for statistical computing. The R foundation. http://www.R-project.org/. Accessed 8/10/2012.
24. Legendre, P. "Species associations: the Kendall coefficient of concordance revisited." Journal of Agricultural, Biological, and Environmental Statistics. 2005;10(2):226–45.
25. Oksanen J, Blanchet FG, Kindt R, Legendre P, Minchin PR, O'Hara RB, Simpson GL, Solymos P, Stevens MHH and Wagner H. vegan: Community Ecology Package. 2014.
26. Diao X. Economywide impact of avian flu in Ghana. A dynamic CGE model analysis. Washington D.C.: International Food Policy Research Institute; 2009.
27. Paul MC, Figuie M, Kovitvadhi A, Valeix S, Wongnarkpet S, Poolkhet C, Kasemsuwan S, Ducrot C, Roger F, Binot A. Collective resistance to HPAI H5N1 surveillance in the Thai cockfighting community: Insights from a social anthropology study. Prev Vet Med. 2015;120(1):106–14. https://doi.org/10.1016/j.prevetmed.2015.02.021.
28. Baumgartner A, Felleisen R, Gut C. Campylobacter in Switzerland. Risk factors and measures for dealing with the problem. Bern: Federal Office of Public Health; 2012.
29. Berezowski J, Akkina J, Rio V Del, DeVore K, Dorea F, Dupuy C, Maxwell M, Singh V, Vial F, Streichert L. Do we need one health surveillance? One Health Newsl; 2015.
30. Stärk KDC, Kuribreña MA, Dauphin G, Vokaty S, Ward MP, Wieland B, Lindberg A. One Health Surveillance—more than a buzz word? Prev Vet Med. 2015;120:124–30. https://doi.org/10.1016/j.prevetmed.2015.01.019.
31. Babo Martins S, Rushton J, Staerk KDC. Economic assessment of zoonoses surveillance in a "One Health" context: A conceptual framework. Zoonoses Public Health. 2016;63:386–95.

32. Babo Martins S, Rushton J, Stärk KDC. Economics of zoonoses surveillance in a 'One Health' context: an assessment of Campylobacter surveillance in Switzerland. Epidemiol Infect. 2017;145:1148–58. https://doi.org/10.1017/S0950268816003320.
33. Murray C, Lopez A. Global Burden of Disease: a comprehensive assessment of mortality and disability from diseases, injuries and risk factors in 1990 and projected to 2020. Cambridge, MA; 1996.
34. Monteiro Pires S. Burden of disease of foodborne pathogens in Denmark; 2014.
35. Häsler B, Cornelsen L, Bennani H, Rushton J. A review of the metrics for One Health benefits. Rev Sci Tech Int Epiz. 2014;33:453–64.
36. Häsler B, Gilbert W, Jones B. The economic value of One Health in relation to the mitigation of zoonotic disease risks. One Health Hum. …; 2013. doi: https://doi.org/10.1007/82_2012_239
37. Herida M, Dervaux B, Desenclos J-C. Economic evaluations of public health surveillance systems: A systematic review. Am J Public Health. 2016:1–7. https://doi.org/10.1093/eurpub/ckv250.
38. Adamowicz W, Boxall P, Williams M, Louviere J. Stated preference approaches for measuring passive use values: Choice experiments and contingent valuation. Am J Agric Econ. 1998;80(1):64–75.
39. Louviere JJ, Hensher DA, Swait JD. Stated choice methods: analysis and applications. Cambridge: Cambridge University Press; 2000.
40. Croissant Y. mlogit: multinomial logit model. R package version 0.2-4; 2013.
41. Mwaura F, Muwanika FR, Okobai G Willingness to pay for extension services in Uganda among farmers involved in crop and animal husbandry. In: 3rd African Association of Agricultural Economists, Cape Town, South Africa, 19-23/09/2010; 2010.
42. Zhang H, Kono H, Kubota S. An integrated epidemiological and economic analysis of vaccination against highly pathogenic porcine reproductive and respiratory syndrome (PRRS) in Thua Thien Hue Province, Vietnam. Asian-Australas J Anim Sci. 2014;27:1499–512. https://doi.org/10.5713/ajas.2014.14060.
43. Elbers ARW, Gorgievski-Duijvesteijn MJ, van der Velden PG, Loeffen WLA, Zarafshani K. A socio-psychological investigation into limitations and incentives concerning reporting a clinically suspect situation aimed at improving early detection of classical swine fever outbreaks. Vet Microbiol. 2010;142:108–18. https://doi.org/10.1016/j.vetmic.2009.09.051.
44. Palmer SE, Sully M, Fozdar F. Farmers, animal disease reporting and the effect of trust: a study of west Australian sheep and cattle farmers. Rural Soc. 2009;19 https://doi.org/10.5172/rsj.351.19.1.32.
45. Oparinde A, Birol E. Farm households' preference for cash-based compensation versus livelihood-enhancing programs; 2011.
46. Otienno DJ, Ruto E, Hubbard L. Cattle farmers' preferences for disease free zones in Kenya: an application of the choice experiment method. J Agric Econ. 2011;62:207–24.
47. MARD. Decision No 60/2008/QD-BNN on prevention and control of Porcine reproductive and respiratory syndrome (PRRS), dated 15/7/2008; 2008.
48. MARD. Decision No 5/2007/QD-BNN on prevention and control of foot and mouth disease (FMD), dated 22/1/2007; 2007.
49. WHO. How to conduct a Discrete Choice Experiment for health workforce recruitment and retention in remote and rural areas: User guide with case studies; 2012.
50. World Bank. Enhancing control of highly pathogenic avian influenza in developing countries through compensation: issues and good practice; 2006.
51. Bronner A, Hénaux V, Fortané N, Hendrikx P, Calavas D. Why do farmers and veterinarians not report all bovine abortions, as requested by the clinical brucellosis surveillance system in France? BMC Vet Res. 2014;10:93.
52. Muroga N, Hayama Y, Yamamoto T, Kurogi A, Tsuda T, Tsutsui T. The 2010 foot-and-mouth disease epidemic in Japan. J Vet Med Sci. 2012;74:399–404. https://doi.org/10.1292/jvms.11-0271.
53. Park J-H, Lee K-N, Ko Y-J, Kim S-M, Lee H-S, Shin Y-K, Sohn H-J, Park J-Y, Yeh J-Y, Lee Y-H, Kim M-J, Joo Y-S, Yoon H, Yoon S-S, Cho I-S, Kim B. Control of foot-and-mouth disease during 2010–2011 epidemic, South Korea. Emerg Infect Dis. 2013;19:655–9. https://doi.org/10.3201/eid1904.121320.

Part IV

Qualitative and Semi-Quantitative Methods for Process Evaluation

Qualitative Methods to Evaluate Health Surveillance Systems

7

Marisa Peyre and Flavie Goutard

Abstract

The challenges of priority, sustainability, social acceptance, and communication are at the heart of the concerns for political decision-makers when it comes to defining and implementing health surveillance strategies. In most countries, animal health surveillance is largely based on the structural organization of veterinary services, but most often relies on informal networks that cannot be evaluated with the same tools as formalized surveillance systems. Qualitative methods combined or not with quantitative ones are essential to characterize the system processes and performances in the field and to capture the social, economic, and cultural constraints that often impact the system efficacy. Such elements are critical to ensure development and adoption of effective and adapted corrective actions by all the actors of the system. Engagement of the surveillance system actors within the evaluation process itself by the means of participatory approaches and co-development of solutions for improvement is also key to build up trust between actors from different levels (from field to national) and sectors (public and privates). Innovative methods and tools for the qualitative and quantitative evaluation of surveillance systems have been developed and largely applied in the field of animal health surveillance evaluation over the past decade.

M. Peyre · F. Goutard (✉)
CIRAD, UMR ASTRE, Montpellier, France

ASTRE, CIRAD, INRAE, University of Montpellier, Montpellier, France
e-mail: flavie.goutard@cirad.fr

M. Peyre et al. (eds.), *Principles for Evaluation of One Health Surveillance: The EVA Book*, https://doi.org/10.1007/978-3-030-82727-4_7

The aim of this chapter is to provide an overview of such methods and their field application. To gain more detail knowledge on each method, the readers can refer to published references provided and also to the specific chapters of this book.

Keywords

Evaluation · Qualitative methods · Health surveillance · Participatory approaches

7.1 Introduction

The challenges of priority, sustainability, social acceptance, and communication are at the heart of the concerns of political decision-makers when it comes to defining and implementing their surveillance strategies. The review of health surveillance evaluation methods by Calba et al. highlighted the importance and the need to develop an integrated approach to animal health assessment, taking into account not only the epidemiological and technical aspects but also the social and economic aspects [1, 2]. These tools must allow a relevant framing of the evaluation process, adapted to needs and resources, notably with the definition of a clear objective, and an evaluation question formulated in order to be able to respond to it (value judgment and recommendations). It is therefore necessary to develop quantitative tools to assess the performance of surveillance systems while coupling them with qualitative methods to characterize the functioning of the real system in the field in order to propose effective and appropriate corrective actions. In most countries, animal health surveillance is largely based on the structural organization of veterinary services, but most often relies on informal networks [3–5]. This type of structure can hardly be assessed with the same tools and approaches as formalized surveillance networks. Some assessments might therefore rely more on the institutional organization of the networks and their formalization, while others will have to focus on the actors of the system, their social organization, and specific constraints. However, the notion of formalization of networks is a key element in the performance and sustainability of the systems and must therefore be encouraged. Evaluating the performance of surveillance systems becomes a necessity, on the one hand, in terms of sensitivity, specificity, and predictive value—characterizing the ability to detect a true emergence in a defined space–time framework—and, on the other hand, terms of cost in relation to the desired efficiency. Indeed, it is essential to be able to quantify the performance of systems in order to improve them and adjust the necessary means (actors, budgets, structures) to the needs of a country (detection of emergencies, monitoring of the effectiveness of control such as vaccination). Therefore, qualitative and quantitative methods are intended to be complementary. It is indeed essential to characterize the way the system works in theory in order to be able to compare it with its real functioning in the field in order to propose effective and adapted corrective actions to be implemented.

Box 7.1 Qualitative/Semiquantitative Tools Available (Nonexhaustive List)

- **PVS et PVS Gap Analysis, OIE** () : Tool for evaluating veterinary services, the surveillance component is taken into account in the analysis of national prevention systems in a very global way.
- **Quality criteria evaluation public health surveillance, CDC (2001)** (): Method for evaluating public health surveillance systems according to 10 quality criteria essential for the proper functioning of the system, this method is not associated with a standardized tool and requires the involvement of experts, as well as the development of evaluation protocols adapted to each context.
- **OASIS, ANSES (2009)**: Standardized tool for evaluating the functioning of the system; takes into account the quantitative evaluation method developed by B. Dufour and P. Hendrikx, based on a method of critical point analysis of the system (HACCP) and on the evaluation of the quality criteria developed by the CDC. It is a turnkey tool consisting of a questionnaire, a grid and scoring guide, and an automated tool for scoring and graphical representation of results (on Microsoft Excel) [6].
- **SERVAL, HAVLA/RVC (2012)** () : Conceptual framework for evaluating surveillance systems, does not constitute a turnkey tool but represents a toolbox that allows the user to choose the necessary tools according to the type of evaluation, must be adapted to the context and used by experts in the field. This tool also allows a complete description of the system.

Limits: All the tools mentioned above require the involvement of an expert, previously trained in their use, competent in the field of surveillance and aware of the context of the evaluation field.

Innovative methods and tools for the qualitative and quantitative evaluation of surveillance systems have been developed in order to address the limits of the methods currently available, including

- The adaptation of the OASIS tool to the context of developing countries in order to generate a standardized qualitative/semiquantitative assessment tool for the surveillance system: OASIS has been adapted to context of developing countries with a module for financial analysis of networks under development, which takes into account the cost-effectiveness of the corrective actions identified by the tool and thus prioritizes the actions to be implemented [7]. This tool is presented in the context of this chapter.
- The use of participatory approaches in evaluation:
  - (a) The development of participatory economic evaluation methods in order to measure the economic impact of diseases and the societal costs and benefits of surveillance systems, and thus considering social issues critical for the proper functioning of systems (Chap. 7, Sect. 7.3).
  - (b) The development of a method for assessing the acceptability of surveillance systems—AccEPT (Chap. 8, Sect. 8.4).

- The adaptation and validation of quantitative evaluation methods for the performance of animal health surveillance systems: Capture/recapture and Decision Tree analyses [8, 9], which especially allows to assess the importance of under-detection (Chap. 11, Sect. 11.5).
- The adaptation and application of social network analysis (SNA) to the analysis of the process of sharing health information and of the socioeconomic factors impacting this health information sharing (Chap. 12, Sect. 12.5).

The aim of this chapter is to provide an overview of the qualitative methods currently used in the field of health surveillance evaluation. To gain more detail knowledge on each method, the readers can refer to published references provided and also to the specific chapters of this book.

7.2 OASIS: A Tool Adapted to the Evaluation of the Surveillance Process

The OASIS tool is a standardized tool for evaluating the quality and operating efficiency of surveillance systems, which was initially developed for a regional surveillance project (Caribbean, Maghreb and Indian Ocean). This tool was then adapted in 2007 by the CaribVet team and was then taken up in 2009 by a team from ANSES in order to adapt it to European working methods. In 2010, the tool was translated in English and further adapted by CIRAD to be applied to the evaluation of surveillance systems in South East Asia [7]. The tool and its applications have been the subject of numerous scientific publications and/or reports and its operation will only be briefly described here to facilitate understanding of its potential application [6, 10, 11].

7.2.1 Tool Principles

The OASIS tool is based on the principle that surveillance systems all require more or less the same basic structure to be functional, and therefore compares the surveillance process under evaluation to the process of an ideal system [10].

The tool is made up of three parts:

- A questionnaire that makes it possible to analyze each of the components of the surveillance system, structured in 10 sections: (1) objectives and context of surveillance, (2) central institutional organization, (3) field institutional organization, (4) laboratory, (5) tools for monitoring, (6) monitoring method, (7) data management, (8) training, (9) communication, and (10) evaluation.
- A rating system including 75 criteria defined by expert elicitation, thus ensuring their ability to describe a surveillance network as accurately as possible. A precise scoring guide to score these criteria from 0 to 3 in order to limit the possible interpretations of the assessor and to facilitate scoring work.

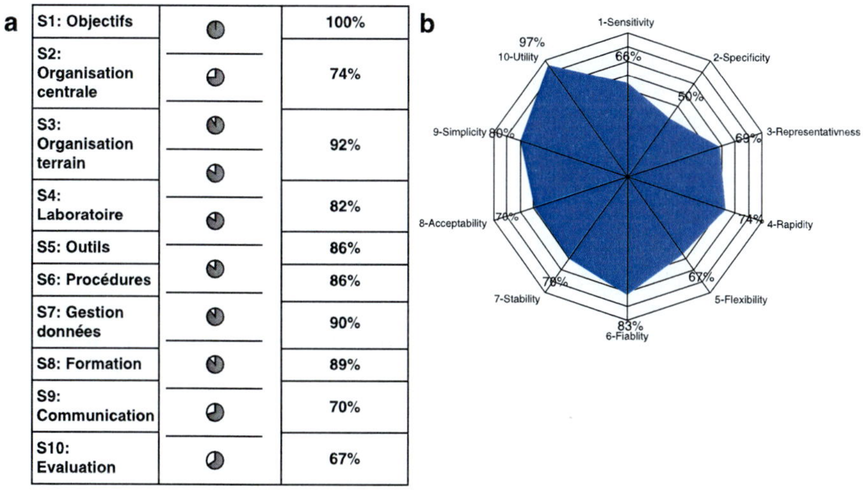

Fig. 7.1 OASIS evaluation of CSF surveillance in Germany: (**a**) strengths and weaknesses of the surveillance system; (**b**) qualitative analysis of the impact of the organization of the system on its performance

- Automated results on an Excel spreadsheet, which include (1) a descriptive analysis of the strengths and weaknesses of the system presenting the level of satisfaction of the 10 sections evaluated (Fig. 7.1a); (2) a critical point analysis based on the principles of HACCP (Hazard Analysis Critical Control Points), which measures seven critical points (network objectives, sampling, animation, tools, data collection and circulation, data analysis and interpretation and dissemination of information) weighted by the experts according to their importance in the performance of the surveillance process [12]; this result makes it possible to identify the margins for possible improvement for these seven critical points of the system; (3i) a qualitative analysis of the impact of the surveillance process on 10 evaluation attributes (sensitivity, specificity, representativeness, speed, flexibility, reliability, stability, acceptability, simplicity, and usefulness) (Fig. 7.1b), the nature of the criteria used, and their weights was also defined by expert elicitation.

7.2.2 Practical Use

The OASIS tool could be used to perform internal or external evaluations of surveillance systems. For external evaluation, it needs to be applied by an independent expert working in close collaboration with the system coordinator to gather the required information (Box 7.2). The expert can also involve other actors of the system to collect evidence of its implementation in the field. In order to do so, the expert must define a representative number of the different type of actors to be interviewed in order to have the most objective view of the network operation.

Internal evaluations are based on the same principle using the tool without the involvement of independent expert. It is, however, recommended to get prior training and/or to require technical support by relevant evaluation expert to ensure best use of the tool and meaningful recommendations.

As the financial aspect often represents a major obstacle, especially in developing countries, it is essential to estimate the cost-effectiveness of the corrective actions proposed to prioritize the improvements and forecast the necessary budgets and their viability over time. However, the cost-effectiveness evaluation of the surveillance (and control) of animal diseases remains a complicated exercise, on the one hand, because of the difficulty of access to these financial data considered as sensitive and, on the other hand, because of the methodological limits of performance evaluation of these systems (Parts III and V). Under its latest version, the tool provides an overview of the system financial sustainability over a 6-month to 2-year period according to the origin and duration of funding.

The applications of the tool in the field highlighted the following aspects:

- The importance of financial issues in decision-making in terms of improving the systems process: Cost of the corrective action but also its social impact versus its effectiveness (acceptability and performances).
- The financial sustainability of the surveillance system: Often essential surveillance activities are funded ad hoc as part of fixed terms internationally funded project. This could impair greatly the performance of the system that will not provide similar type and quality of data in a continuous manner—questioning the capacity of such system to address its objectives weather it is early detection of emerging disease or case detection for control. The questions that arise are: (1) What is the real impact of these ad hoc activities on the quality and performance of the system in the long term; (2) What are the differences in performances at regional and international level and how does this impact the ability to prevent emergence and pandemic spread?

Box 7.2 Evaluation of the Classical Swine Fever Surveillance System in Germany [13]

OASIS was applied to the evaluation of the organization of the CSF surveillance system in Germany within the framework of the RISKSUR project [3] .

Weaknesses were identified at the central organizational and field level due to limited material resources. The specificity of tests and surveillance protocols is limited, which makes it possible to promote the sensitivity of the system in order to demonstrate free status. Acceptability at the level of data sources and collectors is low due to the consequences of a declaration of suspicion or confirmation of a case, which also leads to biases in the quality of the data reported. The representativeness of the system is limited, which justifies the need to modify the monitoring protocols. Communication within the system deserves to be strengthened, as well as evaluation with the establishment of relevant performance indicators and external evaluation.

A surveillance system aimed at demonstrating the disease-free status of a disease must encourage high sensitivity with regard to specificity. However, the analysis of the system by the OASIS tool highlighted a limited sensitivity of the system (66%), which is affected by a low acceptability of this monitoring by the stakeholders (70%) as well as a low representativeness (69%). These elements must be reinforced. Work carried out by Schultz et al. to address such issues is presented as part of this book (Part III) [14].

7.3 The Use of Social Network Analysis to Characterize Health Information-Sharing Systems

The analysis of the structure of health surveillance system could be performed by looking at the social organization of the actors within the system and the information-sharing processes within such social networks (Part V) [3]. This approach allows to analyze the way private or public actors manage the risks linked to animal health, with or without the intervention of the state. The study of these networks also allows to understand to what extent the veterinary authorities are involved in this collective risk management or not and the perceived value of this official surveillance [3, 15]. The approach is based on the graph theory, where relationships between actors are no longer based solely on proximity links but on links of a social nature or commercial [16, 17]. Graph theory analyzes the place of actors in the network, their influence, the attributes determining this influence, or the conformation of the network, the creation of links with certain actors rather than with others [16, 17]. This approach can be combined with participative approach for data collection with the aim of better understanding the role of each actor in the network, as well as its socioeconomic constraints linked to health information sharing (Box 7.3) [18] (Part III).

This innovative approach in animal health has been widely applied with the aim of analyzing the socioeconomic factors that influence the sharing of health information and thus promote underreporting:

- As part of the evaluation of the HPAI surveillance system in Vietnam and Thailand with the analysis of health information-sharing networks between actors in the poultry sector ([3, 19, 20], n.d.) (Part III).
- In the context of the evaluation of the pig disease surveillance system in Vietnam with the analysis of networks for sharing health information between actors in the pig sector [21] (Part III).
- But also with the aim of better targeting surveillance as part of the evaluation of the surveillance system for swine influenza (PI) in Vietnam with the analysis of the risk of spread of PI through the movements of pigs within the production chain and the identification of risk concentration "nodes" to target surveillance [22].

Box 7.3 Comparative Analysis of Health Information-Sharing Network Among Poultry Farmers in Vietnam Using Structured Questionnaire Surveys or Participatory Approaches for Data Collection

Health information-sharing network among poultry farmers in Vietnam was analyzed using social network analysis (SNA) method and comparing two approaches for data collection, one based on classical structured questionnaire survey and the other on participatory semi-structured interviews [3]. Both data collection methods confirmed the importance of the private sector in the transmission of health information at different local and intermediate scales (village, town, district, and province). Classic SNA surveys are based on a selection of actors whose role in surveillance is defined a priori according to the organizational scheme of the official surveillance system (e.g., the district veterinarian is involved in official surveillance and serves as intermediary between the municipal veterinarian and the provincial veterinarian). This type of study is not concerned with validating the roles of each actor within the network. Participatory data collection studies carried out in parallel, emphasized the predominant role of the private veterinarian activities in the exchange of health information. This information does not always follow the official health events reporting system (Fig. 7.2).

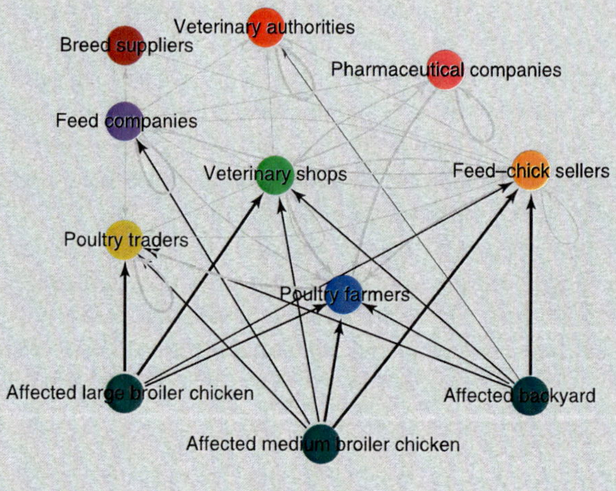

Fig. 7.2 Network for the dissemination of health information between actors in the poultry sector in Vietnam [23]

7.3.1 Importance of Private Actors in the Sharing of Health Information in Vietnam: Impact on the Performance of the Official Surveillance System

Analyses of health information-sharing networks in the swine and avian sectors in Vietnam have highlighted the predominant role of private actors (drug sellers, private veterinarians, food companies) in the dissemination of information and local health risk management [3, 20, 21]. Poultry and pig breeders, when they have a health problem with their animals, first contact drug sellers (veterinary pharmacy), other breeders in their network, and/or private veterinarians from the agrifood companies with which they have trade (Boxes 7.3 and 7.4). Public veterinarians, being part of the community, obtain the information informally and in this context might not always link with the official surveillance network, in particular to avoid damaging the bond of trust they maintain with breeders and the rest of their community [3, 20, 21]. It is critical to understand and acknowledge those social issues that affect the performances of the surveillance systems and to work in collaboration with the field actors of the system (both public and private, including animal producers but also private veterinarians, veterinary drugs sellers, traders, and feed companies) to find adapted solution for improvement.

Box 7.4 Comparative Analysis of the Pig Disease Surveillance System and the Health Information-Sharing Network for Pig Farmers in Vietnam [21]

By combining social network analysis method with participatory approaches, TTH. Pham highlighted the predominant role of private actors in sharing health information on swine diseases in Vietnam at the expense of the official surveillance system and thus the complexity of the what really happens in the field in terms of surveillance system (official versus informal/private) and the challenges linked to socioeconomic factors influencing to the decision to report diseases by or not (Fig. 7.3).

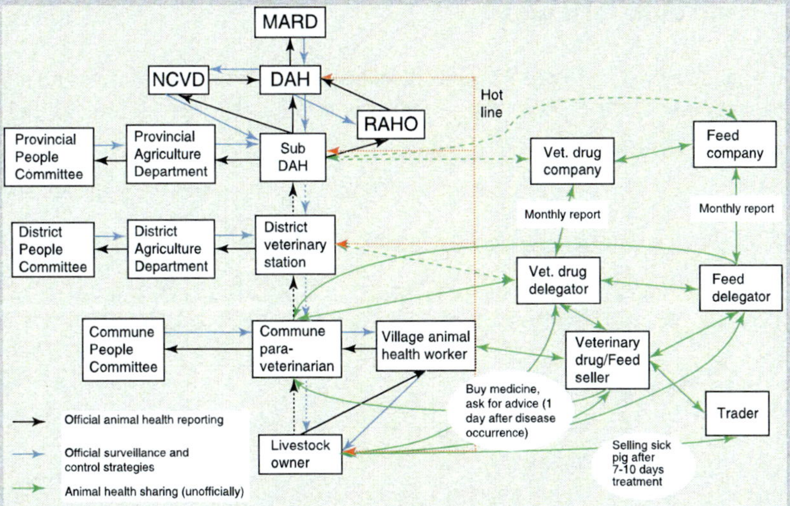

Fig. 7.3 Health information-sharing network on swine diseases in Vietnam: through the official surveillance system (black lines); through the private informal network (green lines)

7.4 Socioeconomic Factors that Impact the Performance of Health Surveillance

7.4.1 Quick Sale of Animals as an Alternative to Reporting

The quick sale of animals in an area where an outbreak is declared is often observed and could impair the effectiveness of disease control to limit the spread of the disease and therefore directly affect the efficacy of the surveillance itself. Moreover, quick sale of remaining live or even sick animals in an infected premise could also be observed and represent an alternative way to disease declaration and official reporting within the surveillance system (Fig. 7.4) [24]. A study performed in Vietnam combining social network analysis and participatory approaches has highlighted some of the rationale behind these kinds of practices: (1) producers limit their economic losses and, above all, recover part of their investment faster than the compensation proposed by the government following a declaration; and (2) this sector is favored by the opacity of private commercial networks, little traceability, and few controls. This type of alternative is more limited in settings where animal production is part of a quality product value chain. These elements highlight the importance of the level of structuring and quality of the production and of the commercial sector on the detection and management of health risks [24].

7.4.2 The Importance of Economic Impact, Trust, and Cultural Issues

Studies on the acceptability of the surveillance system, mixing qualitative and quantitative methods, have shown that animal producers often face significant delays

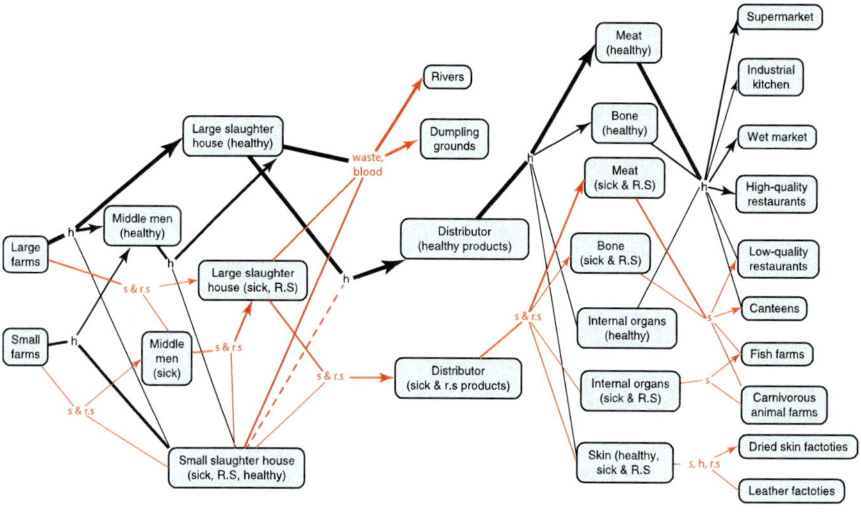

Fig. 7.4 Organization of distribution networks for healthy (black lines) and sick (red lines) pigs, in North Vietnam [25])

before receiving compensation for animals slaughtered during a declaration and thus being able to either restock or repay their debts [20] (Part III). These deadlines are often linked to the complexity of administrative procedures, to issues of conflicts of interest of the actors involved in the declaration procedures but also to trust issues between public and private actors of the surveillance system. These aspects could vary between different settings but could be observed in high- and low- to middle-income countries [1, 26], and these differences are closely linked to the differences in the structure of the veterinary services that set the basis for the surveillance system structure.

In Thailand, cockfighting is a very important cultural, economic, and political practice. There is a strong contradiction between the valuation of fighting cocks and the compulsory slaughter measures in the event of a declaration of a case of HPAI. In this sense, there is a major distrust of practitioners and breeders of cockfighting with the surveillance system as well as a major responsibility of the breeder who declares with their community of interest [20]. In a similar way, Pham et al. have shown that pig producers in Vietnam were more concerned with the slaughtering of their saws, resulting from years of genetic selection, rather than on the level of compensation for culling of their valuable animals when it comes to swine disease declaration in their facilities [27].

7.4.3 The Impact on the Market of a Declaration of Cases of Diseases and Risks of Stigmatization of the Actors

In the event of illness, the dissemination of information via the authorities, collectors, or the media has a direct impact on the animal sales chain, leading to a fall in prices and significant economic losses, including for breeders not affected by the disease [15, 18]. The declaring breeder thus takes significant responsibility vis-à-vis other breeders in his community and/or his network of commercial interest, which could lead to his stigmatization. This reluctance of breeders to harm their networks is difficult to apprehend by conventional approaches and requires the use of experimental econometric methods as described in Part III of this book.

7.5 Conclusion

The use of qualitative methods, especially participatory approaches in the evaluation of animal health surveillance systems, has emphasized the fact that socioeconomic and cultural constraints impact the decision of the actors of the surveillance system to declare or not a case of illness. However, the origin and response to these constraints vary more according to specific socioeconomic and cultural contexts, than according to the level of development of a country. Similarities and differences are more strongly linked to the type and level of structuring of the production and development sectors of the livestock sector concerned. The feasibility of combining innovative methods presented in this book in varied epidemiological, socioeconomic, cultural contexts, and targeting different systems and diseases highlights the great flexibility of participatory evaluation and the added value of qualitative methods as part of the evaluation process.

References

1. Calba C, Antoine-Moussiaux N, Charrier F, Hendrikx P, Saegerman C, Peyre M, Goutard FL. Applying participatory approaches in the evaluation of surveillance systems: a pilot study on African swine fever surveillance in Corsica. Prev Vet Med. 2015a;122:389–98. https://doi.org/10.1016/j.prevetmed.2015.10.001.
2. Calba C, Goutard FL, Hoinville L, Hendrikx P, Lindberg A, Saegerman C, Peyre M. Surveillance systems evaluation: a systematic review of the existing approaches. BMC Public Health. 2015b;15:448. https://doi.org/10.1186/s12889-015-1791-5.
3. Delabouglise A, Dao TH, Truong DB, Nguyen TT, Nguyen NTX, Duboz R, Fournié G, Antoine-Moussiaux N, Grosbois V, Vu DT, Le TH, Nguyen VK, Salem G, Peyre M. When private actors matter: information-sharing network and surveillance of highly pathogenic avian influenza in Vietnam. Acta Trop. 2015b;147:38–44. https://doi.org/10.1016/j.actatropica.2015.03.025.
4. Figuié M, Peyre M-I, Binot A. Surveillance of infectious animal diseases in Southeast Asia. Promoting the multiplicity of information networks. Perspect Cirad. 2013:1–4. https://doi.org/10.19182/agritrop/00040.
5. Goutard FL, Binot A, Duboz R, Rasamoelina-Andriamanivo H, Pedrono M, Holl D, Peyre MI, Cappelle J, Chevalier V, Figuié M, Molia S, Roger FL. How to reach the poor? Surveillance in low-income countries, lessons from experiences in Cambodia and Madagascar. Prev Vet Med. 2015;120:12–26. https://doi.org/10.1016/j.prevetmed.2015.02.014.
6. Hendrikx P, Gay E, Chazel M, Moutou F, Danan C, Richomme C, Boue F, Souillard R, Gauchard F, Dufour B. OASIS: an assessment tool of epidemiological surveillance systems in animal health and food safety. Epidemiol Infect. 2011;139:1486–96. https://doi.org/10.1017/S0950268811000161.
7. Peyre, M., Hendrikx, P., Do Huu, D., Goutard, F., Desvaux, S., Roger, F., others, 2011. Evaluation of surveillance systems in animal health: the need to adapt the tools to the contexts of developing countries, results from a regional workshop in South East Asia. Epidémiologie Santé Anim 59, 415–417.
8. Goutard FL, Paul M, Tavornpanich S, Houisse I, Chanachai K, Thanapongtharm W, Cameron A, Stärk KDC, Roger F. Optimizing early detection of avian influenza H5N1 in backyard and free-range poultry production systems in Thailand. Prev Vet Med. 2012;105:223–34. https://doi.org/10.1016/j.prevetmed.2011.12.020.
9. Vergne T, Del Rio Vilas VJ, Cameron A, Dufour B, Grosbois V. Capture–recapture approaches and the surveillance of livestock diseases: a review. Prev Vet Med. 2015;120:253–64. https://doi.org/10.1016/j.prevetmed.2015.04.003.
10. Dufour B, Hendrikx P. Surveillance épidémiologique en santé animale, 3e éd. Quae; 2011.
11. Hendrikx P, Chauzat M-P, Debin M, Neuman P, Fries I, Ritter W, Brown M, Mutinelli F, Conte YL, Gregorc A. Bee mortality and bee surveillance in Europe. EFSA Support Publ. 2009;6 https://doi.org/10.2903/sp.efsa.2009.EN-27.
12. Dufour B. Original article technical and economic evaluation method for use in improving infectious animal disease surveillance networks; 1998.
13. Häsler B, Peyre M, Bisdorff B, Alexis Delabouglise AC, Schulz K, Bouwer A, Hautefeuille C, Grosbois V. RISKSUR deliverable report 5.22: Completed comparative economic evaluation of different surveillance system designs; 2015.
14. Schulz K, Peyre M, Staubach C, Schauer B, Schulz J, Calba C, Häsler B, Conraths FJ. Surveillance strategies for classical swine fever in wild boar—a comprehensive evalua-

tion study to ensure powerful surveillance. Sci Rep. 2017;7:43,871. https://doi.org/10.1038/srep43871.

15. Delabouglise A, Antoine-Moussiaux N, Phan TD, Dao DC, Nguyen TT, Truong BD, Nguyen XNT, Vu TD, Nguyen KV, Le HT, Salem G, Peyre M. The perceived value of passive animal health surveillance: the case of highly pathogenic avian influenza in Vietnam. Zoonoses Public Health. 2015a; https://doi.org/10.1111/zph.12212.
16. Jackson C. External validity in experimental methods: a social reality check; 2011.
17. Lazega E. Wasserman Stanley, Faust Katherine, social network analysis: methods and applications. Rev Fr Sociol. 1995;36:781–3.
18. Delabouglise A. Les enjeux territoriaux de la surveillance de la santé animale: le cas de l'influenza aviaire hautement pathogène au Viet Nam et en Thaïlande; 2015.
19. Delabouglise A, Antoine-Moussiaux N, Phan TD, Dao DC, Nguyen TT, Truong BD, Nguyen XNT, Vu TD, Nguyen KV, Le HT, Salem G, Peyre M. The perceived value of passive animal health surveillance: the case of highly pathogenic avian influenza in Vietnam. Zoonoses Public Health. 2016a;63:112–28. https://doi.org/10.1111/zph.12212.
20. Delabouglise A, Antoine-Moussiaux N, Tatong D, Chumkaeo A, Binot A, Fournié G, Pilot E, Phimpraphi W, Kasemsuwan S, Paul MC, Duboz R, Salem G, Peyre M. Cultural practices shaping zoonotic diseases surveillance: the case of highly pathogenic avian influenza and Thailand native Chicken farmers. Transbound Emerg Dis. 2016b; https://doi.org/10.1111/tbed.12506.
21. Pham HTT. Development of novel methodologies for the socio-economic evaluation of animal health surveillance system: application to swine disease surveillance in Vietnam. Kasetsart University, Bangkok; 2016.
22. Baudon EM. Sustainable surveillance strategies for the detection of swine influenza in Vietnam. HKU Theses Online HKUTO; 2015.
23. Delabouglise A, Dao TH, Truong DB, Nguyen TT, Nguyen NTX, Duboz R, Fournié G, Antoine-Moussiaux N, Grosbois V, Vu DT, Le TH, Nguyen V.K, Salem G, Peyr, M. When private actors matter: information-sharing network and surveillance of Highly Pathogenic Avian Influenza in Vietnam. Acta Trop. 2015;147:38–44. https://doi.org/10.1016/j.actatropica.2015.03.025.
24. Mai HN, Phuong NT, Tien ND, Ton VD, Peyre M. Diversified chicken farming systems and trading networks in Hai Duong Province, Northern Vietnam, Anim Prod Southeast Asia Curr Status Future 38; 2017.
25. Hoang MN, Nguyen PT, Han HQ, Nguyen TD, Vu TD, Peyre M. Network analysis of the sick-pig commodity chain in Northern Vietnam: Risk of disease dissemination. Rev. D'élevage Médecine Vét. Pays Trop. 2020;73:61–70. https://doi.org/10.19182/remvt.31872.
26. Calba C, Goutard FL, Vanholme L, Antoine-Moussiaux N, Hendrikx P, Saegerman C. The added-value of using participatory approaches to assess the acceptability of surveillance systems: the case of bovine tuberculosis in Belgium. PLoS One. 2016;11:e0159041. https://doi.org/10.1371/journal.pone.0159041.
27. Pham HTT, Peyre M, Trinh TQ, Nguyen OC, Vu TD, Rukkwamsuk T, Antoine-Moussiaux N. Application of discrete choice experiment to assess farmers' willingness to report swine diseases in the Red River Delta region, Vietnam. Prev Vet Med. 2017;138:28–36. https://doi.org/10.1016/j.prevetmed.2017.01.002.

8 The Use of Participatory Methods in the Evaluation of Health Surveillance Systems

Flavie Goutard, Clémentine Calba, Sokha Chea, Nicolas Antoine-Moussiaux, Mathieu Pruvot, Katja Schulz, and Marisa Peyre

Abstract

Surveillance systems rely on a network of stakeholders who share information. Socioeconomics factors have an influence on their decision to share or not the information within the system. Those factors are rarely taken into consideration, especially in the evaluation of surveillance systems.

Participatory approaches derived from social sciences have proven useful to take these factors into account and have been adapted over the past 15 years to the context of health surveillance system evaluation. The "AccePT" (Acceptability Participatory Toolkit) method based on participatory approaches has been developed to assess the acceptability of surveillance systems. The method takes into

F. Goutard (✉) · C. Calba
CIRAD, UMR ASTRE, Montpellier, France

ASTRE, CIRAD, INRAE, University of Montpellier, Montpellier, France
e-mail: flavie.goutard@cirad.fr

S. Chea
Wildlife conservation Society, Phnom Penh, Cambodia

N. Antoine-Moussiaux
Fundamental and Applied Research for Animals and Health (FARAH), University of Liège, Liege, Belgium

M. Pruvot
Wildlife conservation Society, Bronx, New York City, USA

K. Schulz
Friedrich-Loeffler-Institut, Federal Research Institute for Animal Health, Institute of Epidemiology, Greifswald, Insel Riems, Germany

M. Peyre
CIRAD, UMR ASTRE, Montpellier, France

ASTRE, CIRAD, INRAE, University of Montpellier, Montpellier, France

M. Peyre et al. (eds.), *Principles for Evaluation of One Health Surveillance: The EVA Book*, https://doi.org/10.1007/978-3-030-82727-4_8

consideration the adequacy of objectives and operation in the system for the stakeholders, the satisfaction of their roles, and their level of trust within the system. This approach allows stakeholders to freely discuss or think about how they experience working or not working with other partners, and to provide context-based recommendations taking into consideration their perceptions, expectations, and needs.

Keywords

Epidemiological surveillance · Evaluation · Acceptability · Participatory approaches

8.1 Introduction

Surveillance systems in animal health were established during the twentieth century following the increase in international trade in live animals and animal products that contributed to the spread of diseases between countries. These complex strategies are put in place to monitor the progress of diseases and to facilitate their control [1]. They respond to public health issues, by protecting human populations from zoonotic risks; to economic issues, by maintaining the national herd and access to international trade; and also to biodiversity-related issues by ensuring the protection of threatened species. Animal health surveillance systems are decision support tools defined by "the systematic and continuous operations of collection, compilation and analysis of animal health information, as well as their dissemination within a timeframe compatible with the implementation of necessary measures" [1]. The information produced by surveillance systems supports decisions on what measures are appropriate, including prevention, control, and research. Animal health surveillance is carried out by a variety of stakeholders, involved at different scales, organized as networks of actors. Information such as epidemiological data and decisions on disease control measures and animal health management must flow in a multidirectional manner in these networks. Dissemination of information is thus an essential element that determines the motivation of a large number of surveillance actors [2].

Surveillance systems have certain limitations that influence their performance in accurately describing the epidemiological situation of a given population. These limitations are related to underreporting, reporting delays, lack of data management, limited representativeness, or imposed budgetary constraints [3]. It is fundamental to evaluate these systems regularly and appropriately to ensure their performance, but also to determine whether the relevant stakeholders are fully engaged and the resources provided are used optimally. Current evaluation approaches are generally not very flexible and do not always consider the context in which the surveillance system is implemented [4–7]. The socioeconomic aspects of surveillance are also poorly considered despite their impact on surveillance performance [8, 9].

8.2 Importance of Sociological and Economic Factors in the Surveillance System Performances

The proper functioning of surveillance systems depends on technical and economic operating constraints as well as social issues generated by the networks of actors involved [10, 11]. The design of more effective and efficient surveillance systems, as well as their evaluation, requires the application of innovative methods and tools accounting for the perceptions, expectations, and needs of the different actors.

To be functional, epidemiological surveillance must be based on a network of actors who share common (or at least compatible) interests, derive mutual benefit from the network operations, and have a common understanding of the circulating information. In other words, these actors must share a common perception of the disease to be monitored and give the same definition of what is a reportable case. Social factors can have important consequences on the validity and the performance of the surveillance strategies, in particular with regard to the problems of stigmatization of individuals or of a social group. It is therefore necessary to be inclusive of the multiple actors—breeders, veterinarians, consumers, traders—who contribute, more or less autonomously, in the management of risks and crisis situations associated with the emergence of diseases. Therefore, the inclusion of a social dimension not only aims to identify the human factors that promote the circulation of health information, but also supports the definition of the modalities of risk co-management.

Participatory approaches derived from social sciences have proven useful over the past 15 years to integrate social factors into the evaluation of health surveillance system [6, 7, 12–15]).

8.3 Advantages of Using Participatory Approaches in the Evaluation Process

Participatory approaches have been initiated in Southern countries with the aim of responding to development issues facing local communities. After being applied to many areas such as natural resource management or agriculture, participatory approaches began to be applied to veterinary epidemiology in the 1980s [16, 17]. Participatory epidemiology (PE) is often used for animal health surveillance in developing countries, where the human and financial resources of veterinary services are limited. This method essentially makes it possible to collect qualitative or semiquantitative data on animal health and disease occurrence. It has been applied in animal disease surveillance in Africa (notably in the rinderpest eradication program) and Asia [18]. PE could be defined as social sciences applied to health data collection and disease control. It requires interactions between stakeholders and focuses on the understanding of local priorities [12].

Based on local and traditional knowledge, these methods actively involve grassroots stakeholders, mainly herders (key actors in disease reporting) to collect information on the health situation [17]. They can be applied in addition to conventional surveillance methods in the identification of field clinical cases that are not detected by passive surveillance systems if the cases can be confirmed by specific biological tests [19–21]. Their main advantages are to increase ownership of the stakeholders in the surveillance system and to increase sustainability of surveillance by relying on formal and informal stakeholder networks [12].

We have applied these approaches to the evaluation of surveillance systems in animal health in South East Asia and Europe (cf. case studies) [6, 7, 14, 22, 23]. Evaluation processes have been used in many areas, including program, performance, and policies evaluations. Evaluators often find themselves faced with the resistance of actors to engage in evaluation processes, which is perceived as a form of judgment [24, 25]. In order to improve the design and implementation of evaluations, but also to optimize the use of results in decision-making, it is important to pay particular attention to stakeholders and to involve them early on in the process [26]. We therefore propose to shift from a top-down approach, in which no consultation processes are used, to more participatory approaches. Participatory approaches can provide the necessary flexibility for evaluation in different context and allow the collection of complementary and essential information on the socioeconomic aspects of surveillance. This process should enable discussion, communication, negotiation, knowledge sharing, and should provide a strong basis for the common identification of socially acceptable solutions. Participatory evaluation leads to stakeholder empowerment in the process, which could improve the sustainability of surveillance systems.

8.4 Application of Participatory Methods to Surveillance System Evaluation

8.4.1 The AccePT Method to Assess Surveillance System Acceptability

Calba et al. [27] have developed a method to estimate the acceptability of animal health surveillance systems based on the use of participatory approaches: the Acceptability Participatory Toolkit (AccePT). This method combines a series of participatory tools used with stakeholders to measure (i) their perception of system objectives, (ii) their perception of the monitoring process (their role, constraints, and relationships with other actors in the system), and finally (iii) their confidence in the system; three essential elements for the acceptance of the surveillance system by its actors [3, 7, 14].

This method was applied to a pilot study on surveillance of porcine pests in Corsica [6, 7] with the aim of determining the applicability of participatory processes in a developed country context with various actors and to test the methodology in the field. It was subsequently applied to the surveillance of bovine tuberculosis in Belgium [14] and to evaluate the acceptability of a multistakeholder wildlife health surveillance network in Cambodia [23].

8.4.1.1 Definition of the Acceptability of a Surveillance System

Acceptability refers to the willingness of individuals and organizations to participate in surveillance, as well as the extent of involvement of each of these users [28]. This attribute of evaluation is considered to be one of the main qualities of surveillance by the United States Center for Diseases Control and Prevention (CDC) [29].

Health surveillance systems are composed of a broad range of stakeholders, and they all have different responsibilities toward, different perceptions of, and different ways of thinking about the surveillance system. Therefore, one of the biggest challenges within the system is to bring every one of them to a position of mutual interest. Stakeholders' willingness to support the system, their satisfaction of the operation, and of their own roles are strong pillars to an effective surveillance system [23].

In order to limit underreporting, it is crucial to determine the stakeholders' perceptions and expectations regarding surveillance, and thus their level of acceptability. This attribute is all the more important as it can influence the performance of the surveillance system, for example, by influencing the sensitivity and responsiveness of the system [15].

Despite this, this attribute is not always measured or when it is, the methods used (e.g., structured questionnaires) do not always make it possible to highlight the points of view and expectations of the actors [3].

The different elements considered in estimating the acceptability of surveillance systems as well as the questions and participatory tools to document them are detailed in Table 8.1. This approach allows participants to consider and discuss their experience working with other stakeholders, identify potential issues doing so, and possible solutions.

8.4.1.2 General Method Flow

The AccePT method consists of individual face-to-face interviews or focus groups of 5–10 participants. Focus groups are preferred because they allow participants to share their experiences and compare their points of view. Their strength lies in the establishment of a debate until a consensus is reached. Any type of stakeholder involved in the surveillance system targeted by the evaluation should be involved in this participatory process (e.g., breeders, veterinarians, laboratories, government departments, etc.). The selection of participants will depend on the willingness of the actors to take part in the study. Moreover, participants should not combine actors with different experience of the system in one focus group discussion where they are required to produce only one combined ranking even though they play in the same position. Best to separate them into groups with the same experience and knowledge of the surveillance system, that way will help to maintain the discussion and experience sharing without compromising the assessment goal. We should avoid situation where actors are required to discuss or rank stakeholders that they

Table 8.1 Considerations for measuring the acceptability of a surveillance system, associated participatory questions, and tools

Elements	Question	Participatory tools
Objective	Is the objective of the surveillance system in line with the objective expected by the actors of the device?	Flowchart diagram
Process		
Role of each actor	Are stakeholders satisfied with their duty within the surveillance system?	Flowchart diagram
Consequences of information flow	Are stakeholders satisfied with the consequences of information flows?	Impact diagram associated with proportional piling
Relations between actors	Are actors satisfied with the relationships they have with other actors involved in the system?	Relationship diagram associated with rating smileys
Trust		
In the system	Do the actors trust the surveillance system to achieve the objectives?	Flowchart diagram associated with proportional piling
In the other actors	Do actors trust other actors involved in the scheme to fulfill their role in surveillance?	Flowchart diagram associated with proportional piling

have not worked with. Some participants that hold high position in the government might struggle to provide direct response to the interview. In this case, interviewer needs to be mindful of these biases and be prepared to handle the interview at the best of his possibility. It is also essential to obtain approval from the local ethics committee and obtain informed consent from each participant before conducting interviews. In addition to representing large categories of stakeholders, caution should be exercised in the selection process to not inadvertently exclude important groups of individuals in a way that would bias the outcomes (e.g., different ethnic groups, size of the breeding operation, the membership to hunter association, etc.). Indeed, the perception of the surveillance system may vary depending on these elements. The interviews are set up following several steps that are the same for individual interviews and focus groups. Each interview begins with an introduction of the participants, the facilitator, and evaluation team, the project and its objectives, as well as the outline of the interview. Following this introduction, the various tools are used, and results are summarized at the end of the meeting. Finally, the participants are thanked and informed of what feedback they will receive following the result analysis.

8.4.1.3 Presentation of the Tools

Relational Diagrams and Rating Smileys

Relationship diagrams are used to identify the professional network of participants and to define the interactions between them. With this tool, participants are introduced to the evaluation process and asked to qualify their professional relationship with other actors on a 3-point scale: insufficient, sufficient, or more than necessary relationship. The activity does not focus exclusively on relationships within the surveillance network, but extends to other professional relationships participants may have outside the network (Fig. 8.1). Once the chart has been developed, the next step is to determine the level of participant satisfaction with the relationships with each member of their professional network. Colored game tokens, with graded smiley face on one side, are used on the diagram, representing five levels of satisfaction: very unsatisfactory, unsatisfactory, moderately satisfactory, satisfactory, very satisfactory. The goal is to place one and only one smiley per actor or organization identified (Fig. 8.1).

Flow Diagrams Associated with Proportional Piling

Flow diagrams are used to determine participants' perceptions of the flow of information within the surveillance system, for instance, the reporting of a suspected case of the disease under surveillance. This exercise facilitates the identification of the different paths that this information can take, whether official or informal. Once participants have completed the diagram, the proportional piling method is used to estimate their level of trust. This tool is applied in two stages: the first stage provides an estimate of the trust participants have in the surveillance system, the second stage assesses trust between actors of the network. Participants are asked to allocate 100 game tokens in two piles in order to highlight the trust they place in the functioning of the whole surveillance (the higher the number of tokens, the greater the trust). Then, in a second step, to distribute these tokens among the various actors identified, according to the same principle (Fig. 8.2).

Impact Diagrams Associated with Proportional Piling

Impact diagrams are used to determine participants' perceptions of the positive and negative impacts of a particular event and to document the consequences that

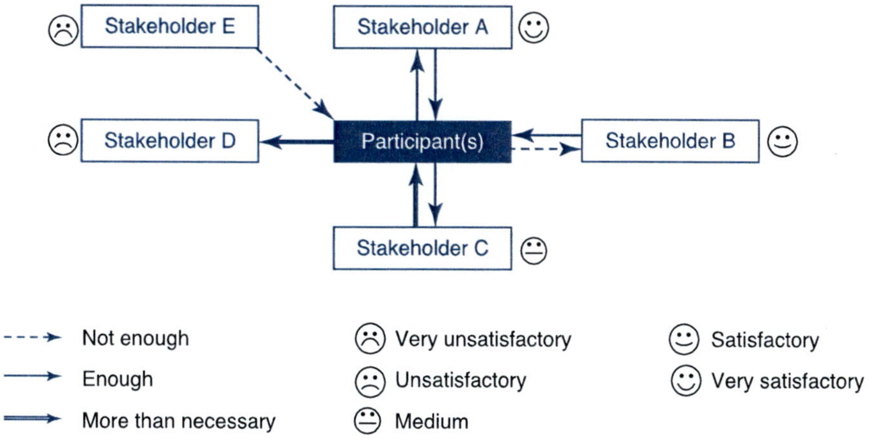

Fig. 8.1 Schematic representation of a relationship diagram associated with rating smileys (AccePT method)

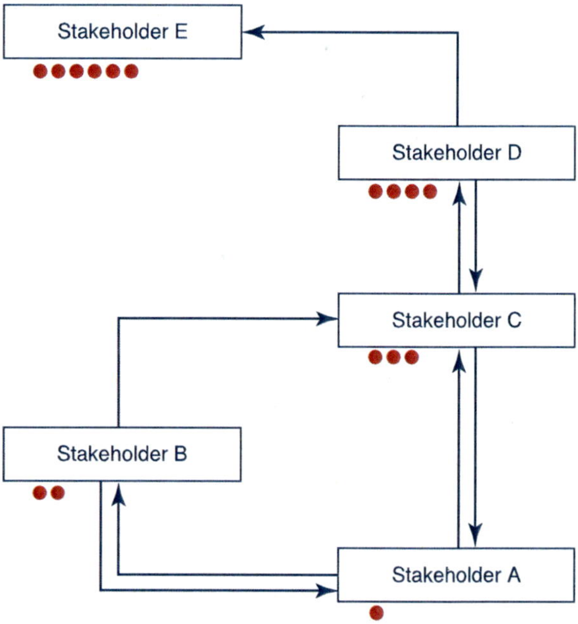

Fig. 8.2 Schematic representation of a flow diagram associated with proportional stacking (AccePT method) (arrows = relation between actors; dots = level of trust; the increase in dots represent increase in trust level)

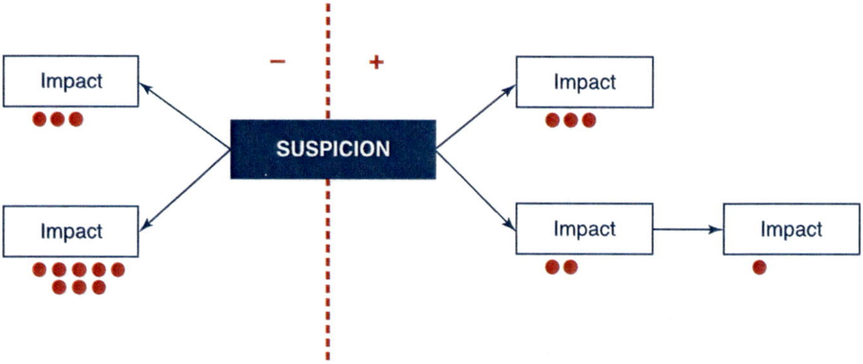

Fig. 8.3 Schematic representation of an impact diagram associated with proportional piling (dots; the highest number = the highest value)

participants directly experience. In our case, the specific event is a suspicion of the disease under surveillance.

Once the diagram has been constructed, the participants will again use proportional piling in two stages: first, they are asked to divided 100 game tokens between positive and negative impact to weight them, then in a second step to distribute each pile of token between the different impacts that have been identified by the participants (Fig. 8.3).

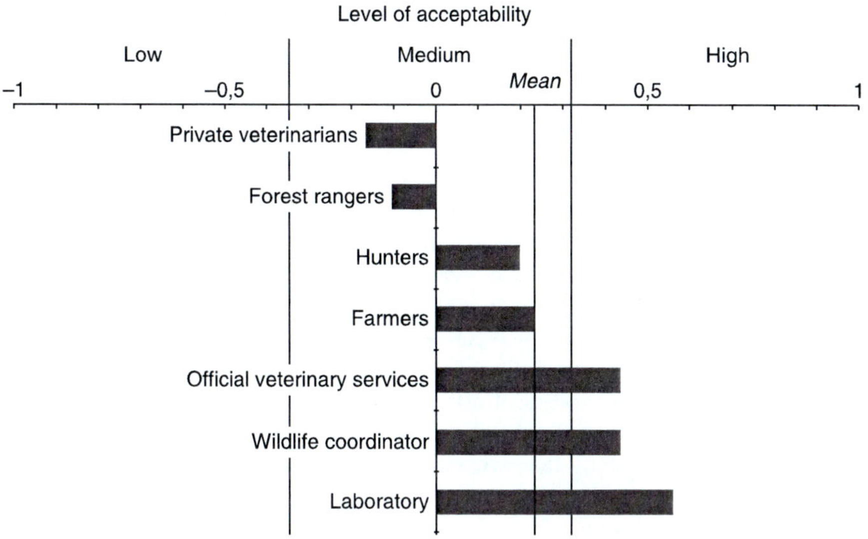

Fig. 8.4 Example of representation of the results of the estimation of the acceptability by the use of the AccePT method (case of the surveillance of bovine tuberculosis in Belgium)

Analysis and Presentation of Results

The results of the Acceptability Estimate are based on the analysis of all the discussions that took place between the participants during the interviews, the diagrams, and the semiquantitative data obtained from smiley scoring and proportional piling.

The analysis is carried out initially for each individual interview and each group discussion. An evaluation grid has been developed presenting scoring criteria based on a semiquantitative scale with the following score according to the different element of acceptability index: "unsatisfied = −1, medium = 0, satisfied = 1" for their satisfaction level in the objective, the operation and the information within the system; "weak = −1, medium = 0, good = 1" for their level of trust. Proportional piling analysis was based on the way that participants divided 100 counters between negative and positive impacts. Based on the scoring guidelines, the scores were then categorized into three levels such as weak [0; 33], which is equal to score −1, medium [33; 66], which is equal to score 0, and good [66; 100], which is equal to score 1. The results can be presented in different formats: by type of actor, by level of surveillance (local, regional, national) or by element of acceptability, or even by the combination of these different elements (Fig. 8.4).

The qualitative data collected during the interviews also includes valuable information for improving the surveillance system. In fact, interviews allow participants to discuss their points of view, expectations, and experiences, which are essential for improving surveillance. Follow-up events to discuss the outcome of the performance evaluation may be very valuable to further discuss the findings and involve additional actors who have not taken part in the process but who may be impacted by the results and the recommendations.

8.4.1.4 Benefits, Limits, and Outlook

The AccePT method is a standardized method for estimating the acceptability of epidemiological surveillance systems in animal health taking via participation of the diversity of actors involved in the network. By using different participatory tools and analyzing the results in the form of a scoring grid, it is possible to determine a general level of acceptability of the system, as well as a level of acceptability by type of actors.

The use of this method makes it possible to formulate recommendations that are context-specific, and most of which can be directly formulated by the participants. It also leads to a better acceptability of the evaluation thanks to the direct involvement of the actors in the process. It offers the opportunity to clearly document the general context of the surveillance and the structure of the surveillance system. It contributes to strengthening the ownership of the stakeholders in the system and provides capacity-building opportunities regarding specific diseases or epidemiological surveillance generally.

Implementing the AccePT method, however, requires specific training in the use of participatory approaches. In addition, there are substantial time requirements related to the organization of interview sessions, participant recruitment, interviews facilitation, and analysis of the results. Biases related to semistructured interview approaches can also influence the outcomes and further justify the need for appropriate training in participatory approaches. The organization of the different focus group should be organized very early in the process of evaluation in order to target homogenous group to avoid power relationships within interview groups and ensure participants freedom of expression during sessions. Cultural factors, such as the tendency to avoid conflict at all cost and also not wanting others to lose face, may significantly influence the dynamic during interview sessions. Some participants may not want to be seen as being too negative toward other partners and may bias their scoring toward the least conflictual options. Particular care should be used to mitigate the influence this may have on the scoring process.

There is a potential for participatory epidemiology to be valuable in the evaluation of other attributes, such as communication, stability, representativeness, or training provision. These methods could also be used for different issues, such as impact studies of research projects or "One Health" projects (see Chaps. 9 and 16).

The three cases studies presented below confirmed the interest of using these approaches to better identify the actors involved in the operation of surveillance beyond the official system and to specify their roles:

- Take into account stakeholders' perceptions/expectations and thereby improve understanding of the system; issue context-dependent recommendations; better understand the organizational and functional attributes.
- Involve stakeholders directly in the evaluation process, thus identifying potential bottlenecks, ensuring greater acceptability of the evaluation process itself, and fostering the sense of ownership of the system.
- Indirectly generate key information related to the general context and external factors.

8.5 Case Study 1: Application of Participatory Approaches to Evaluate Avian Influenza Surveillance in Vietnam

Participatory approaches were applied in a pilot study to evaluate avian influenza surveillance system in Vietnam [30]. The objective of the study was to estimate the performance of the passive reporting system of avian influenza in Luong Dien Commune (located in Cam Giang District, Hai Duong Province) in Vietnam. The specific objective was to assess the occurrence and reporting of sudden death in poultry. The underlying hypothesis was that sudden death is occurring in the community, but is not always reported. The study was conducted in 2012, in three villages of the commune of Luong Dien, Province of Hai Duong, in the Red River Delta of North Vietnam (about 50 km West of Ha Noi). Individual and focus group interviews of local authorities, veterinarians, and farmers were conducted ($n = 160$ participants) to understand how health information was shared in case of high poultry mortality. Participatory tools such as proportional piling, matrix scoring, mapping, transect walks, Venn diagrams, flow diagrams, seasonal calendar, and disease impact matrix scoring were also used to help in characterizing the system.

The flow of information sharing varied according to the mortality levels observed and those thresholds were defined locally (Fig. 8.5). If poultry mortality was higher than what was considered as the "normal" situation (>10–15% mortality in the village overnight), farmers would directly ask advice from private drug and/or veterinarian drug sellers. In case of higher mortality (>30% in the village overnight), the event was considered as "epidemic" by the farmer who would inform the village and/or the commune veterinarian for advice (do they need to slaughter the poultry?)

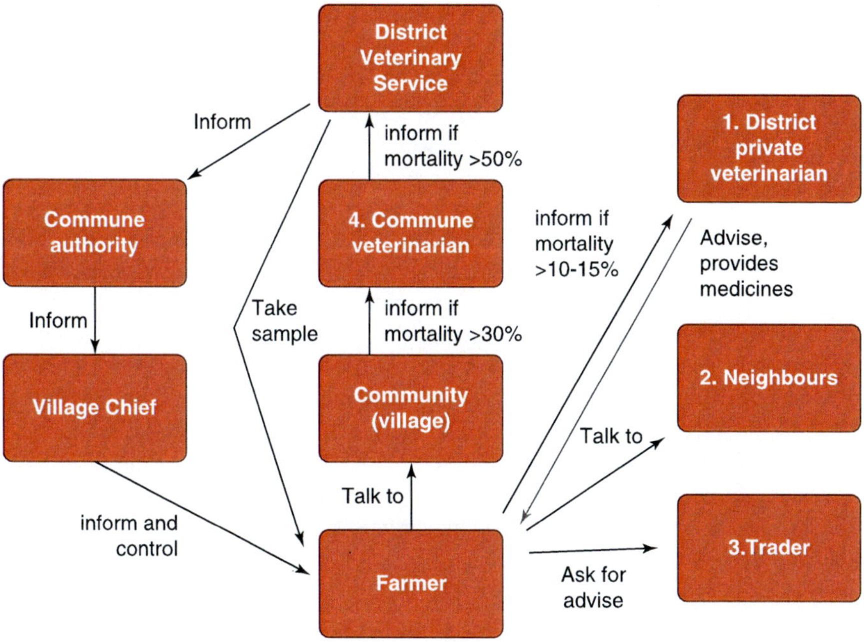

Fig. 8.5 Health information flow of avian diseases at local and intermediate scales in North Vietnam

and investigation. If the village or commune veterinarian considers that the mortality rate is too important to be manage locally (>50% in the village overnight), he will inform the official district veterinarians by sending an official letter when (considering that there is a risk of H5N1). In this case only, the official surveillance network is activated and the control measures are deployed. This pilot work highlighted two important aspects: (i) the definition of an HPAI suspicion case will vary according to the local situation and is far less sensitive than the official system case (>5% of sudden mortality); and (ii) the reporting system at local level does not follow the "vertical" path of the official passive surveillance system but rather a "horizontal" one for reasons of efficiency, speed, and simplicity; the farmers are looking for quick and nonbinding solutions to the health problems facing him and preferentially turn to local providers of veterinary services (pharmacies, suppliers of inputs). According to the same logic, the official veterinary services can be contacted, but personally, as private service providers.

Compared with traditional surveys based on the use of directed questionnaires and a priori sampling of actors, the use of participatory approaches allowed

- To identify some key actors in the surveillance system that were not mentioned in traditional surveys (e.g., drug vendors and veterinary food wholesalers).
- To clarify the role of the actors in the official system, which is certainly predominant in the exchange of health information but essentially in a private capacity (public veterinarians all have a liberal activity) and this type of information does not therefore follow the official path of notification of sanitary incidents.

This pilot work was subsequently validated and extended as part of Delabouglise et al. work (cf. Chaps. 6 and 11; Delabouglise reference papers).

8.6 Case Study 2: Evaluation of the Acceptability of Classical Swine Fever Surveillance System in Germany

The AccEPT method was used for the evaluation of the classical swine fever (CSF) surveillance system in Germany, where analysis of the monitoring process by the OASISTrop tool had revealed significant limitations in acceptability of the system by its actors [22]. In an attempt to enhance the system's sensitivity and representativeness, four new monitoring components were designed and compared to the current surveillance strategy. Only the passive component in place and one alternative component (selection of samples based on the age of the animals) have proved to be acceptable to the hunters, actors at the source of the data of the system (Fig. 8.6). This study highlighted the importance of considering this attribute in the selection of surveillance strategies adapted to the actors to ensure its implementation in the field and improvement of the system.

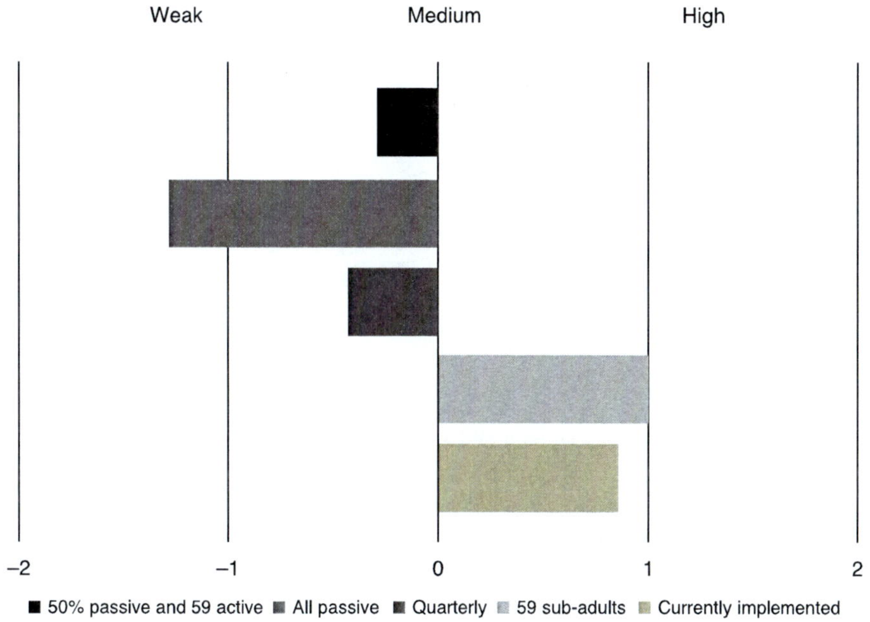

Fig. 8.6 Level of acceptability of different PPPC surveillance strategies in Germany. (From 22]

8.7 Case Study 3: Evaluation of the Acceptability of a Pilot Multistakeholder Wildlife Health Surveillance Network in Cambodia

The AccEPT method was used for the evaluation of the pilot wildlife health surveillance network in Cambodia, established by WCS under the EU-funded LACANET project. The general objective was to understand the level of stakeholders' willingness to cooperate and to keep their support to the surveillance system. For the total scoring, it can be seen that the participants were satisfied with the system objective, system operation, their own role with the system, relations between stakeholders, and had trust with the system (Table 8.2).

However, if we look in detail at the scores between the different stakeholders we can identify some different levels of satisfaction among them:

- Collaboration between the two wildlife rescue centers was highlighted as important and needed, but mechanisms of efficient dialogue between them still need to be established.
- Provincial animal health agents do not know much about the pilot WHSS and are still reluctant to engage with wildlife health problems in some sites.

Table 8.2 Scoring level of every components measured within the AccEPT method for the pilot wildlife surveillance network in Cambodia, evaluation conducted between mid-April to mid-May 2019 [23]

Row labels	Average of acceptability of the objective	Average of acceptability of the operation	Average of satisfaction of own role	Average of consequence of the information flow/Impact	Average of satisfaction of the relations	Averaged trust devoted in the system
Field Actor	0.91	1	1	0.09	1	1
Field Management	1.00	1	1	1.00	1	1
Laboratory	0.50	1	1	1.00	1	1
Grand Total	0.86	1	1	0.14	1	1

- Local authorities are recognized as key partners for wildlife health surveillance. However, field agents in most sites have issue to establish sustainable and efficient collaboration with local authorities because of the lack of direct benefit for them (no clear reward or compensations identified).

References

1. OIE. Code sanitaire pour les animaux terrestres; 2015 [En ligne]. http://www.oie.int/fr/normes-internationales/code-terrestre/acces-en-ligne/, consulté le 18/09/2018.
2. Dufour B, Hendrikx P. Surveillance épidémiologique en santé animale, Ed Quae, Montpellier, 341 pp; 2011.
3. Calba C. Étude des apports de l'épidémiologie participative à l'évaluation des systèmes de surveillance en santé animale, Manuscrit de thèse, Université de Liège, 217 pp; 2015.
4. Drewe J, Hoinville L, Cook A, Floyd T, Gunn G, Stärk K. SERVAL: a new framework for the evaluation of animal health surveillance. Transbound Emerg Dis. 2015;62:33–45.
5. Hendrikx P, Gay E, Chazel M, Moutou F, Danan C, Richomme C, Boue F, Souillard R, Gauchard F, Dufour B. OASIS: an assessment tool of epidemiological surveillance systems in animal health and food safety. Epidemiol Infect. 2011;139(10):1486–96.
6. Calba C, Antoine-Moussiaux N, Charrier F, Hendrikx P, Saegerman C, Peyre M, Goutard FL. Applying participatory approaches in the evaluation of surveillance systems: a pilot study on African swine fever surveillance in Corsica. Prev Vet Med. 2015a;122(4):389–98.
7. Calba C, Goutard FL, Hoinville L, Hendrikx P, Lindberg A, Saegerman C, Peyre M. Surveillance systems evaluation: a systematic review of the existing approaches. BMC Pub Health. 2015b;15(1):448.
8. Reist M, Jemmi T, Stärk KDC. Policy-driven development of cost-effective, risk-based surveillance strategies. Prev Vet Med. 2012;105(3):176–84.
9. Zepeda C, Salman M, Ruppanner R. International trade, animal health and veterinary epidemiology: challenges and opportunities. Prev Vet Med. 2001;48(4):261–71.
10. Delabouglise A, Antoine-Moussiaux N, Tatong D, Chumkaeo A, Binot A, Fournié G, Pilot E, Phimpraphi W, Kasemsuwan S, Paul MC, Duboz R, Salem G, Peyre M. Cultural practices shaping zoonotic diseases surveillance: the case of highly pathogenic avian influenza and thailand native chicken farmers. Transbound Emerg Dis. 2017;64:1294–305. https://doi.org/10.1111/tbed.12506.
11. Figuié M, Peyre M-I, Binot A. Surveillance of infectious animal diseases in Southeast Asia. Promoting the multiplicity of information networks. Perspect. - Cirad 2013;1–4. https://doi.org/10.19182/agritrop/00040.

12. Goutard FL, Binot A, Duboz R, Rasamoelina-Andriamanivo H, Pedrono M, Holl D, Peyre MI, Cappelle J, Chevalier V, Figuié M, Molia S, Roger FL. How to reach the poor? Surveillance in low-income countries, lessons from experiences in cambodia and madagascar. Prev Vet Med. 2015;120:12–26. https://doi.org/10.1016/j.prevetmed.2015.02.014.
13. Delabouglise A, Dao TH, Truong DB, Nguyen TT, Nguyen NTX, Duboz R, Fournié G, Antoine-Moussiaux N, Grosbois V, Vu DT, Le TH, Nguyen VK, Salem G, Peyre M. When private actors matter: information-sharing network and surveillance of highly pathogenic avian influenza in vietnam. Acta Trop. 2015;147:38–44. https://doi.org/10.1016/j.actatropica.2015.03.025.
14. Calba C, Goutard FL, Vanholme L, Antoine-Moussiaux N, Hendrikx P, Saegerman C. The added-value of using participatory approaches to assess the acceptability of surveillance systems: the case of bovine tuberculosis in Belgium. PLoS One. 2016;11(7)
15. Peyre M, Hoinville L, Haesler B, Lindberg A, Bisdorff B, Dorea F, Wahlström H, Frössling J, Calba C, Grosbois V, Goutard F. Network analysis of surveillance system evaluation attributes: a way towards improvement of the evaluation process. 2nd International Conference on Animal Health Surveillance (ICAHS), La havane, Cuba; 2014.
16. Chambers R. The origins and practice of participatory rural appraisal. World Dev. 1994;22(7):953–69.
17. Mariner JC, Paskin R. Manual on participatory epidemiology: methods for the collection of action-oriented epidemiological intelligence. Rome: Food and Agriculture Organization of the United Nations; 2000, 81 pages. http://www.fao.org/docrep/003/x8833e/x8833e00.HTM
18. Mariner JC, House JA, Mebus CA, Sollod AE, Chibeu D, Jones BA, Roeder PL, Admassu B, van 't Klooster GG. Rinderpest eradication: appropriate technology and social innovations. Science. 2012;337(6100):1309–12.
19. Bellet C, Humblet M, Swanenburg M, Dhé J, Vandeputte S, Thébault A, Gauchard F, Hendrikx P, Vos CD, Koeijer AD, Saegerman C, Sanaa M. Specification of data collection on animal diseases to increase the preparedness of the AHAW panel to answer future mandates. 2012.
20. Mariner JC, Hendrickx S, Pfeiffer DU, Costard S, Knopf L. Integration of participatory approaches. 2011;30:653–9.
21. Vergne T, Grosbois V, Durand B, Goutard F, Bellet C, Holl D, Roger F, Dufour B. A capturere-capture analysis in a challenging environment: assessing the epidemiological situation of foot-and-mouth disease in Cambodia. Prev Vet Med. 2012;105:235–43. https://doi.org/10.1016/j.prevetmed.2011.12.008.
22. Schulz K, Calba C, Peyre M, Staubach C, Conraths FJ. Hunters' acceptability of the surveillance system and alternative surveillance strategies for classical swine fever in wild boar - a participatory approach. BMC Vet Res. 2016;12:187. https://doi.org/10.1186/s12917-016-0822-5.
23. Chea S. Assessing the acceptability of a pilot multi-stakeholders wildlife health surveillance network in Cambodia. Master's thesis, InterRisk program, Kasetsart University, Thailand, and Toulouse University, France; 2019.
24. Scriven M. New frontiers in evaluation. Eval Pract. 1986;7(1):7–44.
25. Taut S, Brauns D. Resistance to evaluation, a psychological perspective. Evaluation. 2003;9(3):247–64.
26. Bryson JM, Patton MQ, Bowman RA. Working with evaluation stakeholders: a rationale, step-wise approach and toolkit. Eval Program Plann. 2011;34(1):1–12.
27. Calba C, Peyre M, Roger F, Antoine-Moussiaux N, Hendrikx P, Saegerman C, Goutard F. Approches participatives et estimation de l'acceptabilité des systèmes de surveillance : la méthode AccePT. Epidémiologie et Santé Animale. 2018;73:49–58.
28. Hoinville L, Alban L, Drewe J, Gibbens J, Gustafson L, Häsler B, Saegerman C, Salman M, Stärk K. Proposed terms and concepts for describing and evaluating animal-health surveillance systems. Prev Vet Med. 2013;112(1):1–12.
29. German RR, Lee L, Horan J, Milstein R, Pertowski C, Waller M. Updated guidelines for evaluating public health surveillance systems. MMWR Recomm Rep. 2001;50:1–35.
30. Vu MQG. Evaluation de la sensibilité du système de surveillance de l'IAHP au Vietnam : application des méthodes de capture-recapture et des approches participatives (Master 2 report). Université Paris Est Créteil, Val de Marnes. 2012.

Evaluation of Collaboration in a Multisectoral Surveillance System: The ECoSur Tool

9

Marion Bordier, Camille Delavenne, Dung Thuy Thi Nguyen, Flavie Goutard, and Pascal Hendrikx

Abstract

In line with the One Health concept, international organizations and the scientific community are strongly supporting the implementation of multisectoral surveillance systems in an attempt to improve the management of health hazards at the human–animal–environment interface. Such surveillance systems call for the

The content of the chapter relates to the thesis of Marion Bordier Bouchot [1].

M. Bordier (✉)
Centre de Coopération Internationale en Recherche Agronomique Pour le Développement (CIRAD), UMR ASTRE, Hanoi, Viet Nam

ASTRE, University of Montpellier, CIRAD, INRAE, Montpellier, France

National Institute of Veterinary Research (NIVR), Hanoi, Viet Nam
e-mail: Marion.bordier@cirad.fr

C. Delavenne
Centre de Coopération Internationale en Recherche Agronomique Pour le Développement (CIRAD), UMR ASTRE, Hanoi, Viet Nam

National Institute of Veterinary Research (NIVR), Hanoi, Viet Nam

D. T. T. Nguyen
CIRAD, UMR ASTRE, Bangkok, Thailand

Kasetsart University, Faculty of Veterinary Medicine, Bangkok, Thailand

F. Goutard
ASTRE, University of Montpellier, CIRAD, INRAE, Montpellier, France

CIRAD, UMR ASTRE, Bangkok, Thailand

Kasetsart University, Faculty of Veterinary Medicine, Bangkok, Thailand

P. Hendrikx
ASTRE, University of Montpellier, CIRAD, INRAE, Montpellier, France

France Vétérinaire International, Montpellier, France

M. Peyre et al. (eds.), *Principles for Evaluation of One Health Surveillance: The EVA Book*, https://doi.org/10.1007/978-3-030-82727-4_9

establishment of collaboration across sectors and disciplines that must be evaluated to ensure they are appropriate and functional to produce the expected results. In this context, we have developed a tool, ECoSur (Evaluation of Collaboration for surveillance), to evaluate the organization, functioning, and functionalities of collaboration taking place in a multisectoral surveillance system. ECoSur relies on 22 attributes characterizing the organization of collaboration at the governance and operation level and nine attributes referring to core functions of collaboration to ensure the sustainable operation of an effective multisectoral surveillance system. Along with these attributes, three indexes allow for the characterization of the organization of collaboration at a macro level according to three processes: management, support, and operation. Attributes are evaluated based on the scoring of criteria that contribute to their definition. Once scores are captured in a spreadsheet, evaluation results are automatically generated. Their interpretation supports the identification of strengths and weaknesses of collaboration and the formulation of recommendations for its amelioration.

Keywords

Collaboration · Evaluation · Multisectoral · One Health · Surveillance

Most of the health hazards are complex and need to be addressed with a holistic approach to better apprehend them [2]. When it comes to surveillance, many multisectoral surveillance systems are being developed under the One Health paradigm, with the strong support of governments and the scientific community [3]. To create relevant multisectoral surveillance systems, collaboration needs to be established or strengthened across relevant sectors, professions, disciplines, and decision-making scales. However, there is no single organizational model for multisectoral surveillance system and collaboration must be consistent with the collaborative context and objective(s) to be effective and sustainable [4]. Furthermore, there is no clear evidence that performance and cost-effectiveness of surveillance is directly proportional to the level of integration achieved in a multisectoral surveillance system [5]. Finally, collaboration is time and resource consuming, and needs to be properly designed and organized to ensure stakeholders' commitment in the long term [6]. In this context, the ECoSur tool (Evaluation of Collaboration for Surveillance) allows for the evaluation of the quality and appropriateness of multisectoral collaboration through an in-depth analysis of its organization and functions. The final purpose is to assess if collaboration as planned and implemented is relevant and functional to produce the expected collaborative outputs and to identify its strengths and weaknesses to formulate recommendations for its improvement.

By collaboration we mean interactions between actors operating in different surveillance components and that have been established to improve the surveillance value, mainly in terms of performance and cost-effectiveness, in such a way that the outputs of the surveillance would not be possible without collaboration.

ECoSur can be used independently if there is a need to focus on collaboration only or combined with existing evaluation tools for an overall assessment of the multisectoral surveillance system.

What ECoSur is not doing:

- This tool does not consider collaboration between actors operating in the same surveillance component.
- This tool does not evaluate the overall performance of the multisectoral surveillance system itself; however, the evaluation of certain collaborative attributes uses data on sectoral surveillance components.
- At this stage of development, this tool does not evaluate the impacts and cost of collaboration and so it does not intend to measure the relation between the quality of collaboration and the effectiveness of the multisectoral surveillance system.
- The tool is not intended to measure the extent of integration achieved in the multisectoral surveillance system. The aim is to characterize the integration that the multisectoral surveillance system seeks to achieve, to assess if this integration level is coherent with the collaborative context and objective(s), and whether the collaborative activities implemented to achieve the intended integration generate the expected outputs.

9.1 The Conceptual Approach Behind the Development of the Tool

The basic principle behind the development of this tool is that, for multisectoral surveillance systems to be functional and sustainable, collaboration must be planned and organized at three levels:

- The policy level, where the collaborative strategy is stated.
- The strategy describes the desired goals of developing collaboration for surveillance and the course of actions to achieve those goals. It also covers the desired multisectoral organizational model and the areas of action of the main stakeholders within this organization. The strategy may be described in various documents depending on the legal tradition of the country, and on who developed it (government, academia, professional organizations, etc.). These can be policies, strategies, memorandums, laws, etc. Such documents are developed at a high political level when it comes to official surveillance. The collaborative strategy for surveillance can be described in a stand-alone document or in an overarching document (control program for a specific health issue, national One Health strategy, etc.).

- The institutional level, where relevant collaborative modalities for the governance and implementation of surveillance activities are defined to achieve the desired goal of the strategy.
- The collaborative modalities for the governance are described in terms of steering and coordinating mechanisms as well as of scientific and technical support. The collaborative modalities for the operation are usually expressed in terms of area of collaboration (i.e., the steps of the surveillance process where collaboration is implemented) and degree of integration (i.e., the strength of collaboration for each area of collaboration). (See Table 9.1 for the possible collaborative

Table 9.1 Possible collaborative modalities for the implementation of surveillance activities

Area of collaboration during the surveillance process	Different degrees of integration				
Surveillance protocol design	Undertaken by a single sector for all surveillance components	Undertaken separately in each sector and then cross-sectoral consultation to seek for synergies	Cross-sectoral consultation and then undertaken in each sector	Undertaken jointly by the different sectors	Undertaken by a multisectoral body for all components
Data collection (sampling, laboratory testing)	Undertaken by a single sector for all components	Harmonization across sectors but undertaken separately	Joint activities across sectors	Undertaken by a multisectoral body for all components	
Data storage and management	Undertaken by a single sector for all components	Harmonization across sectors but undertaken separately	Joint activities across sectors	Undertaken by a multisectoral body for all components	
Data sharing	Exchange[a] of raw data (partial or complete) for unusual events only	Exchange[a] of all raw data (partial or complete) at a low frequency	Ongoing exchange[a] of all data (partial or complete)		
Data analysis and interpretation	Undertaken separately (with or without cross-sectoral harmonization) and then compared by a single sector	Jointly undertaken by a single sector for all components	Undertaken separately (with or without cross-sectoral harmonization) and then compared by the different sectors	Undertaken jointly by the different sectors	Undertaken by a multisectoral body for all components

Table 9.1 (continued)

Area of collaboration during the surveillance process	Different degrees of integration				
Results sharing	Exchange[a] of results (partial or complete) for unusual events only	Exchange[a] of all results (partial or complete) at a low frequency	Ongoing exchange[a] of all results (partial or complete)		
Dissemination to decision-makers	Joint dissemination in separate sectoral activities	Undertaken by a single sector for all components	Undertaken jointly by the different sectors	Undertaken by a multisectoral body for all components	
Communication to surveillance actors and end-users	Joint communication in separate sectoral activities	Undertaken by a single sector for all components	Undertaken jointly by the different sectors	Undertaken by a multisectoral body for all components	

Note: (i) Areas of collaboration do not always occur in this order depending on the collaborative modalities. For instance, if information is shared among sectors on an annual basis, it is more likely that data analysis and interpretation have been undertaken earlier within each sector, before sharing. (ii) We are only referring to the collaborative dimension related to sector; nevertheless, other dimensions can be present in these modalities

[a]One-way or two-way exchange

modalities in a multisectoral surveillance system.) The modalities are usually described in implementing texts, such as regulations, agreements, or charters.

- The operational level where surveillance activities are implemented to ensure the routine operation of the collaborative modalities.
- These activities are conducted at the ground level by surveillance actors to make the collaboration happen. They are usually supported by operational procedures.

Figure 9.1 describes the three levels of collaboration.

The three levels of collaboration must be clearly formalized and endorsed by stakeholders and be relevant to each other. Collaboration for surveillance is generated by stakeholders' expectations regarding the multisectoral surveillance system and is under the influence of a broad range of contextual elements, such as socioeconomic and epidemiological factors, international guidance, and sectoral surveillance capacities. Collaborative activities throughout the surveillance process lead to the production of outputs (harmonization of methods, comparison of data, on-time results sharing, etc.) that must meet the collaboration's objective and purpose.

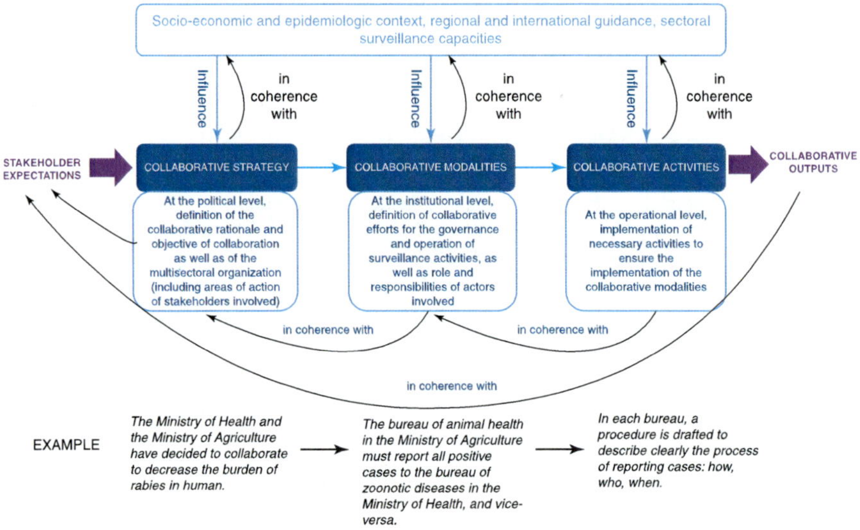

Fig. 9.1 Conceptual framework for the organization and functioning of collaboration in a multisectoral surveillance system. (Adapted from [7])

9.2 The Evaluation Process Used in ECoSur

To evaluate collaboration in a multisectoral surveillance system, attributes and indexes were defined as below:

- A list of 22 organizational attributes that aims at evaluating core characteristics for the organization of collaboration for the governance and implementation of surveillance activities.
- A list of nine functional attributes that aims at evaluating core functions of collaboration for an effective and sustainable multisectoral surveillance system.
- A list of three organizational indexes that aims at evaluating organization of collaboration at a macro level.

The structure of the evaluation process is summarized in Fig. 9.2.

The level of satisfaction of these attributes and indexes is then measured using 74 evaluation criteria, which are scored following a four-tiered scoring grid. The same criterion can be used to evaluate several functional attributes. On the contrary, each organizational attribute and index is evaluated with a set of specific criteria without any overlap.

The list and definitions of attributes and indexes, as well as criteria that support their evaluation, are available in the second sheet of the evaluation matrix (see below).

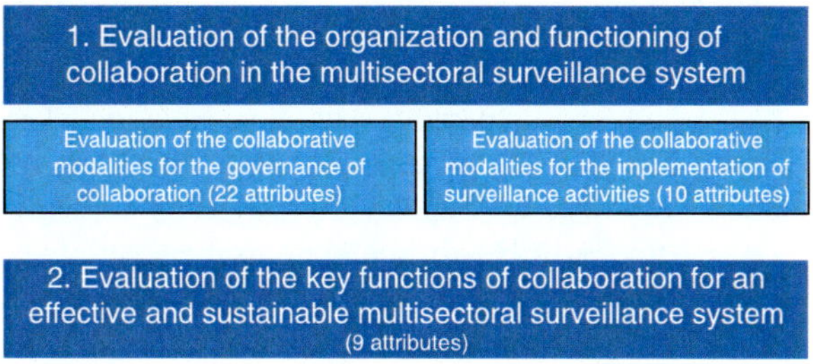

Fig. 9.2 Structure of the evaluation process

9.3 The Structure of ECoSur

ECoSur is composed of four elements.

- A spreadsheet file, referred to as "Data collection file," allows for the collection of preliminary information on all the different surveillance actors and components of the multisectoral surveillance system being evaluated. It includes two sheets, one specific to the surveillance components and one to actors.
- A text file, referred to as "Data collection form," allows a synthesis of all data describing precisely the governance and operation of collaboration in the multisectoral surveillance system that will be used to score the evaluation attributes. This form is divided into three sections: contextualization, governance, and operation of collaboration.
- A spreadsheet, referred to as "Evaluation matrix," consisting of four distinct sheets:
  - The first sheet ("Criteria Scoring") contains the scoring grid for the 74 evaluation criteria. Four grades are defined: Grade 3 indicates that the situation complies fully with the criterion while Grade 0 indicates a total absence of compliance. Grades 2 and 1 are intermediate grades depending on the level of compliance. In some cases, the value "Non-relevant" can be used if the criterion is not relevant to the multisectoral surveillance system under evaluation. A scoring guide was developed to describe the situation in which grades should be awarded.
  - The second sheet ("Attributes Indexes") displays the list of attributes and indexes as well as the criteria contributing to their evaluation.
  - Once the scoring is completed in the first sheet, the third sheet ("Evaluation Results") automatically produces three graphical representations of the evaluation results. Different chart types help to differentiate easily the three levels of evaluation obtained: organization at a micro level, organization at a macro level, and functions.

    The first display represents the evaluation results for the 22 organizational attributes (12 governance and 10 operational attributes). The result for each attribute can be visualized in a pie chart. Each colored area within a pie chart represents the attribute's level of compliance regarding a nominal situation where all evaluation criteria score 3.

The second display represents the evaluation results of the indexes. Results of the three indexes are expressed as percentages of compliance of the situation as compared to a nominal situation where all criteria score 3.

The last display represents the evaluation results of the nine functional attributes on a spider chart. Results are expressed on a five-tiered scale, from A to E corresponding to the level of satisfaction for each core collaborative function. Grade A corresponds to a level ranging from 76 to 100%, meaning that almost all criteria supporting the evaluation of the attribute scored 3, while grade E corresponds to 0%, meaning that they all scored 0. Grades B, C, and D are intermediate levels of satisfaction, representing ranges of 51–75, 26–50, and 1–25%, respectively.

- The fourth sheet ("Calculation") contains all the formula to obtain the scoring of attributes and indexes and displays the numerical results of evaluation for each of them. The same formula is used for all calculation: the sum of the grade awarded to the criteria contributing to their definition, divided by the sum of the highest score obtained by these criteria when the ideal situation is met (i.e., all criteria scored 3).

The development of the matrix is detailed in [7].

All documents related to the tools are free access at: https://survtools.org/wiki/surveillance-evaluation/doku.php?id=quality_of_the_collaboration.

A summary of the structure of the tool is presented in Fig. 9.3.

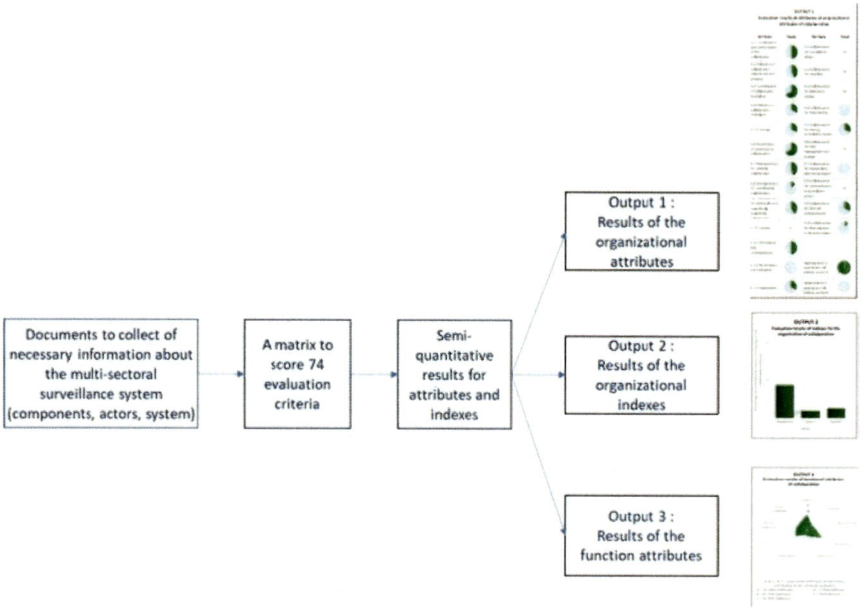

Fig. 9.3 Summary of the structure of ECoSur

9.4 The Application of ECoSur

ECoSur is meant to be applied by an evaluation team. It is recommended that the team members are not involved in the governance of the multisectoral surveillance system, meaning that they are not in charge of steering or coordinating sectoral or collaborative surveillance activities. Team members should be epidemiologists with at least one experimented in surveillance. At least one team member should be familiar with ECoSur while all others should follow a quick training prior the evaluation exercise.

Along with the evaluation team, one or two stakeholders of the multisectoral surveillance system should be identified and involved in the whole evaluation process. This will favor the acceptability of the evaluation process.

9.4.1 First Step: Defining the Evaluation Question and the Evaluation Boundaries

The aim of ECoSur is to answer the overall question: Is collaboration appropriate to produce the expected results in the given context?

However, the rationale and objective for conducting the evaluation might differ from a situation to another and should be clearly defined with stakeholders requiring the evaluation to adjust the evaluation process as well as the report's format and contents.

Depending on the context, the boundaries of the surveillance system may be blurred, and the surveillance efforts might be spread across several components, operating independently or with very few connections. Additionally, some programs continuously collecting data about the hazard under surveillance may exist without being considered a surveillance component (e.g., monitoring programs). Consequently, it is highly important that the evaluation team defines the boundaries of the system under evaluation and the type of collection programs that will be included, and then adheres to this definition throughout the evaluation process.

Finally, in very complex systems with more than 20 components, some components may be more connected than others, creating subsystems within the whole system. For certain attributes, it may be necessary to evaluate the entire system and then each subsystem independently. If this methodological approach is adopted, the evaluation team will have to set a clear scoring protocol to ensure consistency.

Before launching the evaluation process, it is recommended to organize a meeting with the evaluation team and selected stakeholders to present the evaluation exercise and to agree on the evaluation objective and expected outputs. Stakeholders here consist of people initiating the evaluation and people involved in the sectoral and multisectoral governance mechanisms.

9.4.2 Second Step: Collecting Data

A preliminary desktop study should be done to collect all necessary data to complete the data collection file as much as possible, both the actors and components sheets, and the data collection form. This study can be completed with interviews of informants identified as having an extensive knowledge about the surveillance system.

In the data collection file, notes at the top of each column provide guidance about the type of information expected. In the actors' sheet, only information related to activities of the actor within the surveillance system under evaluation must be captured. Be aware that some of the major actors of a multisectoral surveillance system may have no role in any given component within that system. For instance, some governance bodies may have been specifically established for steering or coordinating collaboration and may include actors who are not otherwise involved in any specific surveillance component. Some information may appear redundant between the actors and the components sheet, especially when it comes to the characterization of collaboration. However, filling information in those two sheets is helpful for the further scoring of the criteria.

Some sections of the collection form do not collect additional information compared with the one in the data collection file, but they provide the opportunity to summarize specific information necessary for the scoring of certain criteria, which will ease the scoring process.

It is recommended to start filling out the data collection file before the data collection form. However, the data collection step is not linear and a back-and-forth process between the tables and the form will most realistically occur.

Once all the information available is captured in both the form and the file, a list of missing or unreliable information should be drawn up. Interviews with informants must be conducted to clarify and collect additional information. All the surveillance component coordinators should be interviewed. Additional informants to be interviewed depend on the multisectoral surveillance system under evaluation (including the rationale behind its establishment), the evaluation context (time and resources allocated, evaluation objective), and the sought information. For instance, if the surveillance component relies on effective intermediate units, a representative sample of those should be interviewed (with regards to activity volume, local context, etc.). For passive surveillance components, actors in charge of reporting positive cases (laboratories, medical practitioners, farmers, etc.) should be also interviewed and their representativeness ensured.

The time required to complete this step is dependent on the evaluation team's knowledge about the system, the availability and reliability of data in the literature, the number of surveillance components comprising the system, and the number of required interviews. It may take one or two weeks (full time) on average.

Tip:

- It is highly recommended to harmonize information captured in the different columns of the data collection file, so filters can be applied and information easily extracted for filling the data collection form.
- It can be useful to map the system simultaneously as the information is retrieved to get a graphical representation of the interactions among actors and collaboration across components.

9.4.3 Third Step: Scoring the Criteria of the Organizational and Function Attributes

To score the criteria, the evaluation team uses the first sheet of the evaluation matrix. For each criterion, evaluators analyze the information available in the data collection file and form and choose the most appropriate grade. To help evaluators in this process, the column "scoring guidance" indicates which information is useful to score the criterion. The grade is chosen in a concerted manner among the evaluation team and then entered in the cell of the spreadsheet named "grade." The justification for selecting this grade is detailed in the adjacent cell. This justification is ultimately much more important than the grade itself and should be filled in carefully. It will then support the drafting of the report.

If the data collection form and file have been appropriately filled, the scoring process can be completed within the relatively short time of 2 days. However, if the surveillance is complex with many components involved, it can take more time as evaluation might be conducted both at the system and at the subsystems levels.

Tip:

- It is advised that, where not all required elements for a grade are met, the grade below should be given in order that improvements be clearly noticeable in the future.
- There are 74 criteria to be scored in total. Each criterion is very specific in addressing a characteristic of collaboration at one of the different collaborative levels, namely collaborative strategy, modalities, and activities. Evaluators should go through all the criteria once before starting the scoring to get an overview of the full process. This may help prevent them from evaluating at the wrong stage a characteristic that is addressed in a later criterion.
- Some criteria address the collaboration only while others evaluate the multisectoral surveillance system as a whole (sectoral surveillance and collaborative efforts). Evaluators should clearly identify the evaluation level each criterion is considering when scoring.

9.4.4 Fourth Step: Interpreting Evaluation Results

Once the scoring is done, the spreadsheet will automatically produce three graphical outputs on the third sheet, which correspond to the evaluation results of the organizational attributes and indexes, and functional attributes.

- Output 1 provides the individual results of the 12 organizational attributes in independent pie charts. It allows the easy identification of the weak parts of the collaborative organization. Evaluators can refer to the second sheet of the matrix to track back the criteria that contribute to the scoring of each attribute. It helps to better understand the reasoning behind the scoring and to determine how the different criteria impact the attribute's grade.
- Output 2 displays the results of the organizational indexes in a single histogram. This graphical representation illustrates the level of satisfaction regarding the collaborative effort's organization at a macro level, from the management, support, and operational points of view. The use of the histogram allows for the visualization of these three highly aggregated evaluation results at a glance and enables an easy comparison.
- Output 3 shows the efficacy of the collaborative effort within the multisectoral surveillance system. It facilitates the analysis of the balance between the different collaborative functions. It can help to identify the specific collaborative functions that need to be strengthened to make the system more effective.

These outputs need to be analyzed and interpreted according to the justification of the scoring. They should support the identification of the strengths and weaknesses of collaboration and provide the foundation for drafting of recommendations for its improvement, if deemed necessary.

9.4.5 Fifth Step: Organizing a Workshop to Validate the Evaluation Results

Once the scoring has been completed and evaluation results interpreted by the evaluation team, a workshop must be organized with key actors of the multisectoral surveillance system under evaluation. Key actors might be coordinators of the surveillance components or informants who were interviewed during the data collection step. The number of participants should not exceed 10 people to ease facilitation of discussion. The aim of this workshop is to discuss, revise if necessary, and validate the scores, as well as the justification provided. On this basis, recommendations can be refined. To review all the criteria, the workshop will need to take one day, or one-and-a-half days if the system is large.

9.4.6 Sixth Step: Drafting the Report

All evaluation results and recommendations should be released in a report drafted by the evaluation team. Evaluation results should always be communicated with relevant explanation and contextualization.

References

1. Bordier M. Comment mettre en œuvre le concept « One Health » pour améliorer la surveillance des dangers sanitaires à l'interface homme-animal-environnement ?. Médecine humaine et pathologie. Université Paris-Est. Français NNT: 2019PESC0101. tel-028900399; 2019.
2. Jeggo M, Mackenzie JS. Defining the future of one health. Microbiol. Spectrum. 2012;2(1):OH-0007-2012. https://doi.org/10.1128/microbiolspec.OH-0007-2012.
3. Destoumieux-Garzón D, Mavingui P, Boetsch G, Boissier J, Darriet F, Duboz P, Fritsch C, Giraudoux P, Le Roux F, Morand S, Paillard C, Pontier D, Sueur C, Voituron Y. The one health concept: 10 years old and a long road ahead. Front Veter Sci. 2018;5 https://doi.org/10.3389/fvets.2018.00014.
4. Bordier M, Uea-Anuwong T, Binot A, Hendrikx P, Goutard FL. Characteristics of one health surveillance systems: a systematic literature review. Prev Vet Med. 2018b; https://doi.org/10.1016/j.prevetmed.2018.10.005.
5. Aenishaenslin C, Häsler B, Ravel A, Parmley J, Stärk K, Buckeridge D. Evidence needed for antimicrobial resistance surveillance systems. Bull World Health Organ. 2019;97:283–9. https://doi.org/10.2471/BLT.18.218917.
6. Bordier M, Binot A, Pauchard Q, Nguyen DT, Trung TN, Fortané N, Goutard FL. Antibiotic resistance in Vietnam: moving towards a one health surveillance system. BMC Public Health. 2018a;18 https://doi.org/10.1186/s12889-018-6022-4.
7. Bordier M, Delavenne C, Nguyen DTT, Goutard FL, Hendrikx P. One health surveillance: a matrix to evaluate multisectoral collaboration. Front Veter Sci. 2019;6:109. https://doi.org/10.3389/fvets.2019.00109.

Part V

Statistical and Modeling Approaches to Evaluate and Inform Surveillance Design

10 Quantitative Methods to Evaluate Health Surveillance Effectiveness

Vladimir Grosbois, Guillaume Fournié, Raphaël Duboz, Timothée Vergne, Marisa Peyre, and Flavie Goutard

Abstract

Decisions regarding the implementation of prevention and intervention measures rely on the assessment through the analysis and interpretation of surveillance data of the epidemiological status of target populations or of focal units in target populations. Because they are generated through imperfect reporting, diagnosing, sampling and testing processes, surveillance data are most of the time non-exhaustive, partially distorted and, sometimes, non-representative. Therefore, even when perfectly tailored response mechanisms are planned, ineffective sur-

V. Grosbois
UMR "ASTRE",CIRAD-INRAE-University of Montpellier, Montpellier, France
e-mail: Vladimir.grosbois@cirad.fr

G. Fournié (✉)
Veterinary Epidemiology, Economics and Public Health Group, Pathobiology and Population Sciences Department, Royal Veterinary College, Hawkshead Lane, Hatfield, UK
e-mail: gfournie@rvc.ac.uk

R. Duboz
UMR "ASTRE",CIRAD-INRAE-University of Montpellier, Montpellier, France

UMI "UMMISCO", Sorbonne Université, IRD, Bondy, France

T. Vergne
UMR "Host—pathogen interactions" ENVT-INRAE, National Veterinary School of Toulouse, Toulouse, France

M. Peyre
CIRAD, UMR ASTRE, Montpellier, France

ASTRE, CIRAD, INRAE, University of Montpellier, Montpellier, France

F. Goutard
UMR "ASTRE",CIRAD-INRAE-University of Montpellier, Montpellier, France

Faculty of Veterinary Medicine, Kasetsart University, Bangkok, Thailand

M. Peyre et al. (eds.), *Principles for Evaluation of One Health Surveillance: The EVA Book*, https://doi.org/10.1007/978-3-030-82727-4_10

veillance can result in misjudging an epidemiological situation and adopting inappropriate intervention measures. There is thus a widely recognized need for effective animal health surveillance. In this chapter, we focus on the quantitative methods to evaluate the effectiveness of actual or potential surveillance programs, and their applications. We first introduce the different attributes that reflect surveillance effectiveness. We then briefly describe the methods available to assess these attributes by covering methods that rely on the statistical modelling of the data generated by surveillance programmes (data-based methods) as well as on methods that imply the formalization of the surveillance process through probabilistic, mathematical or simulation models (process-based methods). We finally discuss the relevance of these methods with regard to the type of evaluation (*ex-ante*, *in-itinere*, *ex-post*), the evaluation question (effectiveness evaluation, effectiveness optimization) and the objective of the surveillance programme (early detection, case detection, freedom from disease, prevalence monitoring).

Keywords
Quantitative evaluation · Health surveillance · Effectiveness · Modelling · Surveillance systems

10.1 Introduction

To fight against animal diseases, resources must be allocated to surveillance, prevention and intervention efforts that could otherwise be used for alternative purposes [1, 2]. While the need for effective animal health surveillance is widely recognized for the management of animal health threats, investment is being constrained due to financial budget restrictions. Therefore, there is strong demand for frameworks that allow assessing the economic value of surveillance programmes that inform decision about investments for surveillance. Surveillance has been defined as the systematic measurement, collection, collation, analysis, interpretation, and timely dissemination of animal-health and welfare data from defined populations essential for describing health-hazard occurrence and to contribute to the planning, implementation, and evaluation of risk-mitigation actions [3]. In other words, surveillance provides information for decisions regarding the implementation of interventions. Together surveillance and intervention achieve loss avoidance through the process of making the effects of disease less severe by avoiding, containing, reducing or removing it—the outcome decision-makers are ultimately interested in [1].

Decisions regarding the implementation of prevention and intervention measures rely on the assessment through the analysis and interpretation of surveillance data of the epidemiological status of target populations or of focal units in target populations [1, 2]. Because they are generated through imperfect reporting, diagnosing, sampling and testing processes, surveillance data are most of the time non-exhaustive, partially distorted and also sometimes non-representative. As a consequence, even when perfectly tailored response mechanisms are planned, ineffective surveillance can result in misjudging an epidemiological situation and adopting inappropriate intervention measures. There is thus a widely recognized need for effective animal health surveillance and thus for methods and tools to evaluate the effectiveness of animal health surveillance. In this chapter, we introduce the different methodological approaches to quantitatively assess surveillance effectiveness and identify modifications in surveillance systems and strategies that can lead to effectiveness improvements. We start by presenting the surveillance system attributes that are relevant with regard to effectiveness. Then we focus on approaches to assess effectiveness that rely on the analysis of the data produced by surveillance systems (data-based approaches). Finally, we cover approaches that use modelling of surveillance processes to assess effectiveness. Following this overview, the Chap. 11 will focus on a specific innovative approach to quantitatively assess effectiveness of animal health surveillance: network modelling.

10.2 Surveillance Effectiveness

In broad terms, effectiveness can be understood as the ability of surveillance systems and strategies to reach their objectives. Because different systems can have differing objectives, the attribute best reflecting effectiveness will depend to a large extent on the objective of surveillance (see Part II). Four broad categories of surveillance objectives are usually distinguished: (1) demonstrating that a population is free from a disease; (2) detecting the circulation in a population of an exotic, emerging or re-emerging disease; (3) identifying the cases of a disease in a population; and (4) assessing the prevalence and the distribution of a disease in a population where that disease is endemic:

1. For systems aiming at demonstrating freedom from disease, effectiveness is the ability of the system to detect the disease in the focal population even when it circulates at a very low intensity. The most relevant attribute is then system-level sensitivity, which is the probability of detecting at least one case of the disease when the disease is actually present in the focal population at a (usually very low) prevalence level defined in the surveillance strategy and referred to as the "design prevalence".
2. For systems aiming at detecting the circulation in a population of an exotic, emerging or re-emerging disease following the introduction of that disease in the population, effectiveness is the ability of the system to detect as soon as possible the disease or the pathogen responsible for the disease following its introduction in the focal population. The related attribute is referred to as timeliness, which is the length of the time period between the introduction of the disease in the population and its first detection by the surveillance system (also referred to as the high-risk period [4]).
3. For systems aiming at identifying the cases of a disease in a population, effectiveness is the ability of the system to detect any one of the diseased units in a

focal population (the unit refers to the epidemiological unit, which can be an individual animal or, more often, an animal production unit). The most relevant attribute is then unit-level sensitivity (sometimes referred to as the detection fraction).

4. For systems aiming at monitoring the prevalence or incidence of an endemic disease, effectiveness is the ability of the system to provide accurate and precise estimations of prevalence and incidence rates. The most relevant attributes are then bias and precision of the prevalence and /or incidence estimations derived from the data produced by the surveillance system (e.g. [5]).

The above-listed attributes reflect the ability of surveillance systems to detect and/or correctly characterize a genuine health issue (see Part II for a full list of evaluation attributes). Surveillance systems that do not perform well with regard to such attributes could fail to control the health issue with harmful sanitary and economic consequences. Attributes that reflect the ability of surveillance systems to generate false detections of disease cases or of a health threat (e.g. the introduction of an emerging disease) are also relevant to its effectiveness. These attributes are system-level specificity, also referred to as the False Alarm Rate, for systems that aim at demonstrating/substantiating freedom from disease or at detecting the emergence of a disease and unit-level specificity for systems aiming at identifying all the cases of a disease in a population. Poor performances with regard to such attributes imply that costly mitigation measures are unnecessarily activated. A rationale to unify all the effectiveness attributes into two types of errors to which surveillance systems are prone has been recently proposed [6]. It is briefly presented below (Case Study 1). Moreover, as surveillance is an important component of the strategy to reach the ultimate objective of controlling the spread of diseases, outcomes such as epidemic size, number of infected units at some point in time (e.g. at the end of the high-risk period) or prevalence in an endemic equilibrium situation are also sometimes used as a measure of surveillance effectiveness evaluation.

10.3 Methods to Quantitatively Assess Surveillance Effectiveness

The effectiveness attributes introduced above can be estimated through the analysis of the data actually produced by surveillance or by modelling surveillance processes. Beyond the estimation of surveillance effectiveness parameters, assessment can also aim at identifying gaps and weaknesses in the surveillance system (e.g. population strata that escape surveillance, flawed processes) and link back to the evaluation of the quality of the surveillance process itself (see Sect. 10.4). Such assessment can lead to improvements in the surveillance systems effectiveness and process. Below, we introduce the methods used to quantitatively assess effectiveness of surveillance systems.

10.3.1 Methods Relying on the Analysis/Statistical Modelling of the Data Generated by the Surveillance Systems (Case Study 2)

10.3.1.1 General Principles

This type of methods can only be applied in *ex-post* or *in-itinere* evaluations because they require that the surveillance system under evaluation is or has been operating so that surveillance data have been produced and can be analysed. There are two broad categories for this type of methods:

1. Multilist Capture-Recapture (CR) models, the principle of which is to confront the information on infected epidemiological units derived from the surveillance data with information on infected epidemiological units originating from at least another distinct source. It is worth noticing that the different information sources can be different components of the same surveillance system.
2. Unilist Capture-Recapture (CR) models, which consists in fitting statistical models to multiple detection data for surveillance systems that generate multiple detections of infected epidemiological units (e.g. each animal infected by a disease detected in an infected herd represents a distinct detection event for that infected herd). Note that CR methods are described in more detail in a recent review paper [7].

10.3.1.2 Type of Inference Obtained

The most common purpose of CR models is to assess the ability of a surveillance system to identify infected epidemiological units (i.e. to assess the unit-level sensitivity of surveillance systems). These methods are thus particularly relevant for surveillance systems aiming at detecting all the cases of a disease in a population and, to a lesser extent, for surveillance systems aiming at monitoring prevalence because failure to identify infected epidemiological units could result in negatively biased prevalence estimations. The general principle of evaluating a surveillance system through the confrontation of information generated by the surveillance system with the information provided by a distinct independent source has also been used (rarely though) to assess timeliness. Beyond the estimation of unit-level sensitivity, CR models can also be used to evaluate heterogeneity in sensitivity among epidemiological units. This can be achieved by stratifying the analysed surveillance data according to factors that are suspected to underlie heterogeneity, so that a distinct statistical model is fitted for each stratum and thus estimation of unit-level sensitivity is obtained. This type of inference is important to identify strata in the population in which surveillance sensitivity is comparatively low and resource allocation to surveillance activities could consequently be enhanced. Finally, when information from multiple sources is available, multilist CR models can also address questions on the interdependency among sources (e.g. communication among distinct surveillance systems or distinct components of a surveillance system that can result in the probability of detecting an infected unit through one system or component varying depending on whether or not the same unit has already been detected by the other systems or components). It can thus provide information on the surveillance process from the sole analysis of the surveillance data.

10.3.1.3 Strengths

The main advantage of CR methods is that they do not require any knowledge/description of the surveillance process and nor do they require setting values for parameters that depict the surveillance process. In other words, these are data-oriented statistical methods in contrast with the process-oriented methods described hereafter.

10.3.1.4 Weaknesses

The main weakness of CR methods is that they do not allow the estimation of surveillance attributes other than unit-level sensitivity. For instance, these methods do not allow the estimation of the specificity of surveillance systems and do actually often rely on the assumption of perfect specificity (no epidemiological unit falsely identified as infected/diseased). Another important weakness is that they require data that are often not available for animal diseases (i.e. case detection data from distinct sources or multiple detection data generated by a single source).

10.3.2 Methods Relying on the Modelling of the Surveillance Processes Only (Case Study 3)

10.3.2.1 General Principles

Contrary to statistical approaches described in the previous section, modelling approaches translate surveillance processes into mathematical/probabilistic terms. The modelled processes depend on surveillance type. Passive surveillance would require reporting and confirmation process to be modelled, active surveillance would require sampling, screening and confirmation processes to be modelled and syndromic surveillance would require data generation and analysis/interpretation process to be modelled. In approaches where only the surveillance process is modelled, the epidemiological states of animal populations are set by assumptions either because they are informed by field data or prior knowledge, or because one wants to assess surveillance effectiveness for a particular epidemiological scenario. They are thus referred to as non-dynamic models, in contrast to mathematical models of disease transmission which will be presented in the next section.

The most common form for non-dynamic models used to assess surveillance effectiveness are the so-called scenario tree models which are very similar to risk analysis models and have been introduced and described in great detail by Martin et al. [8, 9]. This type of model is referred to as scenario tree because the structure of the model can be depicted in the form of a tree. Each branching level of the tree corresponds either to a factor that structures the population in terms of disease risk and/or surveillance modalities or to a step in the surveillance process. The branches represent either the distribution of the units composing the population into distinct risk and/or surveillance strata or the different possible outcomes of the different steps in the surveillance process. A parameter is associated to each branch of the tree model: this parameter is the fraction of the population belonging to a risk and/or surveillance stratum or the probability of a possible outcome at a given step of the surveillance process. The final levels of the tree (i.e. the leaves of the tree) depict the possible final outcomes of the surveillance process for the units that belong to each risk and/or surveillance stratum considered in the model.

It is worth noticing that approaches other than scenario trees have occasionally been used to assess surveillance effectiveness through modelling of the surveillance process only. For instance, simulation models have also been developed for this purpose (e.g. [5]).

10.3.2.2 Type of Inference Obtained

The integration of the parameters along the branches of the scenario tree model in the form of conditional probabilities products produces estimations of the probability that a single unit will yield either a positive or a negative outcome under the modelled surveillance process. Moreover, integration of the model outputs allow obtaining estimations of stratum-level sensitivity (probability of detection at least one infected unit in a specific stratum from the focal population) and system-level sensitivity (probability of detecting at least one infected unit in the focal population).

Scenario tree models also allow taking into account uncertainty in values of the model parameters. This is done by considering a probability distribution for the different possible values of a parameter instead of a single value and by applying Monte-Carlo procedures in which a large number of scenario trees are produced each of which presents a distinct set of input parameter values that result from independent drawings in the probability distributions. The output parameters are then depicted with distributions that reflect the uncertainty in the outputs resulting from the propagation of the uncertainties in the different input parameters along the model branches.

Beyond the evaluation of effectiveness parameters, the scenario tree models have also sometimes been used as surveillance process optimization tools. In that type of application, different values for some input parameter(s) associated with a specific step in the surveillance process (e.g. sampling effort) are considered and the resulting effectiveness outputs are compared (e.g. [10, 11]).

In terms of surveillance objectives, scenario tree models have been widely used to evaluate the system-level sensitivity in surveillance systems aiming at demonstrating/substantiating freedom from disease, in which case the assumed prevalence in the focal population (referred to as the design prevalence) is very low. The rationale in this type of application is that the scenario tree model allows evaluating the propensity of the surveillance system/component to detect a disease/pathogen whenever prevalence reaches levels considered as problematic in particular for the domestic or the export market. Scenario tree models have also sometimes been used to assess the effectiveness of surveillance systems whose objective is to detect the introduction of a disease in a population that is free from that disease [12] or to survey the prevalence of a disease in a population [5].

10.3.2.3 Strengths

By explicitly modelling the processes implied in the surveillance system, it becomes possible to evaluate the effectiveness of actual (ex-post or ex-itinere evaluation) as well as hypothetical (ex-ante evaluation) surveillance strategies.

These models allow stratifying the population under surveillance into strata that differ in terms of disease risk and/or in terms of surveillance modalities. They are thus able to account for heterogeneity among epidemiological units.

10.3.2.4 Weaknesses

Scenario tree models require an assumption about the prevalence of the disease in the focal population as well as setting the values of input parameters that reflect the risk structure in the population (relative risk for the different population strata considered and proportion of the units from the population belonging to each stratum) and the surveillance process in each stratum (sampling probability or case reporting probability, probability of a positive screening test result for a diseased unit, probability of a positive confirmatory test for a diseased unit, etc.). The values of the input model parameters should be carefully determined because biased input parameter values will result in misleading evaluations of effectiveness (garbage in, garbage out). Alternatively, an interesting approach to deal with uncertainty in model parameter values is to develop a qualitative risk model (e.g. [13]) where parameter values are categorical (e.g. low, medium, high).

10.3.3 Methods Relying on the Simultaneous Modelling of the Surveillance Processes and of Disease Transmission in the Population under Surveillance (Case Study 4)

10.3.3.1 General Principles

In this type of method, as for the type of methods presented in the previous section, surveillance process is explicitly formulated with a mathematical/probabilistic model. However, the model for the surveillance process is coupled with/integrated to a model for disease transmission dynamic in the target population that, most of the time, also integrates the disease control process. Finally, the model also sometimes includes the demographic dynamics of the epidemiological units in the population (i.e. whenever the performance of the surveillance system is assessed over the long term; e.g. [14, 15]). Usually, the model is used to simulate the spread/circulation of the disease in the population under surveillance and control (simulation is usually the only option because this type of model is analytically intractable). The epidemiological status, the outcome of the surveillance process and the implemented control actions are monitored over the simulation for each epidemiological unit in the population. The output of the integrated simulation model is the epidemiological status, the outcome of the surveillance process and the outcome of the control process for each epidemiological unit in the population at each time step of the simulation. These outputs are then used to compute the focal surveillance effectiveness attribute(s).

Different types of models can be used including branching process models (e.g. [4]), spatially explicit models (e.g. [16, 17]), compartmental models and social network models (e.g. [18]) (see Chap. 11). Model designing (identifying all the processes to be integrated in the model, choosing the best adapted formalism for the model, figuring out the architecture of the model, defining the model parameters) and parameterization (i.e. setting the values of the model parameters) are particularly critical steps in the modelling process.

Stochasticity (i.e. the influence of chance in the dynamics of finite size populations) is inherent to most of the dynamic simulation models because they consider a finite number of epidemiological units subjected to random processes (processes with different possible outcomes characterized by their probabilities). So the algorithms of dynamic simulation models usually include several steps where the outcome of a process is randomly drawn in a probability distribution. As a consequence, two independent simulations of a same model (same parameter values and initial conditions) will usually yield different outcomes. In order to account for stochasticity, several simulations (preferably a large number) of the same model are usually required.

As for the models for surveillance processes only, introduced in the previous section, uncertainty in the model parameters' values can be accounted for in the modelling process by considering different sets of input parameter values drawn from distributions that reflect uncertainty.

10.3.3.2 Type of Inference Obtained

Dynamic modelling is clearly the most flexible and versatile method to assess surveillance effectiveness. It can be used to evaluate the effectiveness of any surveillance system, whatever is the surveillance objective, and it can be used for *ex-ante*, *in-itinere* or *ex-post* evaluations (see Sect. 10.1).

A crucial characteristic of this type of methods is that processes resulting in disease transmission among epidemiological units and in changes in the status of epidemiological units are explicitly modelled. Therefore, the epidemiological situation (prevalence, epidemiological status of the units, spatial distribution of the diseased units, etc.) is not fixed, but endogenous to the model so that the simulated epidemiological situation in the focal population is likely to vary along the time line of the simulation (at least transitorily, until a stable disease equilibrium is eventually reached). Therefore, the effectiveness of a given surveillance strategy would also vary over time and surveillance effectiveness can be assessed at different points along the epidemiological dynamics time line. Moreover, it is then possible to assess the effectiveness of adaptive surveillance strategies where the modalities of surveillance can change over the course of an epidemic based on the evaluation, at some point in time, of the epidemiological situation through the surveillance data already collected. Because of these characteristics, dynamic models are often used to assess the effectiveness of surveillance systems/components that aim at detecting as early as possible the emergence of a disease. Indeed, emergence is in essence a transitory, non-equilibrium situation and it would be difficult (if not impossible) to assess the effectiveness of surveillance systems aiming at detecting emergences with a methodological framework that considers a static epidemiological situation.

Beyond the computation of effectiveness, dynamic models can be used for sensitivity (e.g. [19]) and optimization analyses (e.g. [18]). In optimization analyses, one or a combination of outputs (usually closely related to surveillance effectiveness) are optimized by varying the values of one or a combination of input parameters (usually input parameters that represent the surveillance processes). The objective of this type of analysis is usually to identify the modalities of the surveillance process that result in optimal effectiveness of the surveillance system. Sensitivity analyses are very similar in that input parameter values are also varied but the focus of the analysis is not on optimizing an effectiveness output but on the variance in the effectiveness output generated by variation in the input parameters. The objective of sensitivity analyses is most of the time to identify the input parameters (i.e. processes in the surveillance system) that have the strongest influence on the output parameter (i.e. effectiveness). The results of sensitivity analyses can be informative for designing surveillance because they identify key processes that strongly influence effectiveness and should thus be paid particular attention.

In optimization as well as in sensitivity analyses, not only input parameters related to the surveillance process can be varied but also the input parameters related to disease transmission or to the disease control process. For instance, different scenarios for both surveillance and control parameters in an optimization analysis can provide information on the optimal combination of surveillance and control modalities in order to achieve a given disease control objective (e.g. [20]).

10.3.3.3 Strengths

With dynamic models, epidemiological situations (prevalence, epidemiological status of the units, spatial distribution of the diseased units, etc.) are generated by the model. Assumptions regarding epidemiological situations are thus not required.

Because the monitored output parameters can be defined at the model designing step (i.e. the modeller defines the ouputs), carefully chosen output would allow the evaluation of any effectiveness attribute. In addition, because this type of model integrates disease transmission, surveillance and control processes, outcomes such as epidemic size, number of infected units at some point in time (e.g. at the end of the high risk period) or prevalence in an endemic equilibrium situation can be used as the currency to evaluate surveillance effectiveness.

10.3.3.4 Weaknesses

Parameterizing dynamic models that integrate surveillance and control processes requires setting the value of large numbers of parameters. Consequently, developing meaningful models requires good knowledge of the epidemiological, surveillance and control processes in the system under evaluation.

10.4 Synthesis (Table 10.1)

Table 10.1 Comparative analysis of the strengths and weaknesses of the different type of methods for quantitative assessment of surveillance effectiveness

Type of method	Type of evaluation	Objective of the evaluation	Objective of the surveillance system	Effectiveness attribute evaluated	Strength	Weakness
Capture–recapture method	*In-itinere* and *ex-post*	Estimating the value of an effectiveness attribute Characterizing heterogeneity in surveillance effectiveness	Detecting the cases of a disease	Unit-level sensitivity	Based on surveillance data analysis, no assumption regarding the epidemiological dynamics (objectivity)	Low flexibility. Required data often not available
Static modelling of surveillance process only (scenario tree models)	All types	Estimating the value of an effectiveness attribute Characterizing heterogeneity in surveillance effectiveness. Optimizing the surveillance process	Substantiating freedom from disease	Unit-level sensitivity. System-level sensitivity	Can deal with heterogeneity in disease risk and surveillance modalities. Can integrate uncertainty in model parameter values	Requires assumption on epidemiological situation and good knowledge of the surveillance modalities
Dynamic modelling	All types	Any objective	Any objective	Any attribute	Highly flexible. Can deal with any type of heterogeneity. Can integrate uncertainty in model parameter values	Requires setting values for a large number of parameters

10.5 Case Study 1: A Rationale to Unify Surveillance Effectiveness Attributes [6]

Here we introduce a rationale that can be used to assess effectiveness, whatever is the objective of the surveillance system considered. It provides a solid ground for developing optimization studies for any aspect of the surveillance process and it allows straightforward integration of economic and epidemiological components to the evaluation framework.

In this rationale, we propose that effectiveness should be assessed through probabilities that surveillance data generation and interpretation result in the implementation of intervention measures that differ from those that would be implemented given a perfect knowledge of the actual epidemiological situation (Fig. 10.1). We distinguish two broad categories of such probabilities and name them by analogy with statistical hypothesis testing. We refer to these as probabilities of Type I errors and probabilities of Type II errors, the probabilities of implementing intervention measures of respectively higher and lower intensity than the intervention measures that would be implemented given of perfect knowledge of the actual epidemiological situation. Type I errors imply that costly intervention measures are unnecessarily

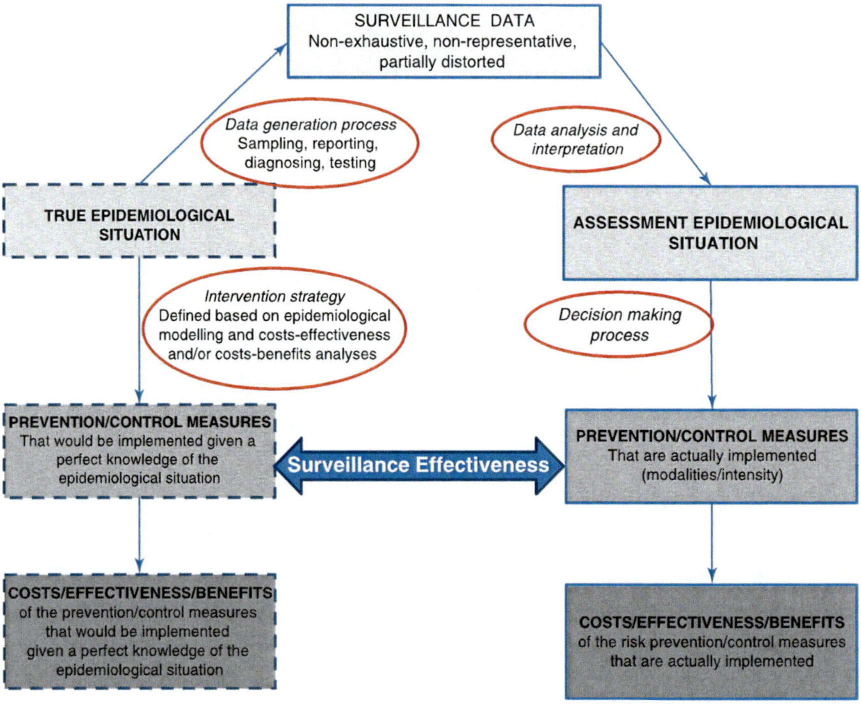

Fig. 10.1 Basis for the effectiveness rationale: comparative analysis of the differences in interventions generated from the current surveillance system and a system with a perfect knowledge of the epidemiological situation

activated while Type II errors result in increased risk of failure to control a genuine disease threat. For a surveillance system to be effective, probabilities of Type I and Type II errors should thus be as low as possible. The computation of probabilities of Type I and Type II errors requires reviewing several aspects of mitigation strategies and processes, as highlighted in Fig. 10.1. Below we detail these aspects using a hypothetical example of an active surveillance system aiming at monitoring prevalence of a cattle disease to inform decision-makers on which vaccination strategy to implement at the national level.

10.5.1 Information Required for the Evaluation of Surveillance Effectiveness (Table 10.2)

First, the state variable that reflects the current epidemiological situation, and the value which determines the intervention measures considered as appropriate by stakeholders and decision-makers have to be defined. The scale at which this variable is assessed through surveillance and at which intervention measures are implemented has also to be determined. Typical state variables are prevalence and incidence. The scale can be animal, herd, country, regional or global level. In our hypothetical example, the relevant state variable is prevalence and the scale is the country.

The proposed rationale relies on the comparison of intervention decisions likely to be made based on the information produced by surveillance with intervention

Table 10.2 Type of information required for the evaluation of surveillance effectiveness

Surveillance objective	Knowing how prevalent is an endemic disease to inform decisions about vaccination strategy		
Relevant scale	Country		
Relevant epidemiological variable	Individual level prevalence (p)		
Intervention strategy	$p \leq 0.1$	$0.1 < p \leq 0.2$	$p > 0.2$
	No vaccination	Vaccination is implemented only in high risk areas	Vaccination is implemented in all areas
Surveillance data generation process	$n = 100$ randomly chosen individuals are sampled over a 1 month period. Each sample is tested using a test with sensitivity $Se = 0.90$ and specificity $Sp = 0.95$. The number of samples testing positive is denoted n_p		
Statistics computed from surveillance data	Proportion of sampled units testing positive (n_p/n)		
Decision rule 1 (test performances not accounted for)	$n_p/n \leq 0.1$	$0.1 < n_p/n \leq 0.2$	$n_p/n > 0.2$
	No vaccination	Vaccination is implemented only in high-risk areas	Vaccination is implemented in all areas

decisions that would be made given a perfect knowledge of the epidemiological situation. One important step is thus to describe the intervention decisions that would be considered as appropriate by stakeholders and decision-makers for a set of possible epidemiological situations. Such intervention strategies consist of a gradation of potential epidemiological situations according to their seriousness and of the intervention measures considered as appropriate by stakeholder and decision-makers for each of these situations. From an analytical point of view, they can be described through the relationship between the value of the epidemiological state variable that characterizes an epidemiological situation and the intervention measures considered as appropriate for that epidemiological situation. In the hypothetical example, possible epidemiological situations are categorized according to three prevalence levels: at low prevalence (lower than 0.1), it is considered that vaccination is not necessary; at intermediate prevalence (between 0.1 and 0.2), it is considered that vaccination should be limited to high-risk areas; at high prevalence (over 0.2), it is considered that vaccination should be implemented in all areas of the country.

It is then necessary to describe the surveillance data-generation process. It involves reporting (e.g. underreporting rate, factors influencing reporting probability), diagnostic (e.g. case definition, probability of misclassifying an epidemiological unit), sampling (e.g. coverage, stratification, intensity, frequency), and sample testing (e.g. sensitivity and specificity of the tests used). In our hypothetical example, surveillance data are assumed to be generated through random sampling of 100 individuals over a month and assessment of individual disease status with a test of known sensitivity (0.90) and specificity (0.95).

Finally, the process of interpretation of surveillance data that results in a decision regarding the implementation of intervention measures needs to be described. In most instances, it involves the computation from the surveillance data of some statistics that provide an assessment of the current epidemiological situation and a decision rule whereby an intervention option is selected depending on the value of such statistics. In our hypothetical example, the data interpretation process simply consists in computing the proportion of samples testing positive and the decision rule is to do nothing if this proportion is lower than 0.1, implement vaccination only in high-risk areas when it is between 0.1 and 0.2 and implement vaccination in all the areas in the country when it is higher than 0.2.

10.6 Case Study 2—Results of the Sensitivity Evaluation of the Avian Influenza Surveillance System in Vietnam: Application of the Unlisted Capture–Recapture Method [21]

The overall objective of this study was to apply capture and recapture methods to quantitatively evaluate the sensitivity of the HPAI surveillance system in Vietnam. The specific objectives were to estimate the sensitivity of the surveillance system using the zero-inflated model by comparing periods with and without vaccination against HPAI H5N1.

This study showed that the sensitivity of surveillance ranged from 34% (CI = 33–100) to 74% (CI = 50–100) at the provincial level and from 48% (CI = 13–100) to 61% (CI = 40–91) at the district level. A significant difference in the probability of detecting at least one infection in a province was observed between the 2009/10 and 2010/11 periods (Pdet = 34% (CI = 21–53) and Pdet = 74% (CI = 56–89), respectively).

- The results of the study confirm that recapture analyses allow more accurate estimates to be obtained at a finer scale such as the district level compared to the province level.
- The different levels of sensitivity observed across the study periods could be correlated to the surveillance-strengthening activities implemented during that period (e.g. the highest level of sensitivity observed at the provincial scale corresponds to the period 2010–2011 when a strengthening of passive surveillance was implemented [22].

In addition, the study shows a significant positive association between a district's risk level (predefined by the veterinary services based on the combination of different risk factors) and its model-estimated probability of infection in the absence of vaccination but not during the vaccination period. However, it is impossible to conclude from these data alone that vaccination has a positive impact because it reduces the risk of infection or a negative impact because it limits the number of notifications (for this it would be necessary to be able to compare general sensitivities as well). It has been observed in other studies that vaccination can have a negative effect on the case notification rate [23]. In this case, stakeholders either do not want to report cases (showing the ineffectiveness of vaccination in their region), or they consider that suspected cases are not HPAI since the poultry have been vaccinated.

This study demonstrated the validity of the model through the positive correlation between the probability of infection estimated by the model and the a priori defined risk of infection; but also an indirect effect of vaccination on the sensitivity of the HPAI surveillance system in Vietnam through its action on the probability of infection.

10.7 Case Study 3—The Use of Models of the Surveillance Processes Only: Quantitative Assessment of the Sensitivity of Avian Influenza Surveillance Systems Using the Scenario Tree Approach [24]

We developed a stochastic scenario tree to model and assess the surveillance system of HPAI H5N1 in Thailand in backyard and free-range poultry production systems. The objective was to estimate the sensitivity of each of the surveillance components using the appropriate parameters for the study period (variable period depending on the component: exhaustive or passive surveillance over 1 year, targeted surveillance of the markets over a given period of time disease). The goal is to calculate for each component an individual sensitivity, then combine them to obtain an overall sensitivity of the network. The method uses a tree structure to describe the population and the surveillance organization and to capture the fact that some individuals will be more likely to be infected based on risk factors and some individuals will be more likely to be detected depending on the structure of the surveillance system.

A scenario tree represents the succession in chronological order of the different stages of the component of the surveillance system (CSS) that leads an individual to be declared infected or uninjured. At each step or node of the tree, probabilities or proportions are estimated for each possible branch as well as the associated relative risk. We obtain the individual sensitivity by multiplying, for each path of the scenario tree, the probabilities, proportions and adjusted risks of the branches of this path, and then adding these products for all the paths ending in a positive outcome (Fig. 10.2).

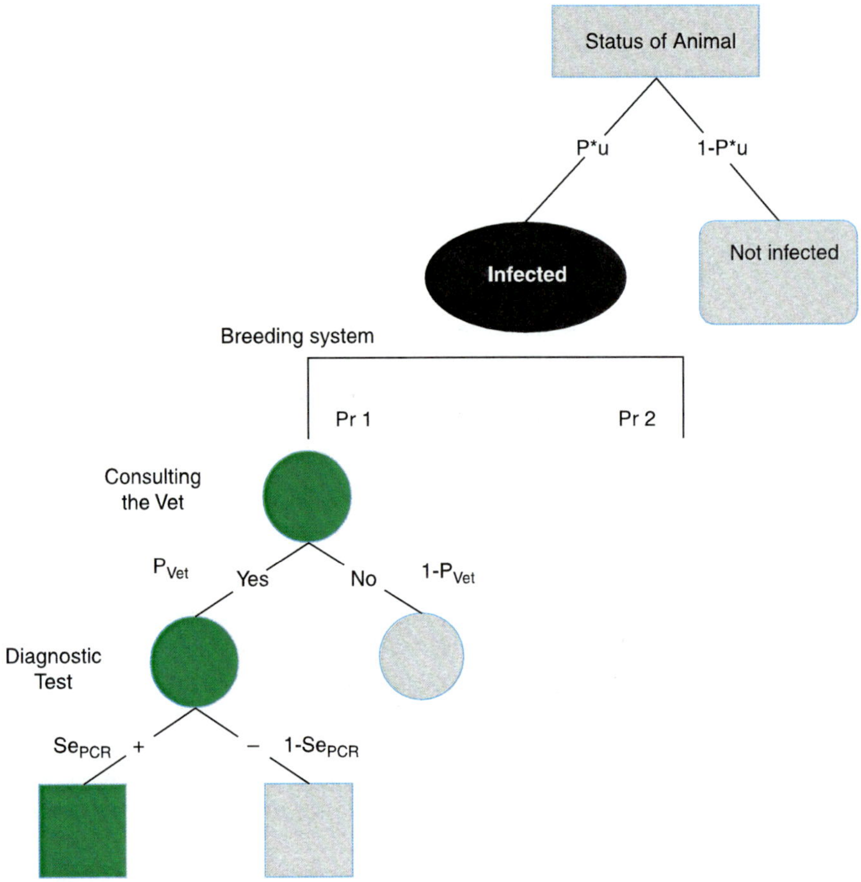

Fig. 10.2 Example of a scenario tree constructed to quantify the sensitivity of an animal health surveillance system

10.7.1 HPAI Surveillance System Organization in Thailand

The surveillance and control of H5N1 avian influenza on farms in Thailand is under the responsibility of the DLD (Department of Livestock), which collects and centralizes all epidemiological information [25]. The aim of the system is to detect outbreaks early and thus ensure a rapid response to maintain the national disease-free status recovered in 2009. The system is based on several complementary components:

- Passive, clinical surveillance based on voluntary reporting of any clinical suspicion of HPAI H5N1 (as officially defined) by breeders at the local DLD office. The agents of the DLD then go into the breeding under 48 h, in order to validate the suspicion, to take samples and to establish a zone of control of the movements around the suspect breeding. All poultry from farms located within a radius of 5 km around an outbreak of HPAI H5N1 confirmed by laboratory analyses are systematically slaughtered and their carcasses burned or buried; livestock equipment is destroyed and buildings are disinfected. Quarantine measures are also in place: any movement of poultry is forbidden within a radius of 60 km around the home, for a period of at least 30 days. Checkpoints are established along the roads and vehicles are checked to ensure that no animals are moved to or from a quarantine area.
- Active surveillance is based on different activities:
  - Active surveillance plan for commercial farms (pre-displacement laboratory tests for short cycles, repeated for long cycles) which are partly based on the private sector
  - The intensive active surveillance (or X-ray) based on clinical signs consisting of compulsory visits of backyard farms by village health volunteers and rapid response teams (RRTs) who actively seek clinical signs of the disease in humans and hens on the farms (Fig. 10.3)
  - The laboratory X-ray surveys consisting in the risk-based collection of samples in chickens and free-grazing ducks (four farms per village) by DLD.
  - X-ray components are both risk-based and run for a period of 2 months twice a year.
  - Market surveillance 2 weeks before the Chinese New Year in 21 high-risk provinces.
  - A positive output of the surveillance is considered when a sample was tested positive for RT-PCR

Evolution of the Definition of the Case of Avian Influenza H5N1, Established by the DLD from January 2004 to December 2012

- January 23, 2004–February 28, 2004 (based on the Hong Kong definition): severe respiratory signs with sinusitis, cyanosis of the ridge, oedema of the head, ruffled plumage or diarrhoea and neurological signs or sudden death of about 100% or 40% in 3 days
- March 1, 2004–February 28, 2004 (adaptation of the case definition to the context of Thailand): mortality >10% in 1 day or mortality >40% in 3 days and respiratory signs or mortality >40% in 3 days and neurological signs

or mortality >40% in 3 days and other signs (diarrhoea, depression, loss of appetite, oviposition, cyanosis of the ridge) or ducks and geese: depression, loss of appetite, oedema of the head, corneal opacity, ruffled plumage

- July 3, 2004–June 30, 2005 (increase in sensitivity, decrease in specificity): mortality >10% in 1 day and respiratory signs or neurological signs or other signs (diarrhoea, depression, loss of appetite, oviposition, cyanosis of the ridge) for ducks and geese: depression, loss of appetite, oedema of head, corneal opacity, ruffled plumage
- July 1, 2005–2012 (increased sensitivity, decreased specificity): poultry in buildings: mortality of 1% in 2 days and drop of water or food consumption by 10% in 1 day; backyard poultry: mortality >5% in 2 days

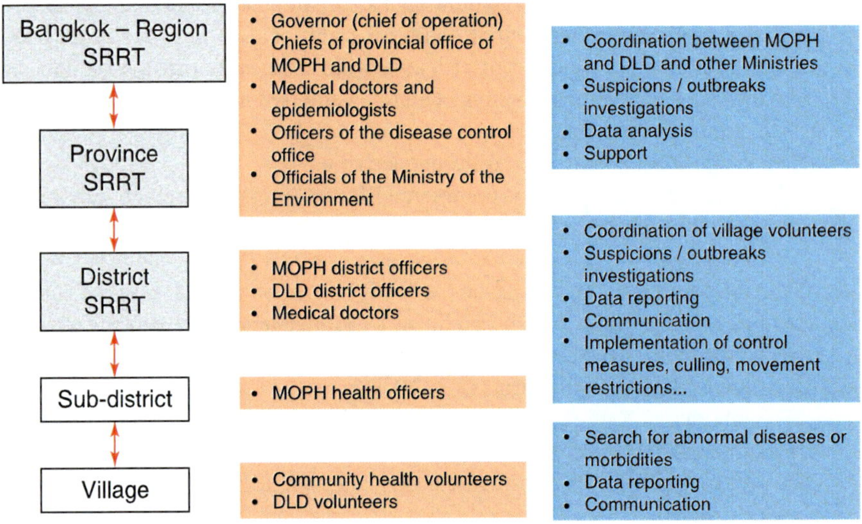

Fig. 10.3 Organization of influenza surveillance and rapid response teams in Thailand (SRRTs) in 2011 [25]

10.7.2 Quantitative Evaluation of HPAI H5N1 Surveillance in Backyard Poultry in Thailand Using Scenario Tree Modelling

During the two most risky months, when X-Ray monitoring is implemented, the current surveillance system has a high probability of detecting disease at an early stage of infection, with a sensitivity of 82% when only three farms are affected. The results show that when all three surveillance components are implemented simultaneously, the most effective is the active search for clinical signs in chicken in mixed farms in high-risk areas. This result is directly related to the case definition used by the DLD to detect suspicions of HPAI H5N1, which is very broad and therefore very sensitive. On the other hand, the poor specificity of this case definition increases the risk of false positives. Outside the X-Ray periods, when only passive surveillance is implemented, the current surveillance sensitivity for the same infection level drops to 50% with a very large confidence interval (95% CI 0.04–0.75). Lack of specificity can create distrust of the DLD, since control measures are often put in place before any laboratory confirmation (Executive Committee for the Prevention and Control of Avian Influenza and preparedness for influenza pandemic, 2007), and may contribute to the lack of sensitivity of passive surveillance. An additional deficiency of this case definition is the 5% level of mortality, which is used as a trigger for suspicions of HPAI H5N1. The basic mortality is difficult to estimate for small farms. However, when looking at the probability of freedom from disease over time (from January 2008 to January 2011), and considering all surveillance components, the median probability of freedom was estimated to be 99.43% (97.82–99.73%) for a low probability of disease introduction and 96.90% (87.25–98.53%) for a risk fivefold higher. These results show that the current monitoring strategy for village livestock systems and ducks is highly sensitive and therefore supports Thailand's declaration of H5N1 status in February 2009.

10.8 Case Study 4—The Use of Dynamic Models [16]

Classical swine fever (CSF) is a porcine viral disease that has severe consequences on animal health, welfare and production. Although Switzerland is currently free from CSF, it is considered that the risk of introduction of the CSF virus is non-negligible. Switzerland veterinary health authorities have thus designed a surveillance and control strategy with the objective of detecting as soon as possible the infected pig farms following the potential introduction of the virus in the pig population. In this strategy, six broad levels of on-farm surveillance and intervention measures are considered depending on the assessment of the epidemiological status of the focal farm, of the neighbouring farms and of the country: there is no intervention as long as CSF remains undetected in Switzerland; reinforced surveillance due to increased awareness is implemented as soon as a first CSF infected farm has been detected in the country; farm isolation during 1 week is implemented in a 10 km radius around each suspected infected farm; unlimited farm isolation is implemented in a 3 km radius around each suspected infected farm; quarantine is implemented in each suspected infected farm and culling is implemented in each confirmed infected farm. In 2014, an exclusion component was added to allow testing for CSF in domestic pig farms with symptoms in line with CSF even in the current situation where the disease has not yet been detected in the country. The objective of this study was to assess the improvement in effectiveness resulting from the integration of this exclusion component in the current system.

A stochastic farm-based simulation model, programmed in R (R Development Core Team and Team R, 2008) was developed. It simulates the spread of CSF virus between farms in space and time. The model accounts explicitly for the spatial distribution of pig farms in Switzerland. The simulation starts by randomly drawing an index case in the list of Switzerland pig farms. Then four successive steps allow the determination of the farms infected by the index case and of the dates at which these farms become infected.

1. The first step of the simulation algorithm for an infected farm is the determination of the date at which the farm becomes infectious, which is deduced from the date at which the farm has become infected and the length of the latent period (hereafter denoted as LLP).
2. The second step is the determination of the length of the infectious period (length of the period between the date at which the farm becomes infectious and the date at which it is detected and confirmed as being infected; hereafter denoted as (LIP) for that farm). At this step, the date at which the farm is detected and confirmed as being infected is deduced from the date at which the farm has become infected (day 0 for the index case), the length of the latent period and the length of the infectious period for that farm. At that date, it is considered that the surveillance and control measures that should be implemented in an infected farm and in its vicinity are indeed implemented.
3. The third step is the determination of the number of other farms infected by that farm (i.e. the effective reproductive rate, hereafter denoted R) during the infectious period.
4. Finally, the farms infected by the infectious farm are selected in the list of Switzerland pig farms and the date at which each of these farms becomes infected is determined. Infected farms are removed from the list of farms from which subsequently infected farms will be drawn so that a same farm cannot be infected twice during a simulated outbreak (in a compartmental model this would imply that there is no transition from the state infectious or recovered to the state susceptible) and the number of susceptible farms decreases as the simulated outbreak develops. The newly infected farms constitute "the next generation of infected farms". The different steps described above are applied to each infected farm of the next generation and then to each infected farm of the second next generation and so on until no newly infected farm is generated by the simulation.

The surveillance and control processes are accounted for in the model by setting different parameter value for farm-level epidemiological parameters (i.e. the weekly number of infected farms for an infectious farm and the length of the infectious period) depending on the surveillance and intervention measures implemented in the farm.

For each simulation run of a given scenario regarding the surveillance and control strategy, the model generates an epidemic. Output information (illustrated on the figure below) includes the spatial locations of the infected farms and the surveillance/intervention measures implemented in each infected farm at the time it becomes infectious.

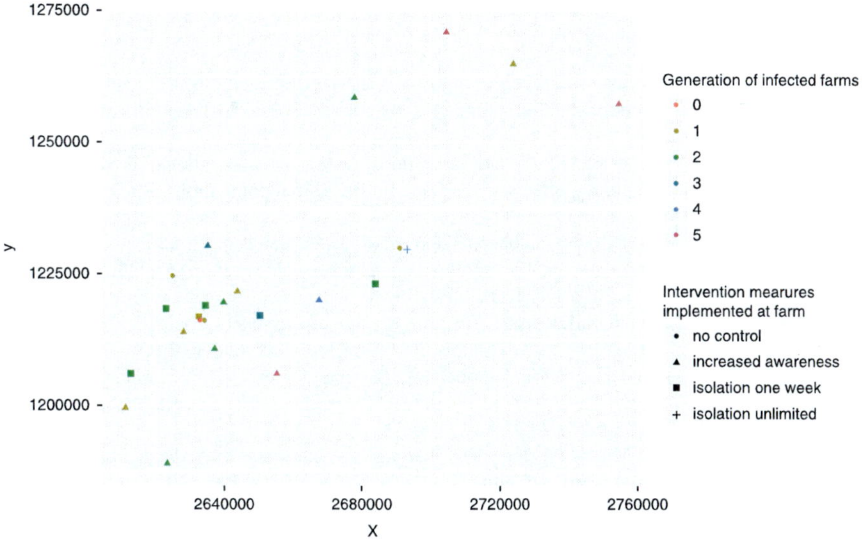

Based on these outputs, two measures of effectiveness of the system with and without the exclusion component were assessed: (1) the number of infected farms per outbreak and (2) the probability of implementing intervention modalities in a farm that are not strong enough given the true epidemiological status of that farm. This is illustrated in the table below.

Simulation model outputs for strategy with or without (italics) the exclusion component

Parameter	Median	Percentile 5%	Percentile 95%
Total number of infected farms	3	1	27
Duration of the outbreak—Days	43	1	158
Total number of infected farms	*4*	*1*	*142*
Duration of the outbreak—Days	*53*	*2*	*364*
Probability of absence of intervention	0.50	0.133	1.00
Probability of implementing reinforced surveillance	0.333	0.0	0.667
Probability of implementing isolation during 1 week	0.0	0.0	0.354
Probability of implementing unlimited isolation	0.0	0.0	0.16
Probability of absence of intervention	*0.50*	*0.016*	*1.00*
Probability of implementing reinforced surveillance	*0.333*	*0*	*0.60*
Probability of implementing isolation during 1 week	*0*	*0*	*0.426*
Probability of implementing unlimited isolation	*0*	*0*	*0.244*

References

1. Häsler B, Howe KS, Stärk KD. Conceptualising the technical relationship of animal disease surveillance to intervention and mitigation as a basis for economic analysis. BMC Health Serv Res. 2011;11(1):225.
2. Howe K, Häsler B, Stärk K. Economic principles for resource allocation decisions at national level to mitigate the effects of disease in farm animal populations. Epidemiol Infect. 2013;141(1):91–101.
3. Hoinville L, Alban L, Drewe J, Gibbens J, Gustafson L, Häsler B, Saegerman C, Salman M, Stärk K. Proposed terms and concepts for describing and evaluating animal-health surveillance systems. Prev Vet Med. 2013;112(1–2):1–12.
4. Klinkenberg D, Nielen M, Mourits M, De Jong M. The effectiveness of classical swine fever surveillance programmes in the Netherlands. Prev Vet Med. 2005;67(1):19–37.
5. Schärrer S, Schwermer H, Presi P, Lindberg A, Zinsstag J, Reist M. Cost and sensitivity of on-farm versus slaughterhouse surveys for prevalence estimation and substantiating freedom from disease. Prev Vet Med. 2015;120(1):51–61.
6. Grosbois V, Häsler B, Peyre M, Hiep DT, Vergne T. A rationale to unify measurements of effectiveness for animal health surveillance. Prev Vet Med. 2015;120(1):70–85.
7. Vergne T, Vilas VJDR, Cameron A, Dufour B, Grosbois V. Capture–recapture approaches and the surveillance of livestock diseases: a review. Prev Vet Med. 2015;120(3–4):253–64.
8. Martin P, Cameron A, Barfod K, Sergeant E, Greiner M. Demonstrating freedom from disease using multiple complex data sources: 2: case study—classical swine fever in Denmark. Prev Vet Med. 2007a;79(2–4):98–115.
9. Martin P, Cameron A, Greiner M. Demonstrating freedom from disease using multiple complex data sources: 1: a new methodology based on scenario trees. Prev Vet Med. 2007b;79(2–4):71–97.
10. Blickenstorfer S, Schwermer H, Engels M, Reist M, Doherr MG, Hadorn DC. Using scenario tree modelling for targeted herd sampling to substantiate freedom from disease. BMC Vet Res. 2011;7(1):49.
11. Nathues C, Hillebrand A, Rossteuscher S, Zimmermann W, Nathues H, Schüpbach G. Evaluating the surveillance for swine dysentery and progressive atrophic rhinitis in closed multiplier herds using scenario tree modelling. Porcine Health Manag. 2015;1(1):7.
12. de Vos CJ, van der Goot JA, van Zijderveld FG, Swanenburg M, Elbers AR. Risk-based testing of imported animals: a case study for bovine tuberculosis in The Netherlands. Prev Vet Med. 2015;121(1–2):8–20.
13. Haesler B, Howe K, Hauser R, Stärk KDC. A qualitative approach to measure the effectiveness of active avian influenza virus surveillance with respect to its cost: a case study from Switzerland. Prev Vet Med. 2012;105(3):209–22.
14. Kudahl AB, Sørensen JT, Nielsen SS, Østergaard S. Simulated economic effects of improving the sensitivity of a diagnostic test in paratuberculosis control. Prev Vet Med. 2007;78(2):118–29.
15. More SJ, Cameron A, Strain S, Cashman W, Ezanno P, Kenny K, Fourichon C, Graham D. Evaluation of testing strategies to identify infected animals at a single round of testing within dairy herds known to be infected with Mycobacterium avium ssp. paratuberculosis. J Dairy Sci. 2015;98(8):5194–210.
16. Léger A, Grosbois V, Simons R, Stärk KD, De Nardi M. Cost-effectiveness of surveillance and biosecurity scenarios for preventing CSF in Switzerland. Microbial Risk Anal. 2019;13 https://doi.org/10.1016/j.mran.2019.07.001.
17. Leslie E, Cowled B, Graeme Garner M, Toribio JA, Ward M. Effective surveillance strategies following a potential classical swine fever incursion in a remote wild pig population in North-Western Australia. Transbound Emerg Dis. 2014;61(5):432–42.
18. Hayama Y, Kobayashi S, Nishida T, Muroga N, Tsutsui T. Network simulation modeling of equine infectious anemia in the non-racehorse population in Japan. Prev Vet Med. 2012;103(1):38–48.

19. Yamamoto T, Tsutsui T, Nishiguchi A, Kobayashi S. Evaluation of surveillance strategies for bovine brucellosis in Japan using a simulation model. Prev Vet Med. 2008;86(1–2):57–74.
20. Gormley AM, Holland EP, Barron MC, Anderson DP, Nugent G. A modelling framework for predicting the optimal balance between control and surveillance effort in the local eradication of tuberculosis in New Zealand wildlife. Prev Vet Med. 2016;125:10–8.
21. Vu MQG. Evaluation de la sensibilité du système de surveillance de l'IAHP au Vietnam: application des méthodes de capture-recapture et des approches participatives (Master 2 report). Université Paris Est Créteil, Val de Marnes; 2012.
22. Duteurtre V, Delabouglise A, Goutard F, Nguyen Viet Khong, K, Duteurtre G, Roger F, Peyre M. Influenza aviaire au Vietnam: état des lieux et complémentarité des activités de surveillance et des études épidémiologiques (2007–2011). Rev. D'élevage Médecine Vét. Pays Trop. 2016;68, 175. https://doi.org/10.19182/remvt.31165.
23. Vergne T, Grosbois V, Jobre Y, Saad A, El Nabi AA, Galal S, Kalifa M, El Kader SA, Dauphin G, Roger F, Lubroth J, Peyre M. Avian influenza vaccination of poultry and passive case reporting, Egypt. Emerg. Infect. Dis. 2012;18:2076–8. k.
24. Goutard FL, Paul M, Tavornpanich S, Houisse I, Chanachai K, Thanapongtharm W, Cameron A, Stärk KDC, Roger F. Optimizing early detection of avian influenza H5N1 in backyard and free-range poultry production systems in Thailand. Prev Vet Med. 2012;105:223–34. https://doi.org/10.1016/j.prevetmed.2011.12.020.
25. Paul M. Géographie d'une épizootie: déterminants socio-spatiaux de la diffusion de l'influenza aviaire en Thaïlande. Thèse de doctorat en Géographie de la santé, Université de Paris Ouest Nanterre La Défense; 2011.

Network Analysis for Surveillance Design and Evaluation

11

Guillaume Fournié, Alexis Delabouglise, Raphaëlle Métras, Younjung Kim, and Raphaël Duboz

Abstract

The way in which an infectious agent or an information is disseminated within an animal production system is influenced by the structure of the network of contacts through which the infectious agent is transmitted between hosts, or information is shared among stakeholders. The analysis of these networks is therefore necessary to comprehensively design and evaluate surveillance programmes. In this chapter, we provide an introduction of key methods to characterise the structural features of a network influencing the diffusion of a disease or an information through it, and we illustrate the relevance of these methods in the context of animal health surveillance design and evaluation. First, we define a network; we present the specific features of network data, how networks are constructed, and the challenges posed by network data collection. Secondly, we introduce metrics used to characterise the position of a node, and the cohesion of

G. Fournié (✉)
Veterinary Epidemiology, Economics and Public Health Group, Pathobiology and Population Sciences, Royal Veterinary College, University of London, London, UK
e-mail: gfournie@rvc.ac.uk

A. Delabouglise
ASTRE, CIRAD, INRAE, University of Montpellier, Montpellier, France

R. Métras
INSERM, Sorbonne Université, Institut Pierre Louis d'Épidémiologie et de Santé Publique (IPLESP), Paris, France

Y. Kim
Centre for Applied One Health Research and Policy Advice, College of Veterinary Medicine and Life Sciences, City University of Hong Kong, Kowloon, Hong Kong

R. Duboz
ASTRE, CIRAD, INRAE, University of Montpellier, Montpellier, France

M. Peyre et al. (eds.), *Principles for Evaluation of One Health Surveillance: The EVA Book*, https://doi.org/10.1007/978-3-030-82727-4_11

the overall network, or a subset of this network. Finally, mathematical models simulating the transmission of infectious agents through a network of potentially infectious contacts are described. Examples of applications of these methods for the design and evaluation of surveillance programmes are provided as case studies.

Keywords
Evaluation · Health surveillance · Social network analysis · Modeling

11.1 Introduction

Surveillance effectiveness depends on the dynamics of targeted infectious agents within the animal production system of interest, and the way in which surveillance-relevant information is shared among stakeholders (see Parts II and III). The factors which require understanding to comprehensively evaluate a surveillance system can be investigated using network analysis. Based on the observation of relevant interactions between a set of actors, this methodology can be used to explore how a given phenomenon may spread among those actors. Applied to animal health surveillance, spreading phenomena and actors in which researchers have been interested are infectious agents and animals or animal populations, on the one hand, and outbreak information and animal production stakeholders, on the other hand.

In veterinary epidemiology, network analysis has been mainly applied to study the transmission of infectious agents through networks of contacts resulting from the movements of animals between livestock premises, regions or countries. Such applications have been promoted by the existence of livestock tracing systems in many developed countries, providing researchers with readily available information on all animal movements occurring between premises (e.g. farms, markets, slaughterhouses) within a given country over time [1–6]. Such studies are less common in developing countries, as detailed movement data are rarely available and require labour-intensive primary data collection [7–11]. Other types of contacts that could also lead to the transmission of infectious agents between animal populations have also been explored, such as the movement of traders and other production stakeholders between premises [12–14]. These studies generally aim (i) to assess the possible course, speed and size of an epidemic following the incursion of an infectious agent in the network; (ii) to identify the most vulnerable and/or infectious premises; and (iii) to assess the effectiveness of surveillance and control programmes. Along the analysis of disease epidemic spreading through networks of contacts, a limited number of studies have been interested in the dissemination of outbreak-suspicion information through theoretical [15] or empirical networks [16, 17]. Assessing the way in which such information are shared among production and animal health stakeholders is however crucial in order to evaluate, and improve, surveillance effectiveness.

The purpose of this chapter is to introduce some key network analytical methods relevant to animal health surveillance evaluation and design. Network analysis has been applied across disciplines to address very diverse theoretical and practical questions,[1] and many textbooks have been written on this topic [18–22]. We refer to them for readers who wish to deepen their understanding of methods presented in this chapter. While we will focus here on methods used to characterise structural features of a network influencing the spread of a disease or an information through it, the methods we introduce are also relevant to the analysis of alternative networks, such as networks of organisations involved in animal health surveillance (Case Study 11.1). The study of such networks can be useful to pinpoint inefficiencies in the management of surveillance activities, to identify barriers to inter-organisational collaboration, and, therefore, to provide recommendations for effective interactions within and between organisations involved in a surveillance system.

11.2 Network Data

11.2.1 Data Structures and Network Construction

Network analysis is concerned with relational data, which consist of *nodes* and *edges*. A node, also referred to in the literature as an actor, a vertex, a site, is a unit connected to other units through edges. In the case of a disease transmission network, a node would be a host, a population of hosts (e.g. a herd) or a physical vector. In the case of an information-sharing network, nodes would usually be people or groups of people, such as farmers, traders, animal health professionals, but could also be communication devices or data servers. An edge represents an interaction between two nodes. The network approach relies on the hypothesis that the structure of the network shaped by those interactions influences the way in which an infectious agent is transmitted, or information disseminated. The interaction should be, therefore, relevant to the spreading phenomenon of interest, i.e., its presence should promote the spread of disease (or information) between nodes. Depending on the nature of the interaction, an edge can be bidirectional, if the phenomenon can spread in both directions, or directed, if the phenomenon can only spread in a given direction. For instance, if the interaction of interest is the commercial movement of small ruminants in the context of Peste des Petits Ruminants (PPR) transmission, the trade of animals from flock A to flock B, but not from flock B to flock A, means that PPR virus, which is transmitted through direct contacts between animals, can only spread from A to B. The corresponding edge should be directed, with flock A as a sender, and flock B as a receiver. In contrast, if we are interested in the mixing of small ruminant flocks on pastures or watering points, two flocks mixing on the same site should be linked by an undirected edge, with A and B as endpoints, as PPR could spread from A to B or B to A, should one or the other flock be infected. All edges in a network usually represent one type of interaction. It is, however, possible to

[1] These include the adoption of behaviours, the distribution of socioeconomic relations and their determinants, cell metabolism, gene regulation, animal food web stability, cascade failures in engineered networks (e.g. power grids).

represent multiple types of interactions occurring between the nodes of a network, which is then referred to as a multiplex network (Case Study 11.1). While we will refer to edges throughout the chapter, they are also called links, ties, bonds, relations, connections, contacts, and, when directed, arcs, in the literature.

Relational data can be completed with node *attributes*. These are individual-level variables. They can either be upstream, independent variables, which may explain the presence of edges (e.g. the type of premises between which animals are moved, stakeholders' occupation), or be downstream, dependent variables, which may be influenced by the position of nodes in the network (e.g. infection status). Likewise, edges can be given attributes, most commonly a *strength* (or weight) characterising the intensity of contacts between nodes (e.g. number of animals moved between farms, frequency of information exchange between stakeholders). Those networks for which the edge strengths are specified are said to be *weighted*.

A network structure is generally presented mathematically as an *adjacency matrix* (Fig. 11.1). It is an $n \times n$ matrix, with n rows and columns, n being the number of nodes in the network. In the matrix $\mathbf{M}$, the element corresponding to the ith row and jth column is denoted m_{ij}. It relates to the existence of an edge between the ith and jth nodes. If the network is undirected (i.e. edges are bidirectional), the matrix is symmetrical and $m_{ij} = m_{ji}$. In such an undirected network, if edge strength is ignored, the network is binary. An edge is either present between two given nodes, $m_{ij} = m_{ji} = 1$, or absent, $m_{ij} = m_{ji} = 0$. In contrast, the adjacency matrix of a directed network is asymmetrical, as it contains information about edge direction, with m_{ij} referring to the existence of an edge from the ith to the jth node. Therefore, if an edge is not reciprocal, $m_{ij} \neq m_{ji}$. In weighted networks, m_{ij} is then equal to the edge strength. For instance, in a network capturing the movement of cattle between premises, m_{ij} would be equal to the number of cattle moved from the ith to the jth premise. A special case arises when $i = j$. m_{ij} relates to the existence of a self-edge—an edge starting and ending in the same ith node. Such an edge is not relevant for the

a

	A	B	C	D
A	0	1	0	0
B	1	0	1	1
C	0	1	0	1
D	0	1	1	0

b

	A	B	C	D
A	0	0	0	1
B	1	0	1	0
C	0	0	0	1
D	0	0	0	0

c

	A	B	C	D
A	0	0	0	1
B	5	0	2	0
C	0	0	0	1
D	0	0	0	0

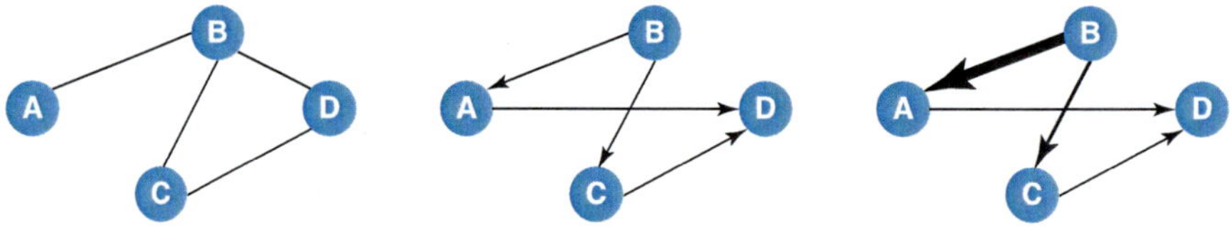

Fig. 11.1 Adjacency matrices and visualisation of (**a**) an unweighted binary network, (**b**) an unweighted directed network and (**c**) a weighted and directed network

types of networks in which we are interested, so all the elements m_{ij} in the diagonal of the matrix $\mathbf{M}$ under discussion in this chapter are equal to 0.

Case Study 11.1 Comparative Analysis of the Swine Surveillance System and the Informal Health Information-Sharing Network of Pig Farmers in Vietnam [23]
The analysis of health information-sharing networks in the Vietnamese hog sector revealed the predominant role of private actors in the dissemination of the information, and in the management of health risk. When they experience unusual morbidity or mortality in their herd, pig farmers generally seek advice from veterinary drug sellers, feed dealers and pig traders. As members of the community, governmental veterinarians may be provided with such information, through informal exchanges. In this context, they are reluctant to disseminate this information through the official surveillance system, as this may affect their relationship with farmers and the wider community (Fig. 11.2). This study highlights the challenges faced by the official surveillance system, and the social factors limiting the system's ability to identify suspected disease outbreaks occurring in swine farms.

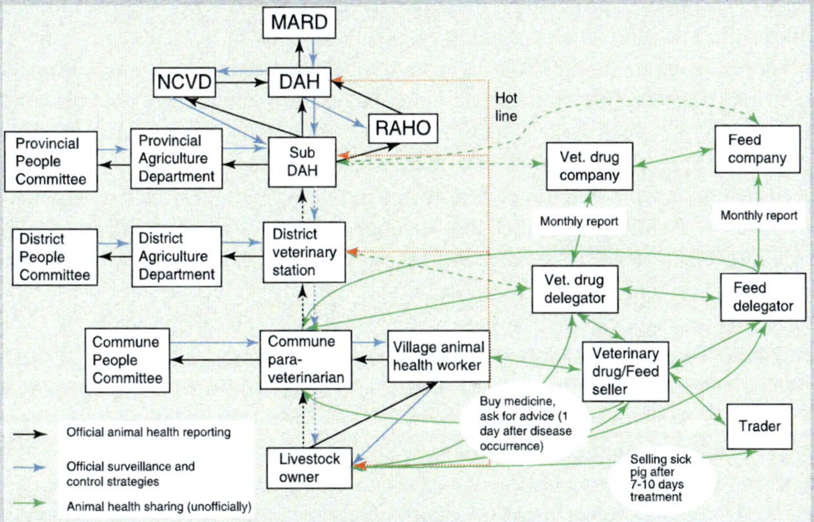

Fig. 11.2 Sharing health information on swine diseases in Vietnam: through the official surveillance system (black lines) and the informal network (green lines) [23]

11.2.2 Study Design and Data Collection

A network is constructed based on the measurement of interactions between a set of elements, or nodes. Therefore, elements, interactions and the way these are measured should be carefully defined, as it will impact on the structure of the resulting network, and, therefore, on the analysis and conclusions drawn from it.

First, a set of nodes, and at least one type of interaction connecting nodes in the system of interest should be identified. For the analysis to be meaningful, nodes need to be comparable. Even when the elements of a network are clearly identified, choices may need to be made about the scale at which nodes would be labelled. For instance, a node may be an individual animal, an animal population on a premise, or an animal population in a given administrative division. Likewise, in an information-sharing network, a node may be an individual stakeholder, a group of stakeholders (e.g. farmers, veterinary health authorities), or an inanimate object, such as a communication device or a data server. If different types of nodes should be represented, *multi-level networks* may be considered [21]. The population of nodes between which connections are studied needs to be delimited. The definition of the limits of the population of nodes is non-trivial, as interactions between nodes rarely have clear boundaries. Practically, geographical locations, memberships to predefined categories, sampling procedures are often used to delimit these populations. As mentioned above, the choice of the type of interactions to be captured in the network depends on the nature of the process to be described and explained. If we aim to construct a disease transmission network, edges need to represent potential infectious contacts between nodes, such as the movements of live animals or fomites between premises. In the case of information-sharing networks, edges would represent the exchange of a given type of information between nodes, such as suspicions of disease events affecting poultry flocks among production stakeholders.

Measurements need to be adapted to the type of interactions under study. They may directly, or indirectly, capture the notion of these interactions. For instance, cattle farmers may be directly asked with whom they talk about mortality events occurring in their herd, or indirectly, by assessing, for instance, their level of trust in other animal production stakeholders. Direct or indirect, any measurement approach is likely to be associated with specific issues—e.g. recall bias, dubious veracity of responses, different interpretations of specific notions by participants and interviewers, uncertain association between measurements and the interaction of interest (see Sect. 11.4). These issues should be identified and accounted for when interpreting the results. While interview-based surveys are widely used to capture a variety of relational data, other approaches may be less labour-intensive, more valid and reliable, depending on the studied system. These may include the use of archives, systematic records of animal movements between premises, lists of suppliers/customers and minutes of meetings. Regardless of the way in which data are collected, the completeness and quality of the information should always be assessed.

In certain cases, such as livestock movement data recorded through a well-established tracing system, relational data can be collected exhaustively, capturing all the interactions occurring among all the elements of a system, or at least within a subset of them. In the latter case, the data would be referred to as partial. In many instances, however, it is not possible, and data need to be collected in the field. If a census of nodes in the system is available, an initial set of nodes can be randomly sampled, and their edges recorded. If the nodes with which those sampled nodes interact are identified, the approach is referred to as *labelled star sampling*; if in-contact nodes are not identified, it is referred to as *unlabelled star sampling*. Unless a high proportion of nodes are sampled, the constructed network may not reflect the actual network. In particular, the network connectivity may be underestimated, and the relative importance of sampled nodes overestimated. In contrast to a random sampling, which ignores the dependencies between nodes, an approach based on *link tracing* may better capture the network structure as its connectivity is used to identify nodes and edges. Such a sampling design, often referred to as *snowball sampling*, is an extension of labelled star sampling. Neighbours of the initial set of nodes (or *seeds*) which were identified and were not among the seeds, constitute the first wave. The edges and neighbours of the first wave nodes are listed, and newly identified nodes referred to as the second wave. The process is reiterated until a predefined number of waves are reached, or until saturation of the node set. As this sampling design relies on link tracing, it is particularly helpful when the system boundaries and elements are unknown, and, therefore, beyond network analysis, to study hard-to-reach populations. It should, however, be noted that the choice of seeds may have a high impact on the structure of the constructed network. For instance, if the network is formed of isolated components or is strongly structured into communities bridged by a limited number of edges, this feature may be missed, and only a given component (or community) may be captured.

It may not always be doable—and suitable—to attempt capturing a whole network and it may be more appropriate to focus on egocentric networks. Such networks are formed by an *ego* (the sampled node), and its *alters* (nodes with which it interacts). It includes edges between the ego and its alters as well as edges reported by the ego among its alters. Egocentric networks can thus be sampled through standard sampling design approaches and treated as independent observations. An obvious limitation of the approach is the lack of assessment of the overall network connectivity. Egocentric networks have been widely used in the study of social networks, in particular to assess the role of the social environment on support and welfare, or to identify stakeholders who could benefit from *structural holes* [24]. Examples in the epidemiology literature include Danon et al. [25] and Fournie et al. [26]. Sampling design and data collection procedures are further discussed in Robins [21].

Instead of capturing all edges existing at a given point in time, or occurring within a given time period, relational data can be captured longitudinally. Adding a temporal dimension to the network data would allow the description of temporal changes in network structures, and the joint evolution of these structures and node attributes [27].

11.2.3 Network Analysis Software

A range of software and programming libraries are available to conduct network analysis. The choice of a particular software should be made based on the type of analysis to be performed. For the visualisation of a network and nodes' attributes, and the measurement of common node- and network-level metrics, several free and open source software exist, such as *Gephi* [28]. They enable the user to navigate graphically within a network, which may account for several thousands of nodes, to zoom, colour and change the layout of the whole network based on network metrics. Its Graphical User Interface (GUI) is intuitive and the user does not need any programming skills. Other user-friendly software exist and include, for instance, *Ucinet* [29], *Pajek* [30] and the *Social Network Visualizer* [31].

For some advanced analyses, however, dedicated programming libraries may be needed. They require to have some knowledge in a statistical and mathematical scripting language such as *R* [32] or *Python*. Libraries also exist in general purpose programming languages such as *C*, *Fortran* or *C++*, requiring even more programming knowledge, and are mainly useful for users wanting to develop their own library. Many advanced network data visualisation and analysis tools exist for R and the *SciPy* ecosystem of libraries written for Python. Available in R, the *igraph* package [33] and the *statnet* suite of libraries [34] are among the most complete. *Statnet* includes, for instance, the *sna* package [35], with a large range of functions for conducting network analysis; the *ergm* packages [36], a collection of functions to fit, simulate, plot and evaluate exponential random graph models; and *EpiModel* [37], to simulate the spread of infectious diseases over a static or dynamic network.

11.3 Network Structural Properties

11.3.1 Node-Level Centrality

A frequent objective of network analysis is the identification of the most important nodes. In animal health surveillance, possible definitions of the importance of a node may include, for instance, its likelihood (or the time required for the node) to become infected (or contaminated) if an infection spread through a network, or the amount of health-related information attracted by an actor. Several metrics have been developed to assess nodes' relative importance, each measuring different aspects of the node position in the network, relying on different assumptions about diffusion processes. There is not a unique measure providing a complete and sufficient assessment of nodes' importance for all contexts. Instead, based on the research objectives and assumptions about the diffusion process of interest, several measures may be selected and compared.

The *centrality measures* proposed by Freeman [38] are the most commonly used node-level metrics: *degree*, *betweenness* and *closeness*. Degree is equal to the number of nodes to which a given node is connected. It is based on the view that the more a node is active and interacts with other nodes, the more central it is in the network. In directed networks, we differentiate in-degree, the number of nodes sending an edge to a given node, and out-degree, the number of nodes receiving an edge from a given node. Similarly, the strength of a node can be defined in weighted networks as the sum of the strengths of the edges received by and/or leaving from this node. Contrary to degree and strength, which assess the direct connection of a node and thus only reflect the local structure of the network, betweenness and closeness take into consideration its global structure. Betweenness informs on the extent to which a node is located between other pairs of nodes, and closeness measures how close a node is from others. Thus, these two measures correspond to two different definitions of being central in a network. While nodes that sit on many paths are more likely to facilitate the diffusion process, nodes close to others may quickly acquire and/or transmit an infection, or an information.

Closeness is classically defined as the inverse of the sum of all the *geodesic distances* from a given node to all others. A geodesic distance g_{ij} is the length of the shortest path between two nodes i and j (i.e. minimal number of edges required to connect nodes i and j), with a path being a sequence of distinct edges and nodes connecting two given nodes. For a node k, the closeness is $(N-1)/\sum_{i \neq k} g_{ki}$, where N is the number of nodes. If two nodes i and j are disconnected, then $g_{ij} \to \infty$ and the closeness is equal to zero. Alternatives may be to assess closeness only within connected components, or, as suggested by Kolaczyk [19], to set up an upper limit on g_{ij}, equal, for instance, to N or the maximal geodesic distance. Similarly to degree, edge directions can be accounted for, leading to the estimation of in- and out-closeness. Betweenness is often defined as the frequency at which a given node lies on the geodesic path between two other nodes. For a node k, it is given by $\sum_{i,i \neq j \neq k} \sum_{j,i \neq j \neq k} g_{ij/k} / \sum_{l} g_{ij/l}$, where $g_{ij/k}$ is the number of geodesic paths between nodes i and j passing by k. This definition of betweenness implicitly assumes that a phenomenon diffusing through the network takes the most direct paths to reach a given node. An opposite assumption would be that phenomena diffuse without any idea of their direction. With random-walk betweenness, the choices of consecutive edges from a given node to another are made at random, a path being formed through a random walk. All possible paths, and not only geodesic distances, thus contribute to the measure [39]. Such a definition may better reflect the stochastic nature of the contagion process [9, 11]. With regard to the spread of information, it is likely that the most suitable definition falls in between these two extremes [20].

Although degree, betweenness and closeness are often found to be positively correlated in empirical networks [13], this may not necessarily be the case, as it depends on the global network structure, in particular its structuration into communities (see 11.3.2) [40]. Degree considers that all neighbours of a given node are equivalent. Some other measures account for the status of those neighbours. They rely on the idea that the centrality of a node increases if it is connected to nodes which are central themselves. *Bonacich's eigenvector centrality* is one of the most commonly used of such metrics [41]. It may not, however, always be computable in directed networks [20]. A variant, *alpha centrality* [42], is described and an application presented in Case Study 11.2.

Several other centrality measures, variants of those abovementioned, or based on other definition of centrality and importance, have been proposed. We refer the readers to textbooks mentioned in the introductory section of this chapter. Worth mentioning here are the two "prestige" metrics *PageRank* [43], one of the key algorithms on which Google relies to rank web pages, and *Kleinberg's hubs and authorities* [44], which could be particularly relevant to explore the flow of information in an animal health surveillance network. In a directed network, PageRank's score of a node increases as it receives edges from important nodes. The contribution of a sender (i.e. a node sending a directed edge towards another node) to the score of a given node is inversely proportional to the sender's out-degree, ensuring that nodes with extremely high out-degree do not pass much centrality on to all receiving nodes, and do not disproportionally influence the ranking. In some situations, it may be more relevant to consider that the centrality of a node should increase as it points towards central nodes. Kleinsberg's algorithm thus defines, for each node, an authority and hub scores; with an authority being a node pointed to by many hubs, and a hub a node pointing to many authorities.

Input and *output domain* sizes, with the latter being sometimes referred to as infection chain, are the number of other nodes that can reach and are reachable by a given node. These measures have been interpreted as an assessment of the number of nodes that could infect or be infected by a given node.

In a weighted network, the computation of geodesic distances depends on the interpretation of edge strengths. In contact and information-sharing networks, edge strength is generally expressed as being inversely proportional to the distance. For instance, the more two farms trade cattle between one another, the closer epidemiologically they would be expected to be. Likewise, we may want to consider that the proximity between two actors increases with the frequency at which they meet and exchange information. The geodesic distance can be then defined as the sum of the inverse edge strengths [45], known as *Dijkstra's algorithm*. It may not, however, exactly reflect the process at play. For instance, if s cattle are moved from premises A to B, the epidemiological distance between these two premises may be better defined by $(1 - p)^s$ than $1/s$, with the former being the probability of the infection not spreading from A to B given that A is infected, and p the probability of a single cattle transmitting the infection. In order to simplify the analysis of weighted networks, Kao et al. [3] proposed to deconstruct networks of potentially infectious contacts and to create epidemiological networks composed by truly infectious edges that would occur if a given node was infected. Practically, for each initially weighted edge, the probability of infection given that the sender is infected needs to be computed (see an application in [13]). An epidemiological network is then simulated by applying a Bernoulli trial on each edge. This network, edges of which can now be considered equally, is thus created and analysed as a binary network. As such a network is stochastically generated, the procedure needs to be repeated a great number of times, such that each centrality measure is not represented by a single estimate, but a distribution.

Depending on the research question, the centrality of edges may be of greater interest than the centrality of nodes, for instance, if surveillance activities target interactions rather than actual nodes, or if the emphasis is on the identification of the most important channels through which information spreads, rather than on the actors receiving or sending information. Centrality measures described above can be then computed for edges by building a dual network in which nodes are changed into edges and edges into nodes.

Case Study 11.2 Use of Bonacich's Alpha Centrality Measure to Assess Information Sharing [17]

The amount of information collected by an actor (node) in an information-sharing network depends on the centrality of its neighbours. It may also depend on exogenous factors, which are independent from the network structure (e.g. geographical proximity to an outbreak location). These aspects are captured by Bonacich's alpha centrality measure [42]. The vector x of nodes' Alpha centrality is given by: $x = \alpha A^T x + e$. A^T is the transpose of the adjacency matrix, e the vector of exogenous influences on nodes, and α a parameter relating to the relative importance of the network topology: The higher the α, the higher the contribution of the network structure (endogenous influence) to node centrality.

When dealing with information on disease outbreaks, one needs to differentiate "primary" information flows, provided by farmers directly witnessing disease signs, from "secondary" information flows (or "hearsay") involving actors sharing an information obtained from someone else. For instance, during an epidemic, a farmer may openly talk about disease events occurring on someone else's farm, while dissimulating cases occurring on their own farm. Hence, the spread of information results from two directed networks: one shaped by "primary" information flows, and another by "secondary" information flows. These two networks have the same nodes (individual actors or categories of actors) but different edges (relating to the primary or secondary nature of the information). A case study was conducted in Northern and Southern Vietnam to assess flows of information on avian influenza (AI) outbreak suspicions between groups of stakeholders (e.g. farmers, government veterinarians, feed industry). It was assumed that each node i had exogenous sources of information e_i that directly came from first-hand witnesses of disease events. In other words, each value e_i was the in-degree of node i when only primary information flows were considered. The obtained centrality measure can be considered as an indicator of the relative likelihood of each node being informed of an AI outbreak suspicion. While poultry farmers were most likely to be informed, other categories of actors (e.g. vet shops, feed dealers) had a privileged access to information on AI suspicions, depending on the farm type and study area (Figs. 11.3 and 11.4).

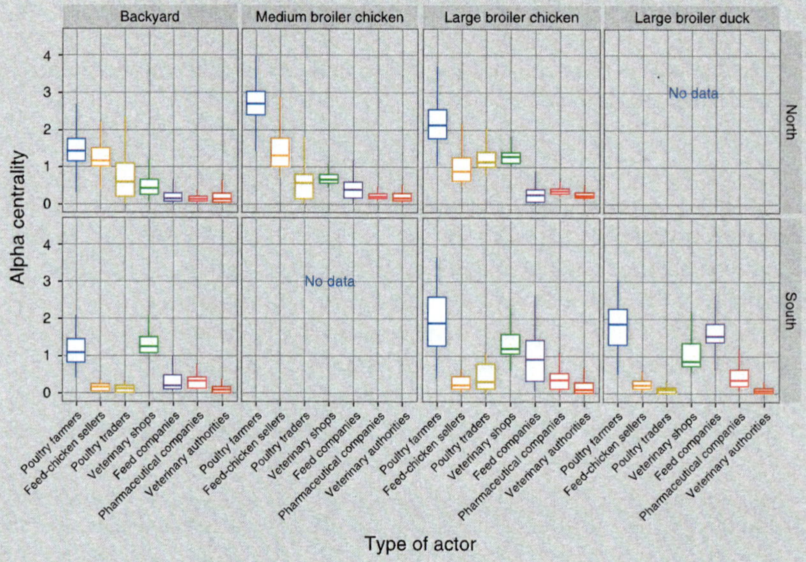

Fig. 11.3 Ranges of alpha centrality for different categories of actors. Results are differentiated according to the primary source of information (production type of affected farms) and the study area (Northern and Southern study areas)

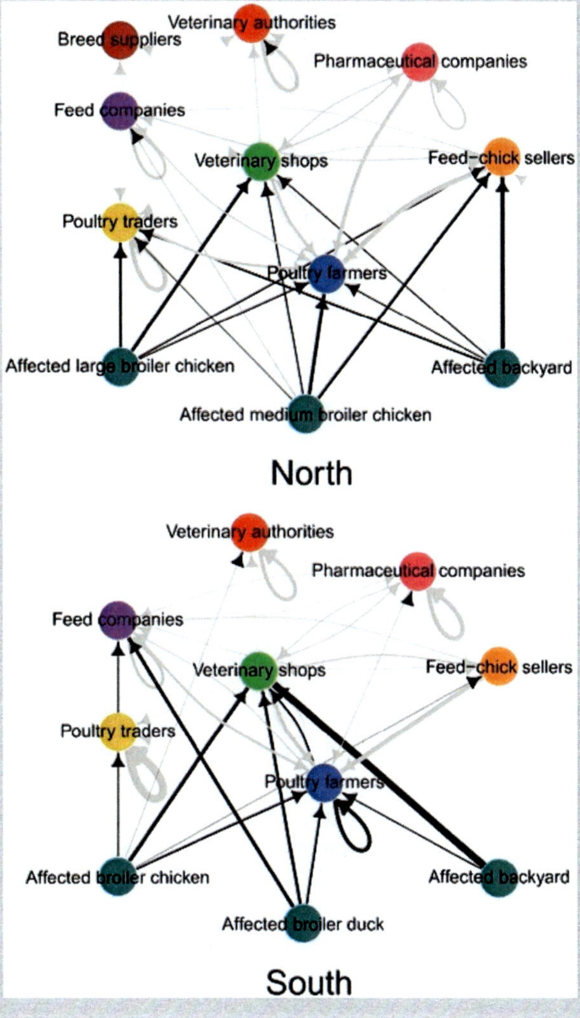

Fig. 11.4 Information-sharing networks of avian influenza suspicion information identified in the two study areas in Northern and Southern Vietnam [17]

11.3.2 Large-Scale Structure of Networks

11.3.2.1 Cohesion

An important question in network analysis is to find out whether nodes in a network can directly or indirectly reach one another—i.e. if there is at least one path between any pair of nodes. Such a network is said to be *connected*. However, empirical networks can be separated in *disconnected components*, each component being a maximal subset of connected nodes. Typically, a single component encompasses most nodes, while the rest of nodes are either isolated or grouped in much smaller components. In the literature, the largest component is often referred to as the *giant connected component*, even though the terms are not actually synonymous in network theory. See Newman [20] for further discussion on this topic. In directed networks, we differentiate *weakly and strongly connected components*, which correspond to the maximal subsets of nodes in which any node can reach any other regardless, or following, edge directions, respectively. The sizes of the largest strong and weakly connected components can be interpreted as estimates of the lower and upper bound of the maximum epidemic size [3]. Directed network are often shaped around one large strongly connected component, which is associated to an *in-* and an *out-component*, respectively defined as the sets of nodes that can reach or from which the strongly connected component can be reached, following network edges. Such representations of network structures are useful to characterise regions of the network according to their potential to spread and/or acquire infection or information [46]. Identifying nodes, or groups of nodes, the removal of which disconnects large components into smaller subsets may allow locating where the network is vulnerable.

The connectivity of a network can be further explored by assessing the *density, clustering coefficient* and *average path length* of its components. The density is the ratio between the observed number of edges among a group of nodes and the total number of possible edges between those nodes. The clustering coefficient measures the degree to which nodes tend to cluster together. Also referred to as transitivity, it is classically calculated as the fraction of closed triplets [19]. A triplet is a group of three nodes, connected by two or three links (i.e. open and closed triplets). It can be interpreted as the probability that two neighbours of a given node are neighbours themselves. The direction and weight of edges can be accounted for [22, 47, 48]. From an epidemiological point of view, clustering may first increase the speed at which a disease spreads within a network, but would then reduce the transmission: as several nodes share many neighbours, the number of susceptible neighbours an infectious node can infect decreases with successive generations [49]. Local clustering coefficient, for each node, can also be computed. Often correlated to betweenness, this measure may indicate the presence of structural holes in a network, i.e. the absence of edges between nodes surrounding a given node. In a social network, structural holes may contribute to the social capital of an individual, providing them with the control of the flow of information (e.g. about disease outbreaks) as this individual becomes an indispensable intermediary between other actors who lack other alternatives [24]. When a network has a high level of clustering and short distances between any two nodes, it is referred to as a *small-world* [50], a concept popularised by the notion of six degrees of separation. In such networks, a disease or an information can rapidly reach any region of the network. This feature can be assessed by comparing the observed clustering coefficient and average path length (i.e. the mean of all geodesic distances within a component) to those of random networks with the same number of nodes and edges. In a small-world network, the clustering coefficient is higher than in random networks, but the average path length is about the same.

11.3.2.2 Degree Distribution

While degree (or strength) was presented above as a node-level metric, its distribution provides information about the overall structure of the network. Most, if not all, networks of interest for animal health surveillance exhibit right-skewed degree distribution: most nodes are peripheral, with low degree, whereas there are a small number of nodes that account for a large proportion of edges. The presence of highly connected nodes, often referred to as hubs, increases the speed at which an infection spreads in a network, and lowers the epidemic threshold—i.e. the minimal transmission level under which infection cannot spread. Indeed, although most nodes are peripheral, they are all close to a hub, and once a hub is infected, a large part of the network becomes exposed. Such properties are even exacerbated for a class of networks, referred to as *scale-free*. The degree distribution then follows a power-law regime [18, 51], appearing as a straight line on a log-log plot. The proportion of nodes of degree k is given by $Ck^{-\alpha}$, with C a constant and α the exponent. In large scale-free networks, hubs dramatically reduce path lengths, making them ultra-small worlds [52], and the epidemic threshold vanishes. An infection can almost instantaneously reach most nodes, and spread despite a very low transmission potential [18]. Due to the relevance of those properties for disease dynamics, networks presented in the animal health literature are often described as scale-free. However, the statistical exploration of these claims is often limited. Estimated exponent values need to be interpreted with caution, and may only be meaningful for very large networks, in which the degree spans over several orders of magnitude. This is important as network properties depend on α, which typically ranges between 2 and 3 in a scale-free regime. Conclusions about a network being scale-free are sometimes drawn for much higher α values, despite the rapid decay of the degree distribution resulting in fewer and smaller hubs, and in network properties difficult to distinguish from those of random networks. Moreover, fitting is further complicated as a power-law regime may not be followed by the entire range of the degree distribution, due to low- and high-degree cut-offs. Algorithms for fitting degree distributions and additional details can be found in Clauset et al. [53], Barabási [18] and Kolaczyk [19].

Networks with similar degree distributions may greatly differ in the way nodes are paired. Degree correlation can be defined as the relationship between the degree of a node and the average degree of its neighbours. A correlation coefficient r can be computed, with $-1 \leq r \leq 1$ [54], and be generalised for directed and weighted networks [47, 54]. In assortative networks ($r > 0$), nodes tend to be connected to other nodes of similar degree. Such pattern leads to the creation of a dense core of high-degree nodes linked together, surrounded by a sparse periphery formed by low-degree nodes. In contrast, high-degree nodes tend to link with low-degree nodes in disassortative networks ($r < 0$), promoting *star* motifs rather than a core/periphery structure. While most social networks are assortative, livestock movement networks are frequently found to be disassortative [5, 55]. These patterns have consequences for the epidemic threshold and the speed at which an infection spreads, both being respectively lower and higher in assortative than disassortative networks. Indeed, as hubs would be rapidly infected during an epidemic, connection between them would further promote the transmission of infection.

11.3.2.3 Partition

A common objective of network analysis is the identification of cohesive groups, within which connections between nodes are frequent. Indeed, the existence of such groups, within which the spread of disease and information would be expected to be intense, would impact on the effectiveness of a given surveillance design. As with the assessment of the importance of nodes, there are many different ways to define, and assess, the cohesion of networks. Several criteria have thus been adopted. Adjacency-based groups, or *cliques*, require that all nodes within the group exchange edges. As most empirical networks are sparse, cliques are generally small, even in large networks. Several variants have been proposed to relax this stringent criterion, including k-core, for which each node is connected to at least k other nodes of the group. Cohesion can also rely on the concept of reachability: nodes do not necessarily need to be directly connected for the rapid diffusion of an infection or information within a group, but they need to be rapidly reachable. n-cliques are thus defined as the maximal subset in which all geodesic distances $\leq n$.

These approaches are based on defining motifs, and then on searching whether they are present in the network of interest. Alternatively, we may aim to partition a network in an unspecified number of *communities*—i.e. a locally densely connected subset, within which nodes are more likely to be linked with other members in the community, than with nodes that do not belong to it. The most common approach to detect communities is to maximise a measure of the quality of the network partition, the *modularity*. It assesses whether the number of edges in each group of nodes is higher than what would be expected by chance. The partition with the highest modularity offers the optimal community structure [56]. There are, however, several limitations with this measure. The modularity function does not have a clear peak, but reaches a plateau around its maximum, making the optimal partition difficult to distinguish from suboptimal propositions. Also, small communities are forced into larger ones. It may therefore be useful to explore whether large communities exhibit an internal community structure. Community detection algorithms generally partition networks by allocating each node to a single community. Yet, we may expect a node to belong to several communities, and therefore communities to overlap. For instance, a layer farm may be provided with feed by a given company, sell its eggs to another, and be visited by a given veterinary practice. Instead, an edge, rather than a node, may be seen as belonging to a specific community. By defining a community as a set of interrelated edges, all the edges, and not the nodes, of a network are partitioned into non-overlapping communities. A node may then belong to as many communities as its edges belong to [57].

Rather than grouping nodes which are intensely connected to each other, we may aim to identify *positions*, subsets of nodes which are similarly embedded in the network. Indeed, two nodes having similar connections to other nodes in the network may have the same influence on the transmission of an infection or an information. Therefore, identifying positions and relationships among them can reveal the underlying network architecture shaping the pattern of spread of a given phenomenon. This may, for instance, be useful to identify premises which are likely to become infected rapidly following the emergence of an infectious agent in a production system, and which should, therefore, be targeted by an early disease detection programme, or, in a surveillance network, to identify stakeholders or organizations controlling the flow of information. The analysis of positions is generally based on the exploration of the *structural equivalence* of nodes (see Wasserman and Faust [22] for alternative definitions of equivalence). An application is presented in Case study 11.3. Two nodes are said to be structurally equivalent if they have the same set of edges with other nodes in the network. As nodes are unlikely to be strictly equivalent, the extent to which nodes are equivalent needs to be measured, using different definition of correlation or distances. Based on these measures, nodes are then grouped into classes (or positions), using, for instance, hierarchical clustering. The edge density within and between those classes can then be assessed, and a *blockmodel* specified. With such a model, rows and columns of an adjacency matrix are permuted such that nodes belonging to the same class are adjacent to each other. A block refers to the submatrix which includes all edges within a class or between two given classes. If nodes were exactly structurally equivalent, each block would either be filled with only 0 or 1 s. As this is never the case in practice, a statement needs to be made about the presence or absence of connections within and between classes by defining a criterion, for instance, based on a block density being lower or higher than the overall network density [22]. An alternative statistical approach to positional analysis can be adopted through *stochastic blockmodelling*. The membership of each node to a class is not predefined but determined independently. The probability of class memberships (i.e. the probability of each node belonging to each class) and intra- and inter-class connections is estimated, and can be used to determine class assignment and relationships [22, 58].

Case Study 11.3 A Positional Analysis to Inform Risk-Based Surveillance [11]
A questionnaire-based cross-sectional study was conducted among poultry traders operating in the Lake Alaotra region in Madagascar in order to identify the fokontanys (fifth and smallest administrative division) where poultry disease surveillance should take place. A positional analysis was conducted on a binary and undirected network resulting from the movement of poultry and their traders between fokontanys. The Euclidean distance was used as the measure of equivalence. For nodes i and j, it was the distance between rows i and j and columns i and j of the adjacency matrix: $d_{ij} = \sqrt{\sum_k \left(x_{ik} - x_{jk}\right)^2 + \left(x_{ki} - x_{kj}\right)^2}$, with x_{ik} being equal to 1 or 0 if an edge is present or absent, respectively, between nodes i and k. Note that $d_{ij} = 0$ if nodes i and j are perfectly equivalent. Based on the pairwise distances, hierarchical clustering was used with Ward's algorithm to partition the network into classes minimizing within-class, and maximizing

between-class variance [59]. A blockmodel was then developed. There was a connection between (within) classes if the inter- (intra-) density was higher than the overall network density. The 347 nodes were distributed into 5 classes. The third class was the smallest ($n = 12$) but its nodes were hubs. It was associated with the highest intra- and inter-class densities, and was the only class connecting all others. This was because a large market was located in each fokontany of that class. This class should therefore be targeted by surveillance programmes (Fig. 11.5).

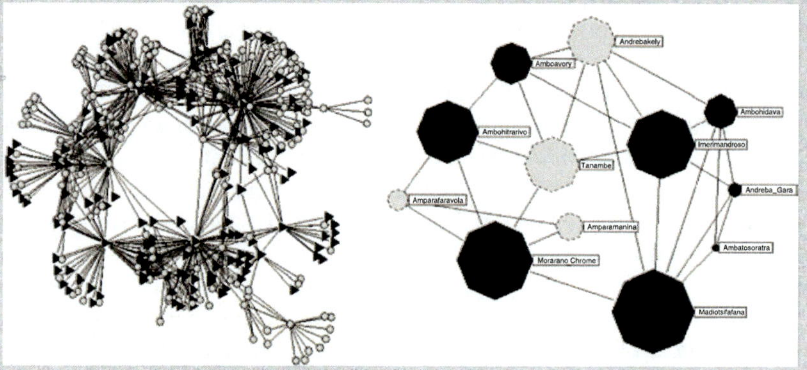

Fig. 11.5 On the left hand, the figure depicts the poultry trading network. The black triangles indicate the nodes which experienced outbreak(s) during the study period (Dec 2009–Dec 2010). On the right hand, the figure shows the connections and the nodes belonging to the third structural equivalence class. This class is the only one connected with all the other classes in the network. The black nodes experienced outbreaks during the study period and nodes sizes are proportional to their random-walk betweenness values. These nodes could be chosen for targeted surveillance

11.4 Models of Disease Transmission

So far, we have focused on the description of network structural features affecting diffusion patterns. By combining network data and mathematical models of disease transmission, it becomes possible to simulate the spread of an infectious agent through a network. Such modelling approaches have been used to assess how network structures influence disease dynamics, and to predict the trajectory and scale of disease outbreaks. Moreover, by explicitly integrating surveillance and control programmes into the model, their effectiveness (e.g. time required to detect the circulation of a new infection) can be quantitatively assessed. Models thus have an increasingly important role in informing policy development in both the public and animal health sectors.

A model conceptualises the spread of infectious agents within single or multiple host populations using mathematical language. Its *unit* refers to the host. It can be an individual host (e.g. a cow), or a host population (e.g. a herd). The infectious agent is not explicitly modelled, but rather the transition of units through a predefined sequence of mutually exclusive health states. In the simplest version, only two health states are considered, *Susceptible* and *Infected*. Susceptible units become infected if they come into contact with an infected unit. Other health states can be considered to reflect the epidemiology of the infectious agent of interest within the studied host population. For instance, infected units may ultimately recover from infection and develop a life-long immune protection, they are then said to be *Recovered*, or the infection may cause their death or culling, infected units are then *Removed*.

In a network-based model, the unit will generally be the network node.[2] As nodes differ in the way in which they are embedded in the network and a frequent objective of such analyses is the identification of nodes to be targeted by risk-based surveillance, models are generally stochastic and individual-based. Each node (or unit) is explicitly represented, and their infection state is tracked over time. The transition of nodes from the susceptible to the infected state is modelled as a random process, a Bernoulli trial with the probability of success being the probability of infection. When assuming random-mixing, i.e. units are equally likely to contact all other units, the probability of infection is the same for all susceptible units. It is expressed as $1-\left(1-\tau c/[N-1]\right)^{I_t}$, with N the number of units, I_t the number of infected units at time t, c the average number of contacts made by a unit per timestep, and τ the probability of a contact being effective (i.e. resulting in infection if involving a susceptible and an infected unit). In a network, a node only comes into contact with their network neighbours. The probability of infection of a susceptible node i between time t and $t + \Delta t$ is then given by $1-\prod_{j}\left(1-\tau\right)^{m_{ji}\mathbf{1}_{jt}}$, where $\mathbf{1}_{jt}$ is an indicator function equal to 1 if node j is infected at time t, and to 0 otherwise. m_{ji} is an element of the adjacency matrix, informing on the absence ($m_{ji} = 0$) or presence ($m_{ji} > 0$) of an edge from node j to i. In a weighted network, m_{ji} is equal to the edge strength, i.e. the number of infectious contacts between j and i. If the network structure changes over time, the actual sequence of edge formation and disappearance can be accounted for, with m_{ji} now referring to the presence of an edge at time t.

As all nodes are explicitly modelled and their infection status tracked over time, different surveillance scenarios can be tested. The infection of a given set of nodes after a predefined time period, or the length of time from disease incursion into the network to the infection of at least one node of that set can be assessed (e.g. Fournie et al. [13] and Case Study 11.4). Further features of surveillance, such as the sampling frequency and the node-level sensitivity can be accounted for. Assuming that the diagnostic test is 100% specific, the detection of the infection in a node i at

[2] When a node is a host population (e.g. a herd), it may be relevant to simulate disease dynamics within a node, as it may impact on the overall infection spread pattern. Individual-based or compartmental meta-population models may be specified [60].

time t is simulated as a Bernoulli trial with the probability of success being $Se\mathbf{1}_{it}\mathbf{1}_{S_t(i)}$, where Se is the probability to detect the infection in a node given that it is infected and tested,[3] and $\mathbf{1}_{S_t(i)}$ is an indicator function equal to 1 if node i is among the set S_t of tested nodes at time t, and 0 otherwise. To learn about different types of mathematical models, readers are referred to the textbooks Keeling and Rohani [61]; Diekmann and Heesterbeek [62] and Vynnycky and White [63].

Case Study 11.4 Modelling Disease Spread and Surveillance Through a Cattle Trade Network [64]

The cattle trade network in Mayotte, an island in the Indian Ocean, was studied to identify which communes should be targeted to detect the incursion of an exotic disease as early as possible. The spread of a hypothetical exotic disease was simulated based on cattle movement data collected from 2007 to 2014. In each simulation, all communes were susceptible until the infection was seeded in a random commune on a random day. Daily cattle movements between communes were then replayed as recorded in the dataset. The probability P_{ijd} that a commune j was infected by commune i on day d was: $P_{ijd} = 1 - (1 - p)^{m_{ijd}}$ if commune i was infected, and $P_{ijd} = 0$ if commune i was not infected. p was the probability that an animal from an infected commune was infectious and transmitted the disease if moved in another commune, and m_{ijd} was the number of animals moved from commune i to j on day d. A total of 20,000 epidemic simulations were generated for different values of p. For each simulation and each commune, the time between the day the infection was seeded on the island, and the day the commune was infected ("time-to-infection") was computed, and its distribution across all the simulations was assessed for each value of p.

Time-to-infection values were compared between central and outer communes classified based on the communes' structural equivalence (see Sect. 11.3.2) in yearly static networks. The stochastic simulations showed that central communes were infected earlier than outer communes when the incursion and spread of a hypothetical exotic disease was simulated on the network. The median number of days from disease incursion to commune infection was about 1.4 times lower for central than outer communes, suggesting that central communes should be targeted by surveillance activities (Fig. 11.6).

[3] If the node is an animal, it is the sensitivity of the laboratory diagnostic test. If the node is a population, it accounts for the laboratory diagnostic test sensitivity and the sample size.

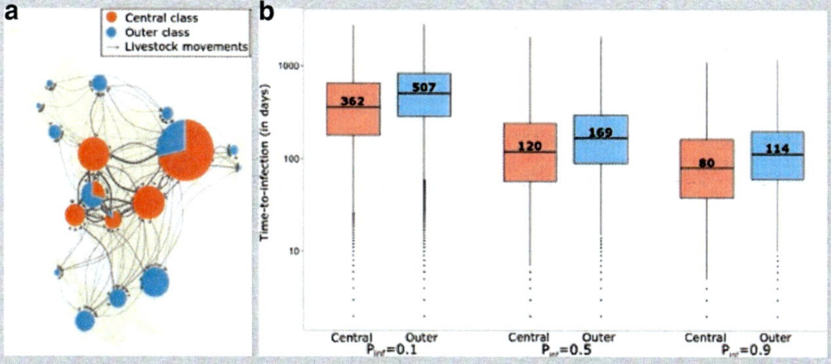

Fig. 11.6 On the left hand side, the Mayotte livestock trade network. The node size is proportional to the number of livestock in 2010. Pie chart: the proportion of communes' cluster membership over the study years (red: central communes, blue: outer communes). On the right hand side, the median and distribution of time-to-infection values (in days) for the two clusters

11.5 Conclusions

By characterising the structural properties of a network, it becomes possible to assess how these properties may impact on the spread of a disease, or the dissemination of an information, through the network of interest. For instance, understanding the way in which the network structure influences the likelihood and speed at which a suspicion of an outbreak reaches the veterinary services, and is communicated to the relevant stakeholders, is directly relevant to the assessment of the sensitivity and timeliness of a surveillance programme. Premises, or group of premises, which may be at higher risk of becoming infected and/or spreading an infection due to their position in the network may be identified; likewise for actors, or groups of actors, which may have a privileged access to animal health-relevant information. The identification of those network nodes which should be or should have been targeted by surveillance activities can thus inform the design and evaluation of surveillance programmes. We introduced here some key methods to explore network structural features which are relevant in the context of animal health surveillance design and evaluation. We focused on methods commonly used in the animal health literature but also touched on some others which have not, or rarely, been used so far, but are nevertheless very relevant to this book topic. There are many more methods, network metrics and algorithms of interest, and we refer the reader to the textbooks mentioned in the introduction for further descriptions. This chapter's focus was on phenomena spreading through networks, and how diffusion patterns are influenced by the network structure. However, a major objective of network analysis, especially in social sciences, is to identify the fundamental processes that govern how network are shaped and organised. Such research questions have started being addressed in the animal health literature, especially through the use of exponential random graph [65] and gravity models [66] to assess the influence of node attributes (e.g. farm type) and edge attributes (e.g. geographical distance between farms) on the presence of an edge. We focused on static networks, for which all edges present during a given time period are considered to be coincidental. However, depending on the speed at which edges are created or disappear and infections or information spread, the length of the time period over which edges are aggregated may impact on the analysis outcome [1]. Accounting for the temporal sequence of edge formation when characterising network structural features impacting on disease dynamics and surveillance effectiveness is an important area of development in network analysis [67, 68].

References

1. Bajardi P, Barrat A, Natale F, Savini L, Colizza V. Dynamical patterns of cattle trade movements. PLoS One. 2011;6(5):e19869. https://doi.org/10.1371/journal.pone.0019869.
2. Dube C, Ribble C, Kelton D, McNab B. A review of network analysis terminology and its application to foot-and-mouth disease modelling and policy development. Transbound Emerg Dis. 2009;56(3):73–85. https://doi.org/10.1111/j.1865-1682.2008.01064.x.
3. Kao RR, Danon L, Green DM, Kiss IZ. Demographic structure and pathogen dynamics on the network of livestock movements in Great Britain. Proc Biol Sci. 2006;273(1597):1999–2007. https://doi.org/10.1098/rspb.2006.3505.
4. Martinez-Lopez B, Perez AM, Sanchez-Vizcaino JM. Social network analysis. Review of general concepts and use in preventive veterinary medicine. Transbound Emerg Dis. 2009;56(4):109–20. https://doi.org/10.1111/j.1865-1682.2009.01073.x.
5. Mweu MM, Fournie G, Halasa T, Toft N, Nielsen SS. Temporal characterisation of the network of Danish cattle movements and its implication for disease control: 2000-2009. Prev Vet Med. 2013;110(3–4):379–87. https://doi.org/10.1016/j.prevetmed.2013.02.015.
6. Ortiz-Pelaez A, Pfeiffer DU, Soares-Magalhaes RJ, Guitian FJ. Use of social network analysis to characterize the pattern of animal movements in the initial phases of the 2001 foot and mouth disease (FMD) epidemic in the UK. Prev Vet Med. 2006;76(1–2):40–55. https://doi.org/10.1016/j.prevetmed.2006.04.007.
7. Baudon E, Fournie G, Hiep DT, Pham TT, Duboz R, Gely M, Peiris M, Cowling BJ, Ton VD, Peyre M. Analysis of swine movements in a province in northern Vietnam and application in the Design of Surveillance Strategies for infectious diseases. Transbound Emerg Dis. 2017;64(2):411–24. https://doi.org/10.1111/tbed.12380.
8. Dean AS, Fournie G, Kulo AE, Boukaya GA, Schelling E, Bonfoh B. Potential risk of regional disease spread in West Africa through cross-border cattle trade. PLoS One. 2013;8(10):e75570. https://doi.org/10.1371/journal.pone.0075570.
9. Molia S, Boly IA, Duboz R, Coulibaly B, Guitian J, Grosbois V, Fournie G, Pfeiffer DU. Live bird markets characterization and trading network analysis in Mali: implications for the surveillance and control of avian influenza and Newcastle disease. Acta Trop. 2016;155:77–88. https://doi.org/10.1016/j.actatropica.2015.12.003.
10. Moyen N, Ahmed G, Gupta S, Tenzin T, Khan R, Khan T, Debnath N, Yamage M, Pfeiffer DU, Fournie G. A large-scale study of a poultry trading network in Bangladesh: implications for control and surveillance of avian influenza viruses. BMC Vet Res. 2018;14(1):12. https://doi.org/10.1186/s12917-018-1331-5.

11. Rasamoelina-Andriamanivo H, Duboz R, Lancelot R, Maminiaina OF, Jourdan M, Rakotondramaro TM, Rakotonjanahary SN, de Almeida RS, Rakotondravao DB, Chevalier V. Description and analysis of the poultry trading network in the Lake Alaotra region, Madagascar: implications for the surveillance and control of Newcastle disease. Acta Trop. 2014;135:10–8. https://doi.org/10.1016/j.actatropica.2014.03.008.
12. Dent JE, Kao RR, Kiss IZ, Hyder K, Arnold M. Contact structures in the poultry industry in Great Britain: exploring transmission routes for a potential avian influenza virus epidemic. BMC Vet Res. 2008;4:27. https://doi.org/10.1186/1746-6148-4-27.
13. Fournie G, Guitian J, Desvaux S, Cuong VC, Dung do H, Pfeiffer DU, Mangtani P, Ghani AC. Interventions for avian influenza A (H5N1) risk management in live bird market networks. Proc Natl Acad Sci U S A. 2013;110(22):9177–82. https://doi.org/10.1073/pnas.1220815110.
14. Rossi G, De Leo GA, Pongolini S, Natalini S, Zarenghi L, Ricchi M, Bolzoni L. The potential role of direct and indirect contacts on infection spread in dairy farm networks. PLoS Comput Biol. 2017;13(1):e1005301. https://doi.org/10.1371/journal.pcbi.1005301.
15. Funk S, Gilad E, Watkins C, Jansen VA. The spread of awareness and its impact on epidemic outbreaks. Proc Natl Acad Sci U S A. 2009;106(16):6872–7. https://doi.org/10.1073/pnas.0810762106.
16. Delabouglise A, Antoine-Moussiaux N, Tatong D, Chumkaeo A, Binot A, Fournie G, Pilot E, Phimpraphi W, Kasemsuwan S, Paul MC, Duboz R, Salem G, Peyre M. Cultural practices shaping zoonotic diseases surveillance: the case of highly pathogenic avian influenza and Thailand native chicken farmers. Transbound Emerg Dis. 2017;64(4):1294–305. https://doi.org/10.1111/tbed.12506.
17. Delabouglise A, Dao TH, Truong DB, Nguyen TT, Nguyen NT, Duboz R, Fournie G, Antoine-Moussiaux N, Grosbois V, Vu DT, Le TH, Nguyen VK, Salem G, Peyre M. When private actors matter: information-sharing network and surveillance of highly pathogenic avian influenza in Vietnam. Acta Trop. 2015;147:38–44. https://doi.org/10.1016/j.actatropica.2015.03.025.
18. Barabási AL. Network science. Cambridge University Press; 2016.
19. Kolaczyk ED. Statistical analysis of network data methods and models, Springer series in statistics. New York: Springer; 2009.
20. Newman MEJ. Networks: an introduction. Oxford: Oxford University Press; 2010.
21. Robins G. Doing social network research: network-based research design for social scientists. Sage; 2015.
22. Wasserman S, Faust K. Social network analysis. Cambridge: Cambridge University Press; 1994.
23. Pham TTH. Economic evaluation of swine disease surveillance system in Vietnam (PhD). Bangkok, Thailand: Kasetsart University; 2016.
24. Burt RS. Structural holes: the social structure of competition. Cambridge: Harvard University Press; 1992.
25. Danon L, House TA, Read JM, Keeling MJ. Social encounter networks: collective properties and disease transmission. J R Soc Interface. 2012;9(76):2826–33. https://doi.org/10.1098/rsif.2012.0357.
26. Fournie G, Tripodi A, Nguyen TT, Nguyen VT, Tran TT, Bisson A, Pfeiffer DU, Newman SH. Investigating poultry trade patterns to guide avian influenza surveillance and control: a case study in Vietnam. Sci Rep. 2016;6:29,463. https://doi.org/10.1038/srep29463.
27. Snijders TA, Van de Bunt GG, Steglich CE. Introduction to actor-based models for network dynamics. Soc Networks. 2010;32(1):44–60.
28. Bastian M, Heymann S, Jacomy M. Gephi: an open source software for exploring and manipulating networks. Paper presented at the International AAAI Conference on Weblogs and Social Media; 2009.
29. Borgatti SP, Everett MG, Freeman LC. Ucinet. In: Encyclopedia of social network analysis and mining; 2014. pp. 2261–2267.
30. Batagelj V, Mrvar A. Pajek-program for large network analysis Connections. 1998;21(2):47–57.
31. Kalamaras DV. Social network visualizer (SocNetV). Social network analysis and visualization software. 2010; Available from: http://socnetv.org.

32. R Development Core Team. R: a language and environment for statistical computing. Vienna, Austria: R Foundation for Statistical Computing; 2015.
33. Csardi G, Nepusz T. The igraph software package for complex network research. Int J Complex Syst. 2006;1695(5):1–9.
34. Handcock MS, Hunter DR, Butts CT, Goodreau SM, Morris M. Statnet: software tools for the representation, visualization, analysis and simulation of network data. J Stat Softw. 2008;24(1):1548.
35. Butts CT. Sna: tools for social network analysis; 2010. http://CRAN.R-project.org/package=sna.
36. Hunter DR, Handcock MS, Butts CT, Goodreau SM, Morris M. Ergm: a package to fit, simulate and diagnose exponential-family models for networks. J Stat Softw. 2008;24(3)
37. Jenness SM, Goodreau SM, Morris M. EpiModel: an R package for mathematical modeling of infectious disease over networks. J Stat Softw. 2018;84
38. Freeman L. A set of measures of centrality based on betweenness. Sociometry. 1977;40(1):35–41.
39. Newman MEJ. A measure of betweenness centrality based on random walks. Soc Networks. 2005;27:39–54.
40. Salathe M, Jones JH. Dynamics and control of diseases in networks with community structure. PLoS Comput Biol. 2010;6(4):e1000736. https://doi.org/10.1371/journal.pcbi.1000736.
41. Bonacich P. Power and centrality: a family of measures. Am J Sociol. 1987;92:1170–82.
42. Bonacich P, Lloyd P. Eigenvector-like measures of centrality for asymmetric relations. Soc Networks. 2001;23(3):191–201.
43. Page L, Brin S, Motwani R, Winograd T. The PageRank citation ranking: Bringing order to the web. Stanford InfoLab. 1999.
44. Kleinberg JM. Authoritative sources in a hyperlinked environment. J ACM (JACM). 1999;46(5):604–32.
45. Dijkstra EW. A note on two problems in connexion with graphs. Numer Math. 1959;1:269–71.
46. Dube C, Ribble C, Kelton D, McNab B. Estimating potential epidemic size following introduction of a long-incubation disease in scale-free connected networks of milking-cow movements in Ontario, Canada. Prev Vet Med. 2011;99(2–4):102–11. https://doi.org/10.1016/j.prevetmed.2011.01.013.
47. Barrat A, Barthelemy M, Pastor-Satorras R, Vespignani A. The architecture of complex weighted networks. Proc Natl Acad Sci U S A. 2004;101(11):3747–52. https://doi.org/10.1073/pnas.0400087101.
48. Opsahl T, Panzarasa P. Clustering in weighted networks. Soc Networks. 2009;31:155–63.
49. Keeling MJ, Eames KT. Networks and epidemic models. J R Soc Interface. 2005;2(4):295–307. https://doi.org/10.1098/rsif.2005.0051.
50. Watts DJ, Strogatz SH. Collective dynamics of 'small-world' networks. Nature. 1998;393(6684):440–2. https://doi.org/10.1038/30918.
51. Amaral LA, Scala A, Barthelemy M, Stanley HE. Classes of small-world networks. Proc Natl Acad Sci U S A. 2000;97(21):11,149–52. https://doi.org/10.1073/pnas.200327197.
52. Cohen R, Havlin S. Scale-free networks are ultrasmall. Phys Rev Lett. 2003;90(5):058701. https://doi.org/10.1103/PhysRevLett.90.058701.
53. Clauset A, Shalizi CR, Newman ME. Power-law distributions in empirical data. SIAM Rev. 2009;51(4):661–703.
54. Newman ME. Assortative mixing in networks. Phys Rev Lett. 2002;89(20):208701.
55. Kiss IZ, Green DM, Kao RR. The network of sheep movements within Great Britain: network properties and their implications for infectious disease spread. J R Soc Interface. 2006;3(10):669–77. https://doi.org/10.1098/rsif.2006.0129.
56. Clauset A, Newman ME, Moore C. Finding community structure in very large networks. Phys Rev E Stat Nonlinear Soft Matter Phys. 2004;70(6 Pt 2):066111. https://doi.org/10.1103/PhysRevE.70.066111.
57. Ahn YY, Bagrow JP, Lehmann S. Link communities reveal multiscale complexity in networks. Nature. 2010;466(7307):761–4. https://doi.org/10.1038/nature09182.

58. Nowicki K, Snijders T. Estimation and prediction for stochastic blockstructures. J Am Stat Assoc. 2001;96(455):1077–87.
59. Manly BFJ. Multivariate statistical methods: a primer, 3rd ed. Chapman & Hall/CRC Press; 2005.
60. Keeling MJ, Danon L, Vernon MC, House TA. Individual identity and movement networks for disease metapopulations. Proc Natl Acad Sci U S A. 2010;107(19):8866–70. https://doi.org/10.1073/pnas.1000416107.
61. Keeling MJ, Rohani P. Modeling infectious diseases in humans and animals. Oxford, UK: Princeton University Press; 2007.
62. Diekmann O, Heesterbeek JA. Mathematical epidemiology of infectious diseases: model building, analysis and interpretation. Chichester; 2000.
63. Vynnycky E, White R. An introduction to infectious disease modelling. Oxford, UK: Oxford University Press; 2010.
64. Kim Y, Dommergues L, M'Sa AB, Merot P, Cardinale E, Edmunds J, Pfeiffer D, Fournie G, Metras R. Livestock trade network: potential for disease transmission and implications for risk-based surveillance on the island of Mayotte. Sci Rep. 2018;8(1):11550. https://doi.org/10.1038/s41598-018-29999-y.
65. Ortiz-Pelaez A, Ashenafi G, Roger F, Waret-Szkuta A. Can geographical factors determine the choices of farmers in the Ethiopian highlands to trade in livestock markets? PLoS One. 2012;7(2):e30710. https://doi.org/10.1371/journal.pone.0030710.
66. Nicolas G, Apolloni A, Coste C, Wint GRW, Lancelot R, Gilbert M. Predictive gravity models of livestock mobility in Mauritania: the effects of supply, demand and cultural factors. PLoS One. 2018;13(7):e0199547. https://doi.org/10.1371/journal.pone.0199547.
67. Bajardi P, Barrat A, Savini L, Colizza V. Optimizing surveillance for livestock disease spreading through animal movements. J R Soc Interface. 2012;9(76):2814–25. https://doi.org/10.1098/rsif.2012.0289.
68. Valdano E, Poletto C, Giovannini A, Palma D, Savini L, Colizza V. Predicting epidemic risk from past temporal contact data. PLoS Comput Biol. 2015;11(3):e1004152. https://doi.org/10.1371/journal.pcbi.1004152.

Part VI

Evaluation in the Policy Cycle

12 Health Surveillance Evaluation in the Policy Cycle

V. J. Del Rio Vilas, M. Arnold, and Marisa Peyre

Abstract

Disease surveillance generates evidence for decision making. Surveillance evaluation focuses on measuring the value of surveillance efforts to take meaningful actions and to inform policy decisions. This value will depend on how well aligned the surveillance efforts are with the fundamental policy question, and on the quality of the surveillance evidence (see Part II). The former relates to strategic relevance, the latter to operational performance. This chapter attempts to explore how evaluation could help improving the strategic relevance of animal health surveillance but also the barriers to the uptake of evaluation recommendations by policy makers, regardless of the surveillance performance itself.

Keywords

Surveillance value · Strategic relevance · Surveillance operationalization · Uncertainty · Forecasting

V. J. Del Rio Vilas
School of Veterinary, University of Surrey, Guildford, UK

Centre for Universal Health, Chatham House, London, UK

M. Arnold
Animal and Plant Health Agency (Weybridge), Surrey, United Kingdom

M. Peyre (✉)
CIRAD, UMR ASTRE, Montpellier, France

ASTRE, CIRAD, INRAE, University of Montpellier, Montpellier, France
e-mail: marisa.peyre@cirad.fr

M. Peyre et al. (eds.), *Principles for Evaluation of One Health Surveillance: The EVA Book*, https://doi.org/10.1007/978-3-030-82727-4_12

12.1 Introduction

12.1.1 Evaluation at the Strategic Level

Whether pursuing a strategic or operational goal, surveillance evaluation is as much a technical endeavour as it is a social one. As such, technical and organizational complexities will be prevalent in the operationalization of the evaluation. Other sections of this book deal mostly with the first type of complexity (see Parts IV and V). In this part, we primarily focus on organizational complexities, although we recognize the often blurred division between the two categories. Within the organizational domain at a strategic level, evaluation of animal health surveillance systems constitutes a multi-dimensional endeavour given the number of decision steps and the need to engage with a diverse stakeholder base with multiple and conflicting values, needs, and expectations.

Most of the existing surveillance evaluation frameworks, and related publications, target until recently surveillance deployment and optimization, i.e. its operational and economic performances. The much higher stakes around strategic surveillance evaluation, its uncertainty in part linked with the long-term horizons considered, and the multiple stakeholders involved may have contributed to the fewer number of publications on strategic evaluation frameworks and efforts. This is worrying. If the question as to why we run a particular surveillance system remains unchallenged, or leads to no measure of the value towards informing the policy, stakeholder or society demand or need (i.e. evaluation to implement meaningful changes), the risk is that surveillance findings, however accurate and precise, may become strategically irrelevant. This is an existential threat to efforts to improve the operationalization of surveillane and its evaluation (Table 12.1).

There are numerous reports of methodologically robust surveillance evaluation exercises that led to imperceptible policy changes [1, 2]. Likewise, examples of surveillance efforts with dubious policy relevance are prevalent, e.g. some forms of dog rabies surveillance where surveillance results provide very little evidence on the extent of disease in the targeted dog populations [3]. For a number of zoonoses, for example echinococcosis granulosus, the primary policy demand is to inform the risk of the disease in the human population. This should set the strategic framework against which all surveillance efforts, including those on the animal hosts (e.g. sheep and dogs), should deliver towards. To the best of our knowledge, there are few reports that measure the relative contribution of animal surveillance sources to the quantification of human risk, independent of the quality of the surveillance operations (as seen in Part III). For tularemia in Finland, Rotejanaprasert and colleagues showed the reduction in risk uncertainty once rodent population data were integrated with human case counts [4].

Table 12.1 Summary of considerations towards implementation of surveillance evaluation to inform policy decisions

#	Considerations	Observations
1	Seek parsimony in the list of surveillance evaluation attributes.	Failure to evaluate all the relevant attributes may lead to added structural uncertainty and limited impact of the evaluation itself. On the other hand, avoid double counting of surveillance evaluation attributes capturing similar underlying performance.
2	If surveillance evaluation is the answer, what was the question?	To stress the importance of a policy-driven evaluation to achieve strategic relevance.
3	No disease surveillance is an island.	Surveillance system evaluations are better conducted within a strategic framework of continuous improvement comprising all health-related capacities.
4	Surveillance evaluation is not the end but a means to an end.	Evaluation must inform a managerial decision, which, if of quality, should lead to a commitment to action [15].
5	Surveillance evaluation must improve things, not correct failures.	If the perceived message by the relevant stakeholders is one of "putting things right or correct existing failures", support from critical stakeholders may dwindle. Improvements on evaluation findings may not materialize entirely due to lack of wide support.
6	Economic benefits are necessary but not sufficient to ensure the implementation of recommendations.	This is due to the multi-dimensional nature of surveillance value. Quantify value as widely as possible encompassing as many attributes and stakeholders as required, in a matrix design, bearing in mind that different attributes will have different relevance to different stakeholders.
7	Quantification over qualification.	To support action via quantification of the evaluation findings (e.g. limited sensitivity) for all variables relevant to the epidemiology of the disease under investigation.
8	Set up regular feedback loops.	They should be clearly described and timed in the evaluation project plan.
9	Consider not just the technical complexities, but the more critical organizational ones.	

12.1.2 The Value of Surveillance and Its Evaluation

Surveillance evaluation focuses on measuring the value of surveillance efforts to inform meaningful actions and relevant policy decisions. It would be restrictive to limit surveillance value to the reduction of disease risk uncertainty, as shown for tularemia. Value is a multi-dimensional concept and other surveillance attributes (e.g. transparency) may be at play which could contribute value to other stakeholders (e.g. farmers surely appreciate ease of reporting while policy actors may allocate greater value to transparency). Until recently, evaluation frameworks had the tendency to focus on effectiveness technical attributes (e.g. sensitivity) while ignoring more qualitative functional attributes (e.g. acceptability), of difficult measurement and aggregation. Not addressing the entire range of attributes leads to partial evaluations that may fail to convene sufficient support across the stakeholders' base for surveillance improvements. In other words, there may be a divide between the strategic evaluation objectives, e.g. to inform the most efficient alternatives towards enhanced surveillance sensitivity, and the operational expectations of field officials that could hamper implementation of the evaluation recommendations [5]. This, in turn, would reduce the impact of the evaluation effort, under the premise that value is only realized through the implementation of the evaluation recommendations (see next section). As advocated in this book, a comprehensive evaluation framework should therefore cover both the strategic and operational demands, and aim to quantify the relative contribution of each relevant operational process towards the strategic goals of the surveillance effort.

Value is unique to each and every stakeholder. Thus, a well-run surveillance effort may be strategically irrelevant but still deliver value to other stakeholders. This value may present itself in the form of enhanced situational awareness for local stakeholders, e.g. the public or local officials responsible for the conduct of the surveillance effort, via the delivery of regular surveillance reports. Methodological challenges remain to enable an evaluation accounting for this wide range of values created by surveillance across society [6]. Value is also context-specific. In a work to assess the relative value of the many rabies capacities that constitute a rabies control programme, e.g. surveillance, dog vaccination, post-exposure prophylaxis, the value of surveillance, relative to the other capacities, changed depending on the endemicity of the disease, and on whether the setting was one of gains (i.e. to support additional capacity building) or losses (i.e. resembling a situation of budget cuts) [7].

An extension of single disease surveillance is the consideration of multiple hazards. In the evaluation of several disease surveillance, led by portfolio managers, the objective is the optimization of resources across disease-specific systems, e.g. via portfolio decision analysis, to deliver the most efficient investment profile [8]. Guo and colleagues present a comprehensive framework that combines a multi-criteria-decision-analysis approach to address stakeholders' preferences with cost–benefit analysis. Given disease relevance as derived from risk assessments, for a specific spatial and temporal setting, different portfolio decision analysis methods can be applied to optimally invest resources across diseases [9]. While prioritizations are gaining popularity to inform the relative relevance of diseases in a specific setting [10], the translation of the prioritization results into resource plans, and within these to specific surveillance improvements across a portfolio of diseases, remains both a technical and organizational challenge.

Prattley et al. [9] proposed the need to consider the risk attitude of decision makers when assessing allocation of surveillance resources across diseases. This consideration also applies to cost-effectiveness analysis of surveillance alternatives for a single hazard. Attema et al. [11] showed that preferences regarding investments to improve surveillance timeliness and false positive rate (FPR) were affected by cognitive biases, namely loss aversion and probability weighing. The authors also quantified the willingness-to-pay (WTP) for such investments and found that, for rabies surveillance, respondents were 2.1 times more willing to pay for improvements in FPR than for those in timeliness. The occurrence of the above biases highlights the need to develop evaluation frameworks that contemplate such biases prior to surveillance investment decisions (see Parts III–V for methods to do so). Failing to do so, for example by ignoring the occurrence of risk aversion, could return biased estimates of the effectiveness of new surveillance streams.

12.1.3 The Delivery of Value Through Implementation of Evaluation Recommendations

What does success look like for a surveillance evaluation? And how do we measure that success? These two questions should be in the mind of anyone planning a surveillance evaluation, from day one. In Box 12.1, we report on a very successful evaluation exercise on bovine spongiform encephalopathy (BSE) surveillance as measured by its policy impact in the UK and the EU. The surveillance changes suggested by the evaluation led to large-scale savings from the abolition of testing of healthy cattle at slaughter in the UK [12], and the reduction of millions of tests in the EU on an annual basis [13]. It is clear from this example that the impact of surveillance evaluation came from the implementation of its recommendations (see Chap. 16).

Ideally, estimation of the impact of recommendations should be part of the evaluation plan once the identification of gaps and surveillance alternatives, to address the gaps, is concluded (see Chap. 16). These alternatives, either to increase overall surveillance capability or to maintain/reduce it in the most efficient manner, are best evaluated under a portfolio approach to account for synergies in both their costs and benefits. This practice, however, is very rare. Most surveillance evaluation efforts tend to describe past accomplishments but fail to formally inform future surveillance performance scenarios. Del Rio Vilas and Pfeiffer [14] stated that "Evaluation of surveillance should be a continuous process rather than an isolated retrospective exercise that highlights past deficiencies with little bearing on the present situation". We now qualify this statement further into two directions linked to the delivery of value: (i) implementation of the evaluation findings, and (ii) into the future, so that the retrospective assessment of the surveillance system is no longer the end but a means to value delivery. Value in a decision setting is an expectation of the probability of the outcome and the "value/impact" of the outcome. It follows that value quantification from surveillance evaluation needs to consider uncertainties associated with the outcome of evaluation, the timing of the possible horizons leading to value realization, and the stakeholders' risk attitudes (see Part II).

The concept of linking surveillance evaluation to policy decisions that are most often forward looking, and demand estimation of decisions impacts, is not prevalent in public or animal health surveillance (Table 12.1). Moreover, current approaches to evaluation of surveillance systems often fail to consider the protracted uncertainty around the input evidence that informs standard surveillance attributes, for instance sensitivity. Subsequent models informing the impact of surveillance improvements based on the evaluation results, calibrated on these data, despite delivering highly accurate outputs, may lead to suboptimal decisions and allocation of resources. The need for surveillance evaluation efforts to allow quantification and propagation of uncertainty to evaluate its impact on the quality of decisions appears evident [5, 16].

Regardless of its focus, strategic or operational, surveillance evaluation requires a clear and relevant question, a framework, and investment to be implemented (e.g.

funding, competences and access to relevant data). From an operational standpoint, the more quantifiable, segmented, and actionable these outputs are, the better are the chances that evaluation outputs would lead to policy action. Early attempts to inform the unobserved number of scrapie affected holdings in the UK failed to provide actionable enough evidence (they merely delivered an estimate of the number of holdings not captured by the existing surveillance system) to lead to policy actions [1, 2]. Later reports tried to increase the policy value of the surveillance evaluation results by means of providing greater detail on the spatial distribution of the missing holdings [17].

12.1.4 Barriers to Implementation of Recommendations from Evaluation

Several motivations may lead to the evaluation of a surveillance system. In general, evaluations can be planned, proactive or reactive. Planned evaluations, i.e. those part of an established programme of ongoing operational improvement and regular strategic review, are not common. Even if a number of organizations may have policies to this effect, their operationalization tends not to follow the letter. Proactive evaluation often originates from internal champions within the organization, both from policy or associated research and executive institutions, and frequently not as a result of a specific policy demand. This type of evaluation, tends to have a scientific motivation, and reduced resource commitment normally constrained to the evaluation exercise, i.e. not expanding to implementation. Lastly, reactive evaluations may stem from responses to enquiries after a failure, or respond to stakeholders' requests.

Surveillance improvements may not see implementation due to the lack of involvement of field staff in the design of the evaluation exercise. The negative effects of this poor early engagement are well described elsewhere and result in a lack of acceptability and recognition of the evaluation results in the field [20, 21] (see Part IV). Also, unless a clear failure in the surveillance system is demonstrated, or significant efficiency gains identified, little appetite by senior management for changes, or other competing priorities, may hamper implementation of evaluation recommendations. Finally, if the perceived deployment costs of the improvements suggested by the evaluation are higher than the expected benefits, it might also stop its implementation. This limitation has been prevalent as until recently evaluation frameworks failed to prioritize the multiple gaps and inform the costs and benefits of the surveillance improvement options. As described in Parts II and III of this book, newly developed evaluation frameworks promoting comprehensive evaluation including technical (e.g. sensitivity, timeliness), functional (e.g. acceptability) and value (e.g. benefits) attributes, should address some of the limitations of the existing surveillance evaluation frameworks: (i) the failure to provide an overall interpretation of the attributes-specific assessments, (ii) the need to incorporate the expectations, perceptions and needs, which would feed into a definition of value, from the multiple stakeholders; and (iii) the need to account for economic value of the different surveillance options [22].

Surveillance is just one element in the range of capacities that constitute disease management programmes. Single surveillance evaluations conducted outside the framework of a portfolio evaluation, whether of multiple disease-specific capacities for one hazard or as part of a portfolio[1] of multiple hazards, may struggle to attract the required resource towards implementation of improvements due to other competing priorities. This of course may also happen within a portfolio approach (as budget constraints will force foregoing of valuable projects, e.g. surveillance improvements for disease A, in benefit of more valuable ones) (see Table 12.2 for the basic principles of portfolio management), but it should lead to no surprises, in an ideal world, given the acceptance by all disease managers of a higher goal: the overall improvement of the portfolio. This uncertain prospect, i.e. whether the identified improvements will be implemented or not, contributes another layer of uncertainty in addition to the parametric uncertainty around evaluation outputs. With this in mind, surveillance system evaluations are better conducted within a strategic framework of continuous improvement comprising all health-related capacities. This helps identification of the relative relevance of surveillance improvements in the overall capacity building effort, and informs the investment boundaries of surveillance-specific improvements.

Table 12.2 Principles of strategic portfolio management

Principle	Observations
Aligned decision forum	A dedicated environment for capacity/disease managers to share their data, evaluation results and assumptions, and discuss the organization's strategic aims.
Value creation focus	The goal is to find the portfolio strategy that maximizes value generation for the organization. This must be accepted by all capacity/disease managers.
Credible, comparable capacity/ disease evaluations	To allow capacity or disease managers to make and accept portfolio-focused decisions.
Embracing uncertainty and dynamics	All uncertainties (parametric around evaluation inputs and outputs, and those relating to implementation success) are addressed explicitly, and updated regularly.
Clear communication and learning between capacity/disease managers within the portfolio	Quality of data, methodologies, and other technical aspects around capacities/diseases evaluations are shared, and performance (of projects or portfolio) is tracked.
Inclusive, collaborative process	All stakeholders participate and derive value from the process.

Adapted from "Strategic portfolio decisions. Strategic decision and risk management. Stanford Center for Professional Development and Strategic Decisions Group, 2009"

[1] a portfolio considers multiple items between which a resource allocation decision has to be made

12.2 The Rest of This Section

Several examples of the integration of surveillance evaluation outputs into the policy cycle are provided in this section. Staerk describes the early detection of animal health hazards in Switzerland as an example of adequate integration of surveillance evaluation and disease mitigation. In this introductory chapter, we also contribute the impactful application of modelling to the evaluation of BSE surveillance data in the UK (Case Study 12.1). The motivation to evaluate BSE surveillance came from European authorities in an attempt to assess whether the levels of testing were proportionate to the risk, given the significant decline in the number of positive samples.

Figuie and Binot argue in Chap. 13 the need for innovation to assess the governance of animal health surveillance. They also highlight the fact that surveillance is not just a technical task and focus on the gap between how surveillance strategies are being defined versus how they are being implemented, trying to bridge the two.

Staerk also describes in Chap. 14 the attempts to conduct cost-effectiveness analyses of different surveillance sources for early detection in Switzerland. This is line with the recent work by Wall et al. [23] who analysed the cost-effectiveness of several surveillance schemes for BSE and scrapie. This last work is much welcomed as it builds on the limited policy value of previous scrapie surveillance evaluation efforts that mostly focused on informing its limited sensitivity [1, 2, 24] or biased spatial representativeness [25].

Peyre et al. present in Chap. 15 a first attempt to evaluate the impact of the evaluation itself, applying the theory of change to assess the relative contribution of the implementation of surveillance evaluation to reaching out disease surveillance wider impacts (e.g. improvement of public health through animal health).

Case Study 12.1 The Methodological Evaluation of Surveillance Evidence: The Case of BSE

Introduction

Bovine Spongiform Encephalopathy (BSE) was first detected in the United Kingdom (UK) in November 1986. The number of cases increased rapidly, and ultimately peaked at over 37,000 in 1992. Epidemiological analysis [26–28] showed that the rendering of cattle to produce meat and bone meal (MBM), and the subsequent inclusion of this MBM in cattle feed, led to the recycling of infection in the cattle population, producing exponential growth in cases. A number of key control measures were introduced in the UK aimed at eliminating the exposure of cattle to feed contaminated with infected MBM. A number of similar measures were taken at different times in EU member states but the use of processed animal proteins was banned in animal feed across the EU from 1 January 2001.

A key element of understanding current trends in BSE prevalence and thus the impact of control measures has been analysis of surveillance data. During the growth of BSE in the UK surveillance was limited to the reporting of clinical suspects by farmers. However, this form of surveillance relies on farmer awareness of clinical signs and on the willingness of farmers to report. This was deemed to produce a biased representation of the distribution of infection and, in an effort to improve our knowledge of the underlying infection load, active surveillance was introduced across the EU in 2001.

The aim of this case study is to look at two examples of how the application of statistical models to the surveillance data has been used to evaluate and improve the surveillance systems and inform policy.

Changes in the age of testing of fallen stock and healthy slaughter

The active surveillance introduced across the EU in January 2001 had required healthy slaughtered cattle to be tested from the age of 30 months of age, with the other "risk" groups (emergency slaughter and fallen stock) being tested from 24 months of age. As the BSE outbreak declined across the EU, there was the question of whether the levels of testing were proportionate to the risk, particularly as the number of positives per 10,000 animals tested had dropped from 1.22 in 2001 to 0.17 in 2007, and was expected to continue to reduce. The European Commission then requested that a modelling study be conducted to determine the impact on the BSE surveillance system of potential changes in the ages of animals tested, i.e. how many positives would be missed and how would this impact the ability to detect re-emergence of BSE if the age at which animals were tested were increased.

The key assumption behind the model was that the observed age distribution of BSE cases in each birth cohort tended to be similar between birth cohorts. Therefore one could predict the number of cases in partially observed cohorts using a normalized "age of onset" distribution. The normalized "age of onset" distribution was obtained from the proportion of fallen stock/emergency slaughter that had been observed in each yearly age range, and similarly for a separate one for healthy slaughtered cattle [29]. This was done using case data from 1994 to 1999. The relative risk of onset for each age group relative to the 7-year age group was calculated for each birth cohort. The average relative risk for each age group was then calculated over all the birth cohorts and this was then normalized to create an "age of onset" distribution for the EU15.

Due to the long incubation period, the prevalence in a birth cohort is problematic to estimate unless the cohort is more than 6 years old. Therefore, at the time of the modelling, there was uncertainty about BSE infection prevalence in post-2000 birth cohorts. Model results were produced using two different assumptions: (i) constant prevalence since 2000 (pessimistic, since control measures had led to a decline in BSE in successive birth cohorts) and (ii) prevalence declining at the rate observed up to and including the 2002 birth cohort. Since retrospectively it is apparent that the latter assumption was more appropriate, only the results from that assumption are reported here.

The models showed that less than two BSE cases per year in healthy slaughtered cattle and in the fallen stock/emergency slaughter stream should be expected from increasing the age of testing from 24 to 60 months. In terms of detecting re-emergence, it was calculated that with an epidemic growth rate of 65% per year (similar to UK in the early 1980s), only 11% of detected cases would be under 48 months. Thus, there would be only a small reduction in the ability of the surveillance system to detect re-emergence of BSE.

These findings were used as the basis for the EU changing the age of sampling of both healthy slaughtered cattle and fallen stock/emergency slaughtered cattle to 48 months. From January 2009, the member states from the EU-15 which could show a declining or low prevalence of BSE and had implemented the EU surveillance for at least six years could apply for the increased age of testing. The same modelling approach was also subsequently applied to provide evidence that the age of healthy slaughtered cattle could be increased to 72 months with little impact on the number of cases detected [30]. Consequently, the age of testing of healthy slaughter increased across the EU to 72 months in 2011.

Revision of the EU surveillance to detect 1 in 100,000

As BSE prevalence continued to decline across the EU, further revisions of the surveillance scheme were agreed [31]. This meant that all member states with the exception of Bulgaria and Romania where surveillance had been introduced later (i.e. the EU-25) would be allowed to test only a minimum annual sample of the healthy slaughtered cattle aged above 72 months.

Therefore, EFSA commissioned a model to calculate the minimum sample size required for healthy slaughtered animals aged over 72 months that would allow detection of BSE with a yearly prevalence of 1 per 100,000 in the adult population (over 24 months of age). It was also to advise on the added value of this minimum sample in terms of monitoring the trend of classical and atypical BSE and for detecting hypothetical re-emergence of BSE. The specific model used by EFSA has been described in full elsewhere [32, 33].

For this study, individual member state level cattle population sizes and the number of positive and tested animals from active surveillance (fallen stock, healthy slaughter and emergency slaughter) were available. These data contained the details of over 91 million cattle tested within the EU-25 surveillance scheme from 2002 to 2011 and have been used to inform previous EFSA scientific opinions [34].

BSE's long incubation period, on average 5–5.5 years [35], and the low sensitivity of the test until late in the incubation period [36], means that the majority of animals die before being detectable by either active or passive surveillance. Therefore, back-calculation approaches were adopted to estimate the infection prevalence of BSE by birth cohort [37], which are able to account for the long incubation period, the age distribution of the standing population, the age at infection and the test sensitivity, in order to calculate the number infected that best accounts for the number detected.

The power of BSE surveillance was evaluated in terms of its ability to detect the prevalence of BSE positives in the standing population. Since the BSE surveillance only directly tests subsamples of the population, i.e. fallen stock/emergency slaughter and healthy slaughter, it was necessary to estimate the standing population prevalence from these active surveillance streams. The basic idea is that the active surveillance enables the prevalence in each birth cohort to be estimated, from which the prevalence in the standing population can be derived. One can then relate the power to detect BSE in the standing population to the number tested in the healthy slaughter stream.

It was found that for the EU25 overall, sufficient cattle were tested in the healthy slaughter stream to meet the target to detecting 1 in 100,000 infected cattle in the standing population. Furthermore, for the member states with the largest cattle populations, this target was also met at member state level: Belgium, Germany, Denmark, Spain, France, Ireland, Netherlands and the UK. This led to a revision of the BSE surveillance of the EU-25 (subsequent use of the model has now meant revision for the EU-28) so that the testing of healthy slaughter is no longer required by member states.

Conclusions

The two cases above are textbook examples of the best use of surveillance evaluation approaches to inform policy in the high-profile area of animal and public health across the EU. The cases show the application of statistical models to surveillance data to generate predictions of the impact of changes in terms of the number that would be missed if the surveillance was reduced.

References

1. Del Rio Vilas VJ, Sayers R, Sivam K, Pfeiffer DU, Guitian J, Wilesmith JW. A case-study of capture-recapture methodology using scrapie surveillance data in Great Britain. Prevent Veter Med. 2005;67:303–17.
2. Del Rio Vilas VJ, Bohning D. Application of one-list capture-recapture models to scrapie surveillance data in Great Britain. Prevent Veter Med. 2008;85:253–66.
3. Del Rio Vilas VJ, Kocaman M, Burkom H, Hopkins R, Berezowski J, Painter I, Gunn J, Montibeller G, Convertino M, Streichert LC, Honoré PA. A value driven framework for the evaluation of surveillance systems. Online J Pub Health Informatics. 2017;9(1):e83.
4. Rotejanaprasert C, Lawson A, Rossow H, Sane J, Huitu O, Henttonen H, Del Rio Vilas VJ. Towards integrated surveillance of zoonoses: Spatiotemporal joint modeling of rodent population data and human tularemia cases in Finland. BMC Med Res Methodol. 2018;18:72.
5. Schulz K, Peyre M, Staubach C, Schauer B, Schulz J, Calba C, Häsler B, Conraths FJ. Surveillance strategies for Classical Swine Fever in wild boar—a comprehensive evaluation study to ensure powerful surveillance. Sci Rep. 2017;7:43,871. https://doi.org/10.1038/srep43871.
6. Antoine-Moussiaux N, Vandenberg O, Kozlakidis Z, Aenishaenslin C, Peyre M, Roche M, Bonnet P, Ravel A. Valuing health surveillance as an information system: interdisciplinary insights. Front Public Health. 2019;7:138. https://doi.org/10.3389/fpubh.2019.00138.

7. Montibeller G, Carreras A, Del Rio Vilas VJ, Franco A. Evaluating capabilities of health systems with multi-criteria decision analysis. Operational Research Society Conference (OR59), Loughborough, UK, September 2017; 2017.
8. Guo X, Claassen GDH, Oude Lansink AGJM, Saatkamp HW. A conceptual framework for economic optimization of an animal health surveillance portfolio. Epidemiol Infect. 2016;144:1084–95.
9. Prattley DJ, Morris RS, Stevenson MA, Thornton R. Application of portfolio theory to risk-based allocation of surveillance resources in animal populations. Prev Vet Med. 2007;81(1–3):56–69.
10. Brookes V, Del Rio Vilas VJ, Ward MP. Disease prioritisation-what is the state of the art? Epidemiol Infect. 2015; https://doi.org/10.1017/S0950268815000801.
11. Attema AE, He L, Cook AJC, Del Rio Vilas VJ. Unbiased assessment of disease surveillance utilities: a prospect theory application. PLoS Neglected Tropical Diseases, 2019;13(5): e0007364. https://doi.org/10.1371/journal.pntd.0007364.
12. Food Standards Agency. Proposed decision to stop BSE testing of healthy cattle slaughtered for human consumption; 2012. https://www.food.gov.uk/sites/default/files/multimedia/pdfs/board/fsa121204.pdf
13. European Commission. Report on the monitoring and testing of ruminants for the presence of transmissible spongiform encephalopathies (TSEs) in the EU in 2013; 2015. Available here https://ec.europa.eu/food/sites/food/files/safety/docs/biosafety_food-borne-disease_tse_ms-annual-report_2013.pdf
14. Del Rio Vilas VJ, Pfeiffer DU. A review on evaluation of bias in scrapie surveillance. Veter J. 2010;185:259–64.
15. Spetzler K, Winter H, Meyer J. Decision quality: value creation for better business decisions. Hoboken, NJ: John Wiley & Sons; 2016.
16. Convertino M. An information theoretic portfolio model for disease surveillance evaluation. GEOMED 2017, Porto; September 2017.
17. Bohning D, Kuhnert R, Del Rio Vilas VJ. Capture-recapture estimation by means of empirical Bayesian smoothing with an application to spatial analysis of hidden scrapie in Great Britain. J Roy Stat Soc Ser C. 2011;60:723–41.
18. World Health Organization. Joint External Evaluation; 2017. http://apps.who.int/iris/handle/10665/204368
19. World Health Organization. International Health Regulations; 2005. http://www.who.int/ihr/about/en/
20. Calba C, Goutard FL, Vanholme L, Antoine-Moussiaux N, Hendrikx P, Saegerman C. The added-value of using participatory approaches to assess the acceptability of surveillance systems: the case of bovine tuberculosis in Belgium. PLoS ONE. 2016;11(7):e0159041. https://doi.org/10.1371/journal.pone.0159041.
21. Schulz K, Calba C, Peyre M, Staubach C, Conraths FJ. Hunters' acceptability of the surveillance system and alternative surveillance strategies for classical swine fever in wild boar—a participatory approach. BMC Vet Res. 2016;12:187. https://doi.org/10.1186/s12917-016-0822-5.
22. Calba C, Goutard F, Hoinville L, Hendrikx P, Lindberg A, Saegerman C, Peyre M. Surveillance systems evaluation: a systematic review of the existing approaches. BMC Public Health. 2015;15:448.
23. Wall TU, Meadow AM, Horganic A. Developing evaluation indicators to improve the process of coproducing usable climate science. Weather Clim. Soc. 2017;9:95–107. https://doi.org/10.1175/WCAS-D-16-0008.1.
24. Böhning D, Vilas V. Estimating the hidden number of scrapie affected holdings in Great Britain using a simple, truncated count model allowing for heterogeneity. J. Agric. Biol. Environ. Stat. 2008;13:1–22. https://doi.org/10.1198/108571108X277904.
25. Birch CPD, Del Rio Vilas VJ, Chikukwa AC, Greene J. A "shotgun" method for tracing the birth locations of sheep from flock tags, applied to scrapie surveillance in Great Britain. Prevent Veter Med. 2010;96:218–25.

26. Wilesmith JW, Wells GAH, Cranwell MP, Ryan JBM. Bovine spongiform encephalopathy: epidemiological studies. Vet Record. 1988;123:638–44.
27. Wilesmith JW, Ryan JBM, Atkinson MJ. Bovine spongiform encephalopathy: epidemiological studies on the origin. Veter Record. 1991;128:199–203.
28. Wilesmith JW, Ryan JBM, Hueston WD, Hoinville LJ. Bovine spongiform encepalopathy: epidemiological features 1985 to 1990. Veter Record. 1992;130:90–4.
29. EFSA Panel on Biological Hazards (BIOHAZ). Risk for human and animal health related to the revision of the BSE monitoring regime in some member states. EFSA J. 2008;762:1–47.
30. EFSA Panel on Biological Hazards (BIOHAZ). Opinion of the Scientific Panel on Biological Hazards on a second update on the risk for human and animal health related to the revision of the BSE monitoring regime in some Member States. The EFSA Journal. 2010;8(12):1946.
31. European Commission (EC). Commission Implementing Decision 2011/358/EU of 17 June 2011 amending Decision 2009/719/EC authorizing certain Member States to amend their annual BSE monitoring programmes (OJ L161, 21.6.2011, p29); 2012.
32. Adkin AL, Simons RRL, Arnold ME. Assessing the sensitivity of European surveillance for detecting BSE in cattle according to international standards. Prevent Veter Med. 2016;135:113–22.
33. Simons RRL, Arnold ME, Adkin AL. Assessing the time taken for a surveillance system to detect a re-emergence of bovine spongiform encephalopathy in cattle. Prevent Veter Med. 2017;138:48–54.
34. EFSA. Evaluation of the revision of the BSE monitoring regime in Croatia. EFSA J. 2016;14:1–27.
35. Arnold ME, Wilesmith JW. Estimation of the age-dependent risk of infection of dairy cattle to BSE. Prevent Veter Med. 2004;66:35–47.
36. Arnold K, Turner N, Barling J, Kelloway K, Mckee M. Transformational leadership and psychological well-being: the mediating role of meaningful work. J. Occup. Health Psychol. 2007;12:193–203. https://doi.org/10.1037/1076-8998.12.3.193.
37. Arnold ME, Wilesmith JW. Modelling studies on BSE occurrence to assist in the review of the Over Thirty Months Scheme in cattle. Proc R Soc B (London). 2003;270:2141–5.

13 Animal Health Surveillance: From Compliance to Real Governance

M. Figuié and A. Binot

Abstract

This chapter focuses on the role of surveillance in the policy process. It promotes a general framework to assess the effectiveness of health surveillance systems from a social science perspective, based on the concept of real governance. Effectiveness of animal health surveillance systems is addressed through the analysis of the gaps between, on the one side, the principles and the "official" rules and norms and, on the other side, their implementation in real life. Practically we suggest to assess the effectiveness of a surveillance system following two stages. First, we expose potential reasons that may explain a lack of compliance, from the informants of a surveillance system, with the "official rules" supposed to drive this system. Second, we identify and assess the "practical rules" that concretely drive the exchange of epidemiological information among local stakeholders (public or private) and the decision-making process (defined as the "practical surveillance system"). These practical rules or norms characterize the "real governance" (that is how, concretely, stakeholders are organized collectively and more or less informally), often associated with informality. Understanding the real governance gives the opportunity to identify alternative solutions built by stakeholders to address the different issues they are facing, and to assess the ability of these stakeholders to organize a collective action, sometimes in order to tackle the failure of the administration.

M. Figuié (✉)
CIRAD, UMR MoISA, Montpellier, France

MoISA, Univ Montpellier, CIHEAM-IAMM, CIRAD, INRAE, Institut Agro, IRD, Montpellier, France
e-mail: Muriel.figuie@cirad.fr

A. Binot
CIRAD, UMR ASTRE, Montpellier, France

ASTRE, Univ Montpellier, CIRAD, INRAE, Montpellier, France

M. Peyre et al. (eds.), *Principles for Evaluation of One Health Surveillance: The EVA Book*, https://doi.org/10.1007/978-3-030-82727-4_13

Evaluation methods described throughout this book contribute to assess the relevance and the quality of the data, information and knowledge produced by the surveillance system. Surveillance besides its technical aspects raises social and political issues and questions. The general framework described in this chapter can bring to the development of innovative pragmatic surveillance tools and methods, as described in this book.

Keywords
Animal diseases · Collective action · Governance · Health · Information · Policy Surveillance

13.1 Introduction

Surveillance of animal health is one of the instruments of animal health public policies. Public policies can be assessed on their relevance, effectiveness and efficiency. Relevance refers to the consistency between the social needs and the policy goal. Effectiveness measures the effects (outcomes and impacts) that can be directly attributed to the implementation of the policy instrument and that contribute to the policy goal achievement. Efficiency compares the effect of a policy instrument with the cost of its implementation [1].

Effectiveness depends on a process that follows in different stages (see Fig. 13.1) from issue identification and framing, to policy measures identification and development, and policy measures implementation [2].[1]

In the case of animal health policies, the epidemiological surveillance provides data, information and knowledge (see Fig. 13.1) that support the different stages of these policies cycle and contribute to their effectiveness. Epidemiological surveillance is also one policy instrument which goes through this policy cycle. Evaluation tools for epidemiological surveillance described in Parts III–V of this book contribute to assess the relevance and the quality of the data, information and knowledge produced by the surveillance system (see Fig. 13.1). Our objective in this chapter is to adress surveillance as a policy instrument.

When it comes to assessing animal health surveillance systems and their governance, the conclusion is often that there is a lack of farmers and local vets' compliance with the official rules designed by the authorities to drive these systems. This lack of compliance contributes to a low level of policy measure implementation. It does not mean necessary that there is not any activities of surveillance. Informal activities may be running, with stakeholders, objectives, rules, norms, decision-making process that can be different from what has been planned by the public

[1] Other criteria may be used for policy assessment such as performance or quality. In France, according to the LOLF (Loi Organique Relative aux Lois de Finances) and with the emergence of the New Public Management, the performances of a public service are defined by effectiveness for the citizen, quality for the service users, efficiency for the taxpayers. http://www.credoc.fr/pdf/Rech/C299.pdf

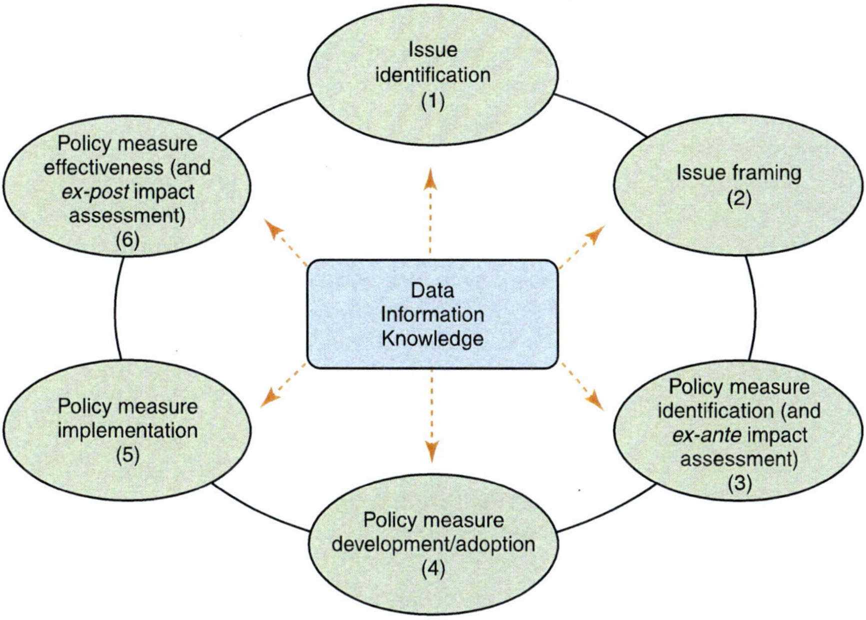

Fig. 13.1 Main stages in the policy cycle, supported by data, information and knowledge [2]

administration. In some cases, this surveillance can be completely independent of the officially designed system and completely informal. Indeed, most of the time, farmers are organized to manage the risks that they have to face [3], and in cases more specific to animal or plant health, professionals (farmers, technicians, traders) exchange information related to disease circulation in more or less formal ways [4–6].

We propose here to go a step further in the approach commonly used to assess animal health surveillance systems by focusing more explicitly on (1) the assessment of the implementation of this policy instrument and its compliance with the rules that are supposed to "officially" drive it (compliance indicates that policy instruments are implemented following the lines defined during the policy measure development stage)(Fig. 13.1) and (2) on the identification and assessment of the "practical rules" that concretely drive the exchange of epidemiological information among local stakeholders (public or private) and the decision-making process. These practical rules and norms can be more or less informal and explicit; they define the "real" governance" of a "practical surveillance system". The term "real governance", coined by Olivier de Sardan [7] *refers to the manner in which public good and services are really delivered. It includes the manner in which the State is really managed and how public policies are really implemented.*

The understanding of the gap between how policy instruments are supposed to function (the official surveillance systems with their official rules and norms) and how they function in practice reveals factors of local realities (technical, economic, social, political). This gap is most of the time supposed to limit the effectiveness of a policy [8]. But it is not always problematic. It may be positive in many situations:

it demonstrates the capacity of local stakeholders to adapt exogenous rules to their specific situation. It reveals elements of the situation that usually remain invisible [7], and it can inspire risk managers willing to set up surveillance systems more pragmatic and adapted to local contexts.

In this chapter, (1) we first clarify some concepts such as governance, compliance, practical rules or norms and real governance. Then (2) we apply these concepts to one policy instrument, the animal health surveillance. In the following sections, we underline (3) the barriers to compliance that may explain the low level of implementation of a policy instrument, in the specific case of surveillance relying on passive farmers' reporting. Then (4) we focus on the gap between how surveillance is supposed to work officially and how it works concretely (the practical surveillance). The understanding of this gap is essential to improve the effectiveness and the governance of the surveillance.

13.2 Governance and Compliance from a Social Sciences Perspective

In political sciences, the concept of **governance** is opposed to the concepts of management and government. "Management" refers to a technical or even technocratic approach; "government" describes the authority of the State, hierarchical and constraining; "governance" entails more flexible forms of power where public and non-public, governmental and non-governmental stakeholders interact [1]. Quite often, this term (governance) is used in a normative way (good governance), by institutions such as the World Bank and development organizations, and refers to "an ideal governance" [7]. This ideal of governance may vary according to the institutions. Social scientists generally characterize it by the integration of different areas of knowledge (multidisciplinary knowledge, experts and laymen's knowledge), inclusion of public values and social concerns in decision-making, rules and norms promoting transparency, inclusiveness and accountability [9].

There are different barriers to complying on the ground with the principles of a public policy (referring to poor or good governance) and in implementing its instruments on daily practices. The consequence is a gap between, on the one side, the principles and the "official" rules and norms (that are generally designed by centralized authorities) and, on the other side, their implementation in real life. Interferences are numerous since a sectorial strategy (e.g. health strategy) is nested in a wider system that determines its real implementation and its effectiveness ([8], see Fig. 13.2).

Lack of compliance with the "official rules" does not mean that there is no rule. "Practical rules" always exist in a social group. They can be endogenous or an adaptation of exogenous official rules to the context (including characteristics of the local public administration system; material, human or financial constraints; cultural and economic local values). Theses practical rules or norms characterize the "**real governance**" [7]. This "real governance" is often associated with informality

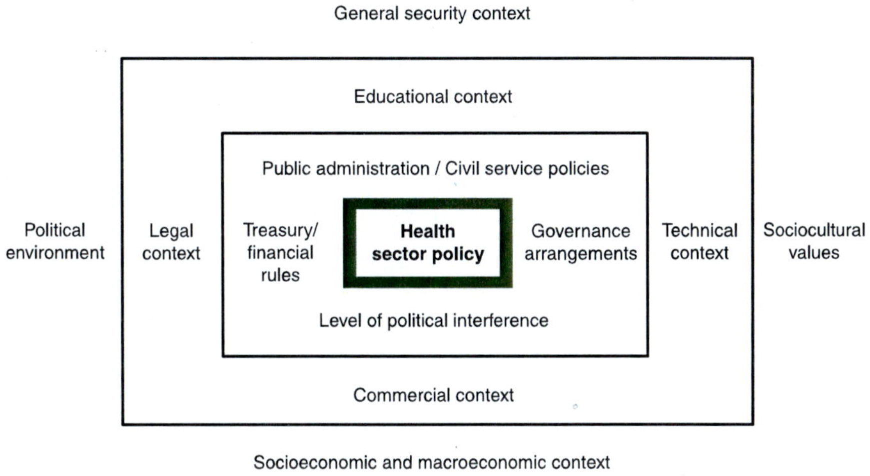

Fig. 13.2 Determinants of policy effectiveness: example from health policy. (Source: Potter, C. C., and J. Harries. 2006. The determinants of policy effectiveness. *Bulletin of the World Health Organization*, 84:843)

and, when it deals with public administration, with corruption or nepotism. But it can also be interpreted in a positive way, as a pragmatic adjustment to the local context (and to the interests, values social norms of the local network of stakeholders) of the rules established by an upper level of governance (or by foreign organizations). Understanding the real governance provides the opportunity to identify alternative solutions built by stakeholders to address the different issues they are faced with, and to assess the ability of these stakeholders to organize a collective action, sometimes in order to tackle the failure of the administration. Some aspects of this real governance could be assisted, supported and encouraged [7].

Assessing a public policy and its instruments requires considering their level of implementation, and the real governance, i.e. how concretely stakeholders are organized collectively (and more or less informally). It supposes the identification of the stakeholders of this network (probably including different stakeholders than the ones considered by the official rules, and can be more or less inclusive). The process of decision-making among these stakeholders should be analysed (more or less explicit, transparent, collective), as well as the way for prioritizing objectives and values to be promoted (public health, economic efficiency), and to organize the share of costs and benefits (Who pays? Who benefits? Who decides of this share?).

This assessment entails mobilizing social sciences, since compliance and real governance deal with psychological concepts such as acceptability and observance but also with socio-political ones such as collective action, norms, interests, power asymmetry, logic and strategy. How can this approach be applied to an animal health surveillance system?

13.3 Assessing the Governance of Animal Health Surveillance System: Available Tools

Surveillance system is an information system designed to support a decision-making process.

As an information system, a surveillance system includes different steps: (1) designing of the surveillance protocols, (2) data collection, (3) data analysis, (4) data interpretation, (5) data dissemination, including feed-back to the actors of the surveillance system and dissemination to decision-makers, (6) data communication to the society [10]. Data collection can be based on different tools, e.g. passive reporting, crowdsourcing, and includes tasks such as gathering, recording, organizing the data; data analysis and data interpretation consist of processing the data and turning it into information that can support decision-making in the framework of risk management process (e.g. isolating a at-risk population). These data can also supply a process of knowledge-building driven by scientist researchers (a process essential to support evidence-based policies). The task of designing of the surveillance protocols is generally assumed by public authorities in the case of health surveillance.

Surveillance systems cannot be reduced to the technical and neutral operation of collecting, managing and analysing information. Surveillance systems include decision-making in order to control risks. In the case of epidemiological surveillance, the decision is related to disease control: the objective of epidemiological surveillance "is to follow regularly the health status or the risk factors of a given population, in particular to detect the emergence of pathological processes and to study their development in time and space, in order to adopt appropriate control measures"[2] ([10] p. 302). Epidemiological surveillance delivers public goods and services, and then puts forward concerns of governance.

Promoting the good governance of an animal health surveillance system raises many challenges. We propose to characterize it by a circular flow of information, based on diverse knowledge, able to support decentralized decision-making process, inclusive, transparent and accountable, and directed towards shared objectives. It supposes an agreement among the stakeholders involved in the system on the question "Who surveys who? And why?" Good governance is an ethical choice but it is also the condition for a greater stakeholders' involvement and for surveillance effectiveness. How far are present surveillance systems from this objective and how to get closer to it?

There is no specific tool available to assess the governance of animal health surveillance, but the World Organisation for Animal Health (OIE) proposes tools for

[2] Our translation of *suivre de manière régulière et prolongée l'état de santé ou les facteurs de risque d'une population définie, en particulier de déceler l'apparition de processus pathologiques et d'en étudier le développement dans le temps et dans l'espace, en vue de l'adoption de mesures appropriées de lutte.*

assessing the governance of veterinary services.[3] The OIE suggests to measure it through the adherence of national vet services with international standards (using the OIE Performance Veterinary Services Tool,[4] OIE website) [11]. This may be useful as a first approximation, but it also presents limits that Msellati et al. [12] underline: this approach relies on rule-based indicators and says little about the performance of the services[5] and the extent of the application of these rules (i.e. their implementation). Msellati et al. note that most of the time the application of these rules is limited in particular by corruption that affects vet services as other public services [12]. Moreover, we can add that this approach does not take into account how these rules have been designed (in a more or less participative and inclusive way), and if these rules are based on shared values and interests, and if transparency and accountability are considered. However, these elements are essential in defining a good governance (see above).

Assessing the adherence of nationally designed surveillance systems with international standards is useful but does not allow understanding how the systems function in real life. We propose here to include two points in the assessment of surveillance systems and of their governance. We do not pretend with these two points to cover all the requirements of such an assessment, but we intend to contribute to improving the current approaches by mobilizing social sciences (most specially sociology and political sciences).

The first point deals with the level of implementation of the official rules and norms that are supposed to drive these systems and the reasons for a potentially low compliance. A starting assumption/hypothesis should be that there might be "good reasons" for this lack of compliance (e.g. "official" rules might be not adapted to local context). Secondly, we propose to take as a second starting assumption that even when compliance is low, stakeholders might be organized nevertheless collectively to deal with animal health information, through "practical" surveillance systems. This organization may be more or less efficient in the view of the objectives shared by their members; objectives may also be heterogeneous and

[3] The OIE defines good governance of vet services as a way to achieve efficiency for preventing, detecting and controlling animal diseases, and for articulating national, regional and international levels of management; good governance of veterinary services requires both legislation and the necessary human and financial resources (OIE website).

[4] PVS is a tool to assess and improve the compliance of a country's veterinary services with OIE standards. The components of the PVS tool are: (1) Human, physical and financial resources to attract further resources and retain professionals with technical and leadership skills; (2) technical authority and capability to address current and new issues, including prevention and control of biological disasters, based on scientific principles; (3) interaction with stakeholders to assist in "staying on course" and carrying out relevant joint programmes and (4) access to markets through compliance with existing standards and the implementation of new disciplines, such as the harmonization of standards, equivalence and zoning [11]. The PVS tools rely on the assessment of 46 areas of competencies, eleven of these competencies can be used to measure governance of veterinary services according to Msellati, L., J. Commault and A. Dehove. (2012). Good veterinary governance: definition, measurement and challenges. *Rev. sci. tech.* Off. int. Epiz. 31:413–430.

[5] The performances of a public service can be defined as effectiveness for the citizen, quality for the service users, efficiency for the taxpayers. http://www.credoc.fr/pdf/Rech/C299.pdf

conflicting; and they may diverge from public interest (and from the objective of the "official" surveillance systems). But this understanding is essential to identify members of these systems, their roles, their interests (and conflict of interests), values, norms and in order to assess the "real" governance that drives concretely the process of producing, sharing and using epidemiological information, as well as the way to improve it.

We examine in the follow-up these two points (compliance and real governance) by focusing on surveillance systems relying on farmers' reporting.

13.4 Compliance of Surveillance Systems Relying on Farmers' Reporting

To overcome one of the limits of an assessment relying on rule-based indicators, the implementation of the official rules should be evaluated and the reasons for a potentially low compliance should be identified. The first step is to identify the official rules (based on administrative documents) and then to assess their compliance based on participant observation (see Part IV). The second step is to conduct in-depth interviews with the stakeholders of the surveillance system (farmers and vets mainly but not only) to identify the reasons for this low level of implementation. Economic evaluation could also be implemented to assess the share of costs and benefits among stakeholders to comply with the surveillance system requirements (cf. Part III).These reasons may be numerous and have their own logic (see our first assumption). Low compliance in animal disease reporting is often underlined and imputed to farmers and field services, as the weak points in the communication channel [13]. The reasons evoked are numerous (lack of resources, interference with economic interests). But most of the times, that is the farmer's lack of incentive in collaborating to animal disease surveillance that is emphasized.

The lack of compliance in "playing the game" (and in following its rules) may have many other sources. Surveillance systems are often centralized and characterized by an asymmetry of information (lack of feedback) and an asymmetry of power between its members (in the decision-making phase). Quite often, these systems organize a kind of bottom-up flow of information from the basis of data providers (e.g. farmers), to decision-makers (e.g. centralized vet authorities). Farmers when they report information to the authorities do not always receive any relevant feedback and do not benefit directly from this surveillance. Farmers may also be more concerned by diseases which are not considered by the existing surveillance systems (see Box 13.1). In these cases, farmers' motivation to report events related to the health of their animal is low. A mix of bottom up and top down approaches are sometimes developed to support the adoption of surveillance national policies in the field (see Chap. 14).

Even if the collection of data is participative (i.e. participatory epidemiology), the decision-making can be authoritarian. In this case, farmers can feel more like objects of surveillance than part of a collaborative network of information.They may be seeking to escape from this surveillance and to the consequences of the decision that information may generate, potentially in opposition with their short-term interests (such as sanitary culling) [14]. Surveillance systems may also voluntarily encompass more than just disease control. Fintz [15] studied avian flu (H5N1) management in Egypt in 2005–2006 and showed how the accompanying rhetoric was conducive to the development of strong dynamics, leading to the imposition of emergency measures, and an agricultural modernization vision. Surveillance can then be seen as a form of "biopolitic" [16], a way for a centralized authority to exert power on population, to control their practices and behaviours. Lack of farmers' collaboration can then be seen as a form of resistance.

If official rules are not implemented, what are the rules that in practice drive the collective action locally organized to deal with animal health issues (following our second assumption)? The identification and assessment of this real governance is the second step of the approach that we propose.

13.5 Real Governance, "Practical" Information Systems and Their Limits

Different studies show that despite a low compliance with official surveillance systems, farmers are interested in sharing epidemiological information and use it for their decision-making. According to these studies, farmers, but also technicians and traders share epidemiological information. This information flows between local actors, mobilizing a categorization of diseases, a "definition of cases", alert thresholds and decision-making processes on their own ([5, 17]; see also [6] for plants diseases). This share of information is driven by practical rules (sometimes implicit) and social values. Information sharing is not limited to animal diseases but may also include market information, innovation, know-how sharing, etc. (see Box 13.1). To identify these practical surveillance systems, experts may adapt methodologies available to analyse network of social actors [18][6] since formalized and specific tools are still lacking.

The discrepancy of these practical systems of information sharing with the officially designed systems reveals social realities: local constraints, knowledges, norms (social, professional), values and concerns, role of traditional authorities, rules of reciprocity, etc. (see Box 13.1). This gap can be interpreted as a local adaptation of the official centralized model to local constraints or as a local response to farmers' dissatisfaction with official systems. It can be interpreted as a sign of the weakness of the administration but also as the autonomy of local levels of governance in relation to centralized authorities.

These "practical" surveillance systems have also strong limits. They can be efficient in protecting local interests (in relation with sanitary but also economic, social, political issues), but they can hardly replace official surveillance systems when it comes to protect public or global goods. The informal systems analysed in the quoted studies have their own logic: they are designed to minimize the local effects (e.g. economic effects by the quick sale of sick animals outside the network) rather

[6] See, e.g. Pham [19] and Delabouglise et al. [21]

[7] The distinction between value/belief and instrumental rationality is not entirely satisfactory. Value/belief rationale actions could serve individual interests in the long term. A calculation and

than to prevent the spatial spread and extension of pathogens. They support individual decisions mainly at farm level that may contribute to export risks outside the community of the members of the network.

Understanding how surveillance systems run in practice is a powerful tool for designing more effective systems. These systems are a kind of social experimentation [20] and as mentioned above, they can inspire risk managers in designing more acceptable instruments. Their understanding gives basis to reshape a surveillance system which may take into account local interests, values and social organizations in order to increase their acceptability and consequently their effectiveness and efficiency.

Box 13.1 Examples of informal surveillance systems

In Vietnam and Thailand, in several villages where poultry rearing was the main activity, farmers reportedly exchanged information on the health status of their animals [5, 17]. This constituted an informal farmer-formed epidemiological monitoring network that was relatively independent of the systems set up by the veterinary health authorities. The information exchanged informed everyone on the poultry diseases present, thus enabling them to take preventive (increased monitoring of their own birds, restricted entry on the farm, cleaning of the premises, etc.) or mitigation (advanced sale of animals) measures.

Farmers are altruistic when they inform their neighbours about the outbreak of an infectious disease causing high mortality, such as avian flu. What drives these farmers is also the hope of being paid back, i.e. to be informed when there is a disease outbreak on a neighbour's farm.[7] Moreover, if the farmers in the case mentioned above adopt altruistic behaviour with regard to other members in their community, then this behaviour is selfish with regard to non-community members. Social (family, professional network) and geographical (within a few kilometres) proximity facilitates information flow within a small network [17]. Disease outbreaks are, however, not revealed to potential buyers outside the collective—it is essential to quickly sell animals exposed to the disease in order to curb economic loss. This comes with the risk of contaminating the livestock of external buyers or jeopardizing consumer health. Moreover, this information is not transmitted to veterinary authorities—livestock farmers expect little support from these authorities and strive to avoid potential coercive measures (sanitary slaughter, set up of a quarantine area, etc.).

Similar examples have been reported by Paul et al. [5], who studied avian flu management by Thai fighting cock breeders; Delabouglise et al. [22] and Pham et al. [19], who studied poultry and swine health information sharing networks in Thailand (2017) and Vietnam (2016), respectively, and by Prete [6] in a study on tomato disease surveillance in France.

the expectation of receiving a return payment could justify solidarity.

13.6 Conclusion

Surveillance, besides its technical aspects, raises social and political issues and questions such as "who keeps who under surveillance and why?" That is a key question when assessing the governance of an information system.

With global emerging infectious diseases and the subsequent globalization of the animal health issue, animal health policies are increasingly focused on cross-border diseases, on pandemics threats and on the objective of building centralized systems, internationally connected, based on standardised tools and recommendations codes. Global health policies push for more harmonized and connected surveillance systems. But "one size does not fit all", in particular in the case of passive farmers' reporting systems depending on farmers' routinized observations of their animals [13]. Global information systems will not function without farmers' reporting. And farmers' reporting will not work without taking into account local issues of health of animals and local concerns [23]. Surveillance systems "must be tailored to meet the needs and fit within the constraints of the different specific contexts" [13]. Otherwise they may lack effectiveness and may be replaced by informal and local surveillance systems that can hardly be performant when it comes to controlling diseases of global scope that threaten the public good. Nevertheless, understanding how animal health surveillance works in real life is essential to improve the collective ability to control animal diseases.

We propose here a general framework to assess animal health surveillance systems as a policy instrument from a social science perspective based on the concept of real governance. We believe that this assessment can contribute to improve the governance of surveillance systems. This general framework still needs to be translated in practice to serve a pragmatic surveillance using some of the innovative tools and methods presented in this book (Parts III, IV and V).

References

1. Boussaguet L, Jacquot S, Ravinet P. Dictionnaire des politiques publiques. Paris: Presses de Sciences Po; 2010.
2. European Environement Agency. Policy effectiveness evaluation. The effectiveness of urban wastewater treatment and packaging waste management systems. Denmark: EEA; 2005.
3. Mormont M. Le sociologue dans l'action collective face au risque. Développement durable et territoires [En ligne], Varia, mis en ligne le 02 novembre 2009, consulté le 08 août 2013:14; 2009.
4. Figuié M, Peyre M, Binot A. Surveillance of infectious animal diseases in Southeast Asia. Promoting the multiplicity of information networks. Perspective. Policy Brief 2013;23.
5. Paul M, Figuié M, Kovitvadhi A, Valeix S, Wongnarkpet S, Poolkhet C, Kasemsuwan S, Ducrot C, Roger F, Binot A. Collective resistance to HPAI H5N1 surveillance in the Thai cockfighting community: Insights from a social anthropology study. Prevent Veter Med. 2015;120:106–14.
6. Prete G. Surveiller en éradiquant : l'importance des "médiateurs de la surveillance" et des réseaux informels dans la surveillance des risques sanitaires et environnementaux. Sociologie du Travail. 2008;50:489–504.
7. Olivier de Sardan J-P. Researching the practical norms of real governance in Africa. Discussion Paper n°5, Africa Power and Politics Programme (APPP)/DFID, London; 2009.

8. Potter CC, Harries J. The determinants of policy effectiveness. Bull World Health Org. 2006;84:843.
9. Van Asselt MBA, Renn O. Risk Governance. J Risk Res. 2011;14:431–49.
10. Toma B, Dufour B, Bénet JJ, Sanaa M, Shaw A, Moutou F. Epidémiologie appliquée à la lutte collective contre les maladies animales transmissibles majeures (3eme ed.). Maison-Alfort: AEEMA; 2010.
11. Schneider HP. Good governance of national veterinary srvices. Rev Sci Tech Off Int Epiz. 2011;30:325–38.
12. Msellati L, Commault J, Dehove A. Good veterinary governance: defintion, measurement and challenges. Rev Sci Tech Off Int Epiz. 2012;31:413–30.
13. Cameron A. Surveillance needs, tools and options: experiences between developed and developing worlds. In: Challenges of animal health information systems and surveillance for animal diseases and zoonoses; 2011.
14. Barbier M. Surveiller pour abattre. Terrains Travaux. 2006;2:101–21.
15. Fintz M. "Cadrage des épizooties et stratégies d'acteurs: le cas de l'influenza aviaire (H5N1) en Egypte." Epidemiol. et santé anim. 2010;58:23–35.
16. Foucault M. Sécurité, territoire, population. Cours au Collège de France, 1977-1978. Paris: Gallimard Seuil; 2004.
17. Figuié M, Desvaux S. Managing global risks: vietnamese poultry farmers and avian flu. In: Morand S, Dujardin JP, Lefait-Robin R, Apiwathnasorn C, editors. Socio-ecological dimensions of infectious diseases in Southeast Asia. Singapore: Springer; 2015. p. 257–73.
18. Lemieux V. Les réseaux d'acteurs sociaux. Paris: PUF; 1999.
19. Pham TTH. Social network analysis of swine surveillance system in Vietnam. in Development of novel methodologies for the socio-economic evaluation of animal health surveillance system: application to swine disease surveillance in Vietnam, PhD Thesis, Kasetsart University, Bangkok, Thailand, Chapter 6; 2016, pp 145–57.
20. Cefaï D, Terzi C, editors. L'expérience des problèmes publics. Perspectives pragmatistes. Les editions de l'EHESS; 2012.
21. Delabouglise A, Antoine-Moussiaux N, Tatong D, Chumkaeo A, Binot A, Fournié G, Pilot E, Phimpraphi W, Kasemsuwan S, Paul MC, Duboz R, Salem G, Peyre M. Cultural practices shaping zoonotic diseases surveillance: the case of highly pathogenic avian influenza and thailand native chicken farmers. Transboundary and Emerging Diseases. 2017;64(4):1294–305. https://doi.org/10.1111/tbed.12506.
22. Delabouglise, Alexis, Choisy M, Phan TD, Antoine-Moussiaux N, Peyre M, Vu TD, Pfeiffer DU, Fournié G. Economic factors influencing zoonotic disease dynamics: demand for poultry meat and seasonal transmission of avian influenza in Vietnam. Sci. Rep. 2017;7:5905. https://doi.org/10.1038/s41598-017-06244-6.
23. International workshop organized by FAO, 23–26 November 2010, Rome, Italy.

Integrating Health Surveillance Evaluation Outputs in the Policy Cycle

14

Katharina D. C. Stärk

Abstract

Policies on animal health are set by government authorities, private organisations and companies, and accordingly, can be compulsory for all or only for certain suppliers. The objective of integrating evaluation in the policy cycle is to provide a mechanism to obtain feedback on the effectiveness and efficiency of policy implementation and—in the case of implementation and/or impact deficiencies—to inform changes to or adaptation of policies, if necessary. This chapter explore the links, often too loose between the strategies defined at the policy level and their practical evaluation in the field; and how this could be improved to promote positive and dynamic changes.

Keywords

Health surveillance · Policy cycle · Decision making · Evaluation

14.1 Introduction

Policies on animal health are set by government authorities, private organisations and companies, and accordingly, can be compulsory for all or only for certain suppliers. Animal health policies can affect farmers, veterinarians and businesses including suppliers, processors and retailers of animal-derived products. The policy-making cycle includes all steps from "agenda setting", over "policy formulation" to "implementation" and finally "evaluation" (Fig. 14.1).

K. D. C. Stärk (✉)
Federal Food Safety and Veterinary Office, Bern, Switzerland
e-mail: Katharina.Staerk@blv.admin.ch

M. Peyre et al. (eds.), *Principles for Evaluation of One Health Surveillance: The EVA Book*, https://doi.org/10.1007/978-3-030-82727-4_14

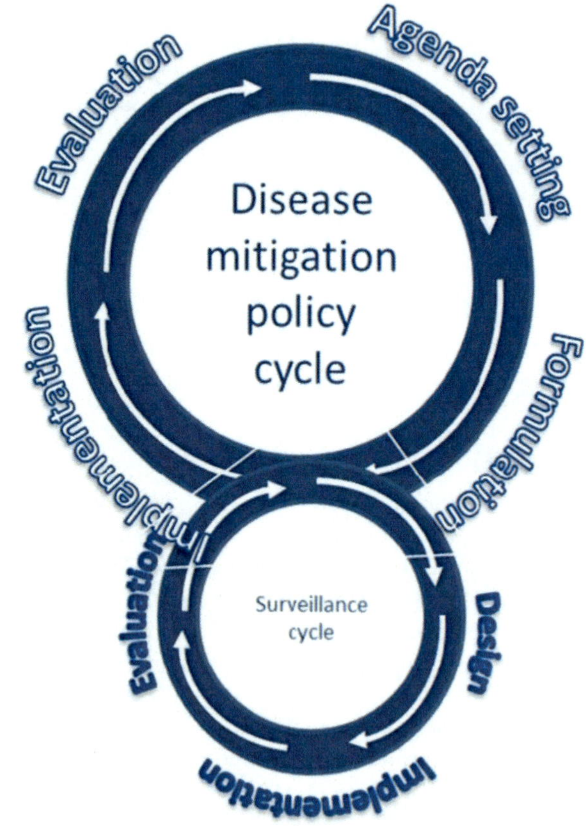

Fig. 14.1 Linkages between the disease mitigation policy cycle and the related surveillance activities

The objective of integrating evaluation in the policy cycle is to provide a mechanism to obtain feedback on the effectiveness and efficiency of policy implementation and—in the case of implementation and/or impact deficiencies—to inform changes to or adaptation of policies, if necessary. For example, in the case of animal health, the policy cycle includes the decision to set a certain pathogen on the animal health agenda, the control objective (e.g. impact mitigation or eradication) and the selection of the appropriate control strategies such as vaccination, stamping out or treatment, if available. Surveillance provides the feedback mechanisms necessary to assess the progress of disease control.

In this chapter, we focus on the evaluation of surveillance activities, but it needs to be remembered that surveillance remains an integral part of disease mitigation [1] and that the economic value of surveillance information needs to be considered in this context [2, 3]. As described in Part III of this book, the link between surveillance and intervention is particularly relevant in the context of economic evaluation of surveillance efforts as both elements are incurring costs while contributing to the joint benefit of disease mitigation.

14.2 Limited Application of the Evaluation of Surveillance System to Inform Policy

Evaluation of surveillance systems should specifically provide feedback on the design, implementation and utility of surveillance (Fig. 14.1). As such, the evaluation includes aspects of the design and implementation of surveillance using methods and tools discussed in earlier chapters of this book. When a formal evaluation of surveillance is conducted, this process forms an integral part of the surveillance cycle. Depending on the governance of a specific disease control programme and its related surveillance, the mechanism of initiating evaluation, conducting evaluation and integrating evaluation results will vary.

Most examples of surveillance evaluation conducted to date were set in the public domain, i.e. the disease control programme, the related surveillance as well as evaluation—if implemented—were designed and executed by government veterinary services. However, the policy framework including evaluation is of course equally applicable to privately run surveillance programmes.

The practical implementation of surveillance evaluation will be easier if envisaged from the start, i.e. planned already at the point of implementing a surveillance activity, and not only after the surveillance programme has been running for some time. Prospective planning will help collect the right data and indicators and therefore allow for an efficient evaluation process with the relevant information readily available. To date, however, this is rarely the case because most surveillance activities have been established at some time in the past and may have been operating for many years while the idea to use evaluation as part of their life cycle is—at least in the animal health context—a relatively recent addition in most countries [4]. The consequence of this is the need to design the evaluation post hoc. The probability that the information needed to inform the evaluation will have been collected is relatively small. Therefore, such evaluations are often much more resource-consuming than evaluations which have been planned from the moment when a new policy was implemented and the related legislation was passed.

At present, there are not yet many examples available to illustrate the interplay between policy setting and evaluation including disease mitigation, surveillance and evaluation. One example is the evaluation of surveillance for early detection of emerging animal health syndromes in Switzerland (Box 14.1). This example illustrates the prospective integration of surveillance evaluation in the cycle: A new surveillance activity was started and from the beginning, evaluation was planned as a milestone to inform the decision whether the activity should be continued or not. Nevertheless, the practical experience in this case demonstrated that the data collected prospectively were not sufficient and more had to be collected to allow for a robust evaluation result. Particularly, economic data are often lacking. These include both simple cost information as well as more complex information to quantify the benefits of surveillance activities [2].

A similar example is the monitoring of antimicrobial usage in livestock in Germany. The relevant legislation was passed in 2014 and requires the recording of all antimicrobials using specified formats. In the legislation, a first evaluation of the legislation after five years was fixed.

Box 14.1 Evaluation of Surveillance for Early Detection of Animal Health Syndromes in Switzerland [5]

A substantial portfolio of activities, tools and programmes was introduced in Switzerland for the early detection of signals caused by emerging animal health hazards. The aim was to generally strengthen prevention. The legal basis for this early warning system was passed in 2013. Since, selected elements of this programme as well as its overall performance were formally evaluated in 2015. The evaluation built on recommended good practice both from the veterinary field as well as from general good practice in evaluation from other sectors.

The early warning activities covered by the evaluation were numerous and diverse. The main focus was on syndrome detection, and all reporting was on a voluntary basis. Most livestock species were included and a very broad range of stakeholders was involved such as practicing veterinarians, meat inspectors and diagnostic laboratories. All reporting of suspect syndromes is made on a voluntary basis. A range of incentives is used in combination with intensive communication and dissemination of data to sustain motivation and awareness among all stakeholders.

The evaluation was meant to be formative, i.e. to inform and improve the next phase of programme implementation and operation. System attributes were used as recommended in most evaluation guidelines. These attributes included among others coverage, representativeness, sensitivity and acceptability. Additionally, economic evaluation was attempted including cost-effectiveness assessment. However, because evaluation attributes had not been specified at the start of programme implementation, the capacity to collect the required data *post hoc* was limited, and the evaluation remained largely qualitative. Assessment of stakeholder opinion was an integral part of the evaluation. Beneficiaries of each early detection component were identified and included as stakeholders. Data were collected using online questionnaires, individual interviews and group workshops.

Performance by attribute varied for individual system components reflecting the diverse nature and approaches implemented. The main challenges were identified in aligning what different stakeholders expected from a system, in quantifying the utility of a component and in assuring the sustainability of voluntary engagement in syndrome reporting. The evaluation of the overall programme demonstrated that system borders were difficult to draw as many activities informed surveillance as well as control. It was also noted that communication of evaluation results requires careful planning. In the final workshop, stakeholders tended to react defensively towards evaluation outcomes that indicated room for improvement. Communication of results should be conducted such that it is perceived as formative feedback rather than criticism.

14.3 Loose Links Between Surveillance Cycle and Policy Cycle: The Need for Evaluation

Most current animal health surveillance programmes have been running for some time and started when the benefits of evaluation were not yet sufficiently recognised to integrate it from the start. Therefore, evaluation is not formally envisaged and not yet systematically integrated in the policy cycle for many programmes. Even worse, many surveillance activities appear to be conducted on a routine basis quite detached from the policy cycle and sometimes even detached from other hazard mitigation activities with which they should be linked. In the absence of evaluation or even regular review, this situation can lead to inefficient use of increasingly scarce surveillance resources. Examples of such surveillance activities can be found in most surveillance portfolios of national veterinary services and also at multi-lateral level.

For some disease control programmes, the lack of systematic review and challenge is understandable as they are founded on international trade standards and therefore considered compulsory and non-negotiable. However, even for such programmes, it would be useful to regularly review their effectiveness and perhaps to challenge their utility. As progress is made in the design and conduct of all aspects of surveillance, existing programmes become outdated and inefficient. For example, when novel diagnostic tools become available the continued use of a test with lower performance should be reflected. As many countries rely on surveillance designs recommended by international organisations such as the OIE, the regular and timely review of relevant codes and standards is essential. The use of evaluation is yet to be integrated in international surveillance standards.

Another critical point in the policy cycle is when control objectives for a specific hazard change and, therefore, surveillance programmes may have to be adjusted or redesigned. These policy transitions occur at the interface of the different stages of hazard mitigation reflected by their respective control objectives [1]. As the control objective for a hazard moves from establishing baseline prevalence estimation to control and subsequently to elimination (i.e. demonstration of freedom), the design of the accompanying surveillance activities needs to be adjusted. Therefore, evaluation is required both at the programme level (i.e. does the control policy achieve its old and/or new objective) as well as at the surveillance level (i.e. does surveillance provide suitable information to inform intervention decisions). This "moving target" of surveillance can be illustrated by the example of bovine spongiform encephalopathy (BSE). More information is provided in Box 14.2.

Box 14.2 Evaluation of Surveillance of Bovine Spongiform Encephalopathy (BSE)

BSE emerged as a novel syndrome in ruminants in the 1980s in the United Kingdom and subsequently led to far-reaching changes in livestock production practices, animal identification and animal health standards in Europe and worldwide [6]. Intensive surveillance activities became a prerequisite for participation in international trade, and most countries introduced or had introduced such programmes by the end of the millennium. Most surveillance designs included testing of very high numbers of slaughter cattle using expensive surveillance protocols. In combination with a range of interventions, BSE occurrence continued to decline to currently very low levels (see www.oie.int). However, most countries have sustained surveillance efforts to minimise the risks of trade disruptions. Because the costs of BSE surveillance are significant, evaluation efforts have started in some countries. For example, as a first step, Germany quantified the economic costs of its programme [7]. Although only direct costs were included, the total costs were estimated to be as high as two billion euros. To fully judge this result, it would have to be set in context of the value of the industry and benefits in general. Economic evaluations of BSE programmes in other countries have been scarce. A formal evaluation of a full BSE programme was only reported for Canada [8] where the evaluation specifically considered the attributes of relevance and performance. The latter also included more qualitative attributes such as information sharing, collaboration between agencies and sustainability of technical expertise. More efforts were dedicated to redesigning sampling strategies in order to reduce efforts and costs while sustaining performance. An example is available for the UK where analyses to increase cost-effectiveness were conducted [9]. As the expected number of cases continues to decrease, the costs of detecting cases increase. A shift of surveillance focus from abattoir testing to farm-based surveillance of suspected cases was found to be most cost-effective. However, policy makers—when presented with the results—were cautious about making changes in active surveillance mostly due to the risk of losing trust among trade partners. An EU-wide evaluation of the technical performance of BSE surveillance showed that the performance exceeded international requirements for the EU as a whole and also for selected individual countries [10]. These results contribute to the policy changes introduced in 2013, lifting the requirement of testing of all healthy cattle at slaughter. An application from Croatia to change its surveillance programme accordingly was subsequently positively assessed by EFSA [11].

A specific policy-related challenge is encountered when international standards or trade agreements specify the design of surveillance. For example, the design of brucellosis and leucosis surveillance in Europe is fixed in European legislation. For other hazards, more flexible designs are allowed in the relevant legislation. This is for example the case for avian influenza surveillance in Europe, where a range of surveillance system components are available including both wildlife and domestic avian populations. If there is a lack of design flexibility, the utility of surveillance evaluation will also be limited as alternative designs will not be acceptable within the legal framework, even if they would be more effective or efficient.

14.4 Practical Implementation of Animal Health Evaluation Versus Standard Requirements

Some legislation focuses on surveillance inputs rather than its outputs. Input mainly refers to the specification of a sample size and the population strata in which sampling needs to be conducted. Such detailed descriptions of inputs can be encountered in numerous surveillance standards and legislations. The impact on standardisation and efficiency was recently discussed for example in the context of antimicrobial residue surveillance [12]. In general, it would be more appropriate to define the performance (or output) that should be achieved by a surveillance activity while leaving the detailed aspects of the design open such that the country or farm can have more flexibility to determine a design that both fits the practical situation in the field as well as meets performance requirements. So-called output-based standards are increasingly being promoted yet remain relatively rare at the moment [13]. One notable example of an internationally standardised programme using such performance indicators was the global rinderpest eradication programme [14].

In a situation where surveillance design is fixed, the impact of surveillance evaluation on policy will be very limited. If there is more flexibility at policy level, a range of outcome options are possible. Depending on the feedback from the evaluation, the design of a surveillance programme can be modified. Simpler adaptations include, for example, the switch to a better diagnostic protocol (i.e. more sensitive, more specific, quicker, less expensive, more practical matrix), the change of the sampling location (farm vs. centralised), or the switch to pooled samples with related sample size adjustments.

14.5 Evaluation to Inform Dynamic Changes

More complex changes may be necessary if the disease control objective has changed, for example moving from prevalence estimation during an eradication campaign towards documenting freedom from disease (or infection). This is an expected change in a successful programme, but can nevertheless be challenging either because the test sensitivity is not sufficient or because of the lack of an accepted prevalence level that is expected to be low enough to reflect acceptable risk.

After disease absence has been documented reliably by surveillance results over some time, it may also be considered to change from active surveillance designs to more passive approaches, i.e. suspect case reporting. This is an option only for diseases with clinical signs that are specific enough for early detection of suspect cases. However, if this requirement is fulfilled, passive reporting is an efficient approach and is internationally practiced and accepted, for example for foot-and-mouth disease. Nevertheless, the decision to stop active surveillance is a big step that has rarely been taken by any government so far. It is likely to be dependent on the economic gains from less testing as well as the alternative needs for surveillance for other, more serious, more prevalent or more costly hazards. The case of BSE is likely to provide a case example for such a scenario soon.

14.6 Conclusion and Way Forward

In summary, the integration of surveillance evaluation into the policy cycle for animal disease mitigation is still in its infancy. Only a few countries have made evaluation a compulsory requirement for renewing budget for disease control programmes. However, in a time of increasingly limited budgets, veterinary services are likely to increase their use of evaluation as it provides a structured and transparent approach to inform policy and budget decisions.

References

1. Häsler B, Howe KS, Stärk KDC. Conceptualising the technical relationship of animal disease surveillance to intervention and mitigation as a basis for economic analysis. BMC Health Serv Res. 2011;11(1):225. Available at: http://www.pubmedcentral.nih.gov/articlerender.fcgi?artid=3189394&tool=pmcentrez&rendertype=abstract. Accessed 18/12/2012.
2. Stärk KDC, Häsler B. The value of information: current challenges in surveillance implementation. Prev Vet Med. 2015;122:229–34. https://doi.org/10.1016/J.PREVETMED.2015.05.002.
3. Stärk KDC, Babo Martins S, Rushton J, Häsler B. Surveillance without intervention: is there a value? BMC Vet Res. in press;
4. Drewe JA, Hoinville LJ, Cook AJC, Floyd T, Stärk KDC. Evaluation of animal and public health surveillance systems: a systematic review. Epidemiol Infect. 2012;140(4):575–90. Available at: http://journals.cambridge.org/abstract_S0950268811002160
5. Stärk KDC, Schuppers M, Brägger M, Balmer S, Nigsch A, Hälser B, Hadornd D. Evaluation of a surveillance system implemented to provide early detection for animal health hazards. Proceedings 14th international symposium of veterinary epidemiology and economics, Merida, Mexico; 2015.
6. Hueston WD. BSE and variant CJD: Emerging science, public pressure and the vagaries of policy-making. Prev Vet Med. 2013;109:179–84. https://doi.org/10.1016/j.prevetmed.2012.11.023.
7. Probst C, Gethmann JM, Heuser R, Niemann H, Conraths FJ. Direct costs of bovine spongiform encephalopathy control measures in Germany. Zoonoses Public Health. 2013; https://doi.org/10.1111/zph.12032.
8. Anonymous. Evaluation of the bovine spongiform encephalopathy (BSE) management programme; 2014. Available online at http://www.inspection.gc.ca. Accessed 21/01/2018.
9. Wall BA, Arnold ME, Radia D, Gilbert W, Ortiz-Pelaez A, Stärk KD, Van Klink E, Guitian J. Evidence for more cost-effective surveillance options for bovine spongiform encephalopathy (BSE) and scrapie in Great Britain. Eurosurveillance. 2017;22:30,594. https://doi.org/10.2807/1560-7917.ES.2017.22.32.30594.
10. Adkin A, Simons R, Arnold M. Assessing the sensitivity of European surveillance for detecting BSE in cattle according to international standards. Prev Vet Med. 2016;135:113–22. https://doi.org/10.1016/J.PREVETMED.2016.10.011.
11. EFSA (European Food Safety Authority). Scientific report on the evaluation of the revision of the BSE monitoring regime in Croatia. EFSA J. 2016;14(2):4399, 27 pp. https://doi.org/10.2903/j.efsa.2016.4399.
12. Alban L, Léger A, Veldhuis A, van Schaik G. Modernizing the antimicrobial residue monitoring programs for pig meat in Europe—the balance between flexibility and harmonization. Food Control. 2018;86:403–13. https://doi.org/10.1016/j.foodcont.2017.11.040.

13. Cameron AR. The consequences of risk-based surveillance: developing output-based standards for surveillance to demonstrate freedom from disease. Prev Vet Med. 2012;105(4):280–6. Available at: http://www.ncbi.nlm.nih.gov/pubmed/22305852.
14. Anonymous. Performance indicators for Rinderpest surveillance. International Atomic Energy Agency, IAEA-TECDOC-1261, 92 pp; 2001. Available online www-naweb.iaea. Accessed 26/01/2018.

Added Value and Impact of the Evaluation Process in Health Surveillance

15

Marisa Peyre, Stéphanie Cong, Vu Dinh Ton, Guy Faure, Eugénie Baudon, Nguyen Viet Khong, Malik Peiris, Ben Cowling, and Flavie Goutard

Abstract

Impact evaluation is increasingly requested from research for both donor and social accountability (Faure et al., Agric Syst 165, 128–136; 2018). Conducting it properly is difficult, especially in the context of a developing country. Quantitative studies are often biased toward expected and tangible impacts. Complementary and more qualitative approaches are focused on understanding causality and are more in line with

M. Peyre (✉)
CIRAD, UMR ASTRE, Montpellier, France

ASTRE, CIRAD, INRAE, University of Montpellier, Montpellier, France
e-mail: marisa.peyre@cirad.fr

S. Cong · F. Goutard
CIRAD, UMR ASTRE, Montpellier, France

ASTRE, CIRAD, INRAE, University of Montpellier, Montpellier, France

V. D. Ton
Faculty of Animal Science, Vietnam National University of Agriculture, Trau Quy, Vietnam

G. Faure
CIRAD, UMR INNOVATION, Montpellier, France

E. Baudon
CIRAD, UMR ASTRE, Montpellier, France

WHO Collaborating Centre for Infectious Disease Epidemiology and Control, School of Public Health, The University of Hong Kong, Sandy Bay, Hong Kong Special Administrative Region

N. V. Khong
National Institute of Veterinary Research, Hanoi, Vietnam

M. Peiris · B. Cowling
WHO Collaborating Centre for Infectious Disease Epidemiology and Control, School of Public Health, The University of Hong Kong, Sandy Bay, Hong Kong Special Administrative Region

M. Peyre et al. (eds.), *Principles for Evaluation of One Health Surveillance: The EVA Book*, https://doi.org/10.1007/978-3-030-82727-4_15

actors' participation in impact evaluation. CIRAD has developed a method (ImpresS) and applied it to assessing 13 case studies, each of them including a cluster of projects involving research and conducted in widely different environments (Faure et al., Agric Syst 165, 128–136; 2018). One of the case studies looked at the impacts of the use of innovative evaluation approaches to strengthening animal health surveillance. This research was implemented by Cirad and its partners between 2009 and 2016 in order to develop innovative evaluation approaches to evaluate animal health surveillance systems in South East Asia (REVASIA: http://revasia.cirad.fr). In this chapter, we present how the impact evaluation approach based on the theory of change can help in framing surveillance programs and also how this approach can be used to assess the impact of the evaluation itself.

Keywords
Impact · Evaluation · Theory of change · Surveillance

15.1 Introduction

Impact evaluation is increasingly requested from research for both donor and social accountability [1]. Conducting it properly is difficult, especially in the context of a developing country. Quantitative studies are often biased toward expected and tangible impacts. Complementary and more qualitative approaches are focused on understanding causality and are more in line with actor's participation in impact evaluation. The impact assessment method developed by Cirad combines both approaches. The method is based on the theory of change, which looks at all the steps required to foster changes in behaviors to reach a specific impact.

15.1.1 What is a Theory of Change?

A theory of change (TOC) presents a roadmap defining all the steps required to bring about a given long-term goal. This set of connected steps usually includes: the **inputs**—the resources (funding, competences, etc.) needed to undertake the activities, the activities could be those done as part of a research program, a health policy program, etc.; the **outputs**—the results generated by the activities (e.g., the development of a cost-effective surveillance protocol); the **outcomes**—the results of the outputs which are taken up by the actors involved in the innovation process with changes in terms of practices (technics and organization) and behavior (e.g., the integration of the new efficient surveillance protocol within the national surveillance system); the **impacts**—the long-term effects generated by the outcomes (e.g., the improvement of animal health due to the implementation of the new efficient surveillance protocol). The impact is defined here as the long-term effects induced by the interventions and could be of multiple nature (economic, social, sanitary, political, etc.), multiple levels (individual, institutional, regional, national, etc.), and of different types (positive or negative; direct or indirect).

The steps of the TOC and the links between them are often depicted on a map known as a **pathway of change/impact pathway**, which is a graphic representation of the change process (Fig. 15.1).

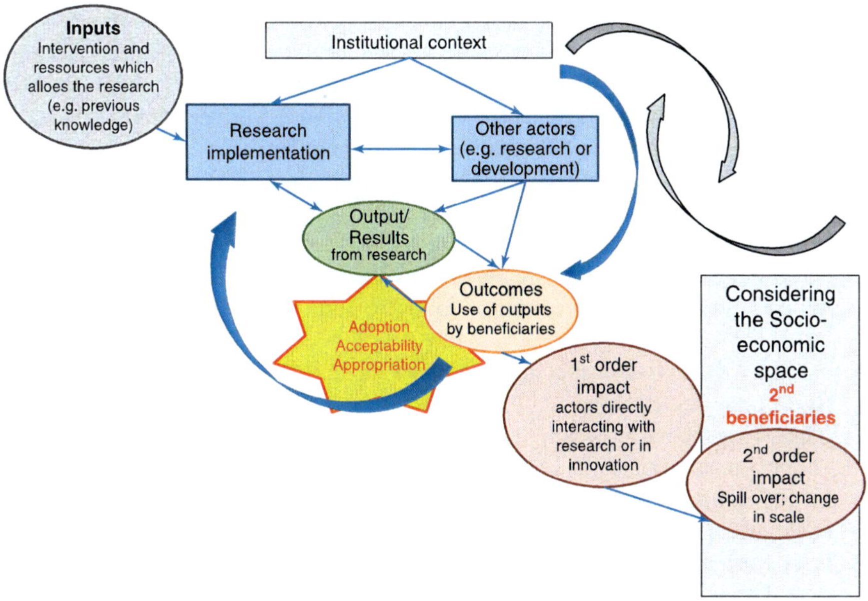

Fig. 15.1 The change or impact pathway: links between inputs, outputs, outcomes, and impact

The theory of change could be used with an ex-ante evaluation perspective (planning), an in-itinere perspective (monitoring), or an ex-post evaluation of research project or development interventions. From an action perspective, the TOC is useful to identify and monitor all the changes required to reach expected impacts [2] (Fig. 15.1). This theory applies to any type of action, which requires behavior and social changes [3].

In order to have an impact, a research invention (i.e., the output, e.g., a cost-effective surveillance protocol generated from an evaluation work) needs to interact with other actors, which use and adapt the research outputs, in order to change things in place (i.e., the outcome, e.g., the implementation of the efficient surveillance protocol in the national strategy). Hence we characterize the contribution of research to the impacts and we do not focus on the attribution to research of the changes. The innovation process is not linear and there are many feedbacks and loops. Between the research outputs and the impact many intermediary outcomes might be required to generate impacts but also might induce the need to produce new research outputs. This complex process will eventually lead to the expected impact (Fig. 15.1, Case study 1).

15.1.2 The Process of Creating a Theory of Change

When undertaking an ex-ante impact evaluation, stakeholders must be clear about what they want to achieve. When considering animal health or one health surveillance, it is likely that the different actors involved will have different views about what their goals are and the level of misunderstanding that exists between them. The first step will be to work with all the stakeholders to identify their expected long-term goals and thus the impacts they want to achieve. The next step is for everybody involved to think about all of the outcomes (including changes of practices and behaviors) that must occur in order to reach those impacts. They then need to consider, in light of this big-picture perspective, which of these outcomes they will take the responsibility to work on—both individually or as a team; and what changes in practices and behavior (if any) are required to undertake these activities.

Six main steps are recommended to follow to build up this change pathway:

1. Writing a **narrative** to explain the logic of the initiative: tell the story of what is trying to be achieved.
2. Identifying the basic assumptions about the **context:** the factors (social, cultural political, institutional etc…) that can enable or limit the achievements.
3. Identifying the **long-term goals:** each actor might have different views on what could be achieved in the long term.
4. Backward mapping and connecting the outcomes and the conditions/risk to make happen. Then defining the outputs, activities necessary to achieve the goal and explaining why these conditions are necessary and sufficient, which will define the outcomes, outputs, and inputs required.
5. Identifying the **interventions** that the initiative will perform to create your desired change, which will highlight the contribution of a specific initiative in reaching those impacts.
6. Developing **indicators to measure your outcomes** to assess the performance of your initiative and **to measure the impacts generated**.

This mapping exercise could be done using participatory approaches and tools such as actor consultation workshops; individual or focus group; convergent interviews (e.g., key informant), questionnaires (e.g., internet), expert reviews (Fig. 15.2).

15.1.2.1 Data Collection and Analysis

Different data collection methods can be used to gather information on the steps described above (Table 15.1).

Analysis could combine both qualitative and quantitative data using:

- **Numeric analysis:** correlation, data mining (looking for patterns), multivariate analysis, time-series analysis
- **Textual analysis:** content analysis (relevant to help defining the evaluation question), thematic coding (indexation into categories), World cloud, Word tree

Combining quantitative and qualitative methods during conducting of the process will provide more insightful understandings by (i) identifying issues or obtaining information on variables not acquired by quantitative surveys; (ii) generating hypotheses to be tested through the quantitative approach; (iii) understanding unanticipated results from quantitative data or (iv) verifying or rejecting results (triangulation).

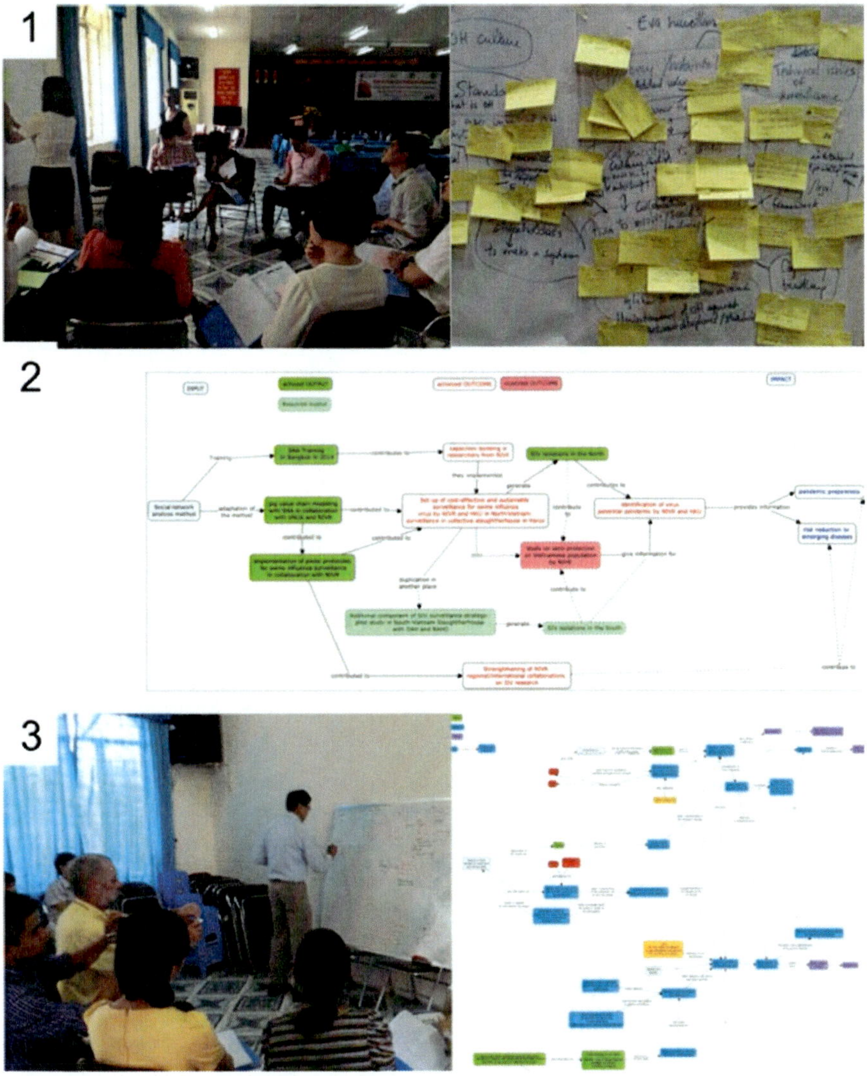

Fig. 15.2 Data collection and analysis process using expert opinion workshops. (1) Actors' consultation, identification of inputs/outputs/outcomes/impacts; (2) building up of pathway and scenarios; (3) validation of pathways and scenarios

15.1.3 The Value of a Theory of Change

Health policies (surveillance and control) are often planned without an explicit understanding of the early and intermediate steps required for long-term changes to occur—especially behavioural changes. A TOC creates an honest picture of the steps required to reach this goal. It provides an opportunity for stakeholders to assess what they can influence, what impact they can have, and whether it is realistic

Table 15.1 Examples of different types of methods used to collect data for impact pathway development

Method type	Definition
Brainstorming	Focusing on a problem and then allowing participants to come up with as many solutions as possible.
Concept Mapping	Showing how different ideas relate to each other—sometimes this is called a mind map or a cluster map.
Dotmocracy	Collecting and recognizing levels of agreement on written statements among a large number of people.
Expert opinion elicitation process	Soliciting opinions from groups in an iterative process of answering questions in order to gain a consensus; e.g., Delphi Study.
Outcome mapping	Measuring deliverables and its effects on primary beneficiaries by looking at behavioral change exhibited by secondary beneficiaries. The outcome-mapping process consists of a design phase (which includes describing the perspective of the actions; identifying relevant partners; defining progress indicators; followed by a cyclic record-keeping phase, reviewing all the previous steps to identify gaps and behaviors change required).
ORID	Enabling a focused conversation by allowing participants to consider all that is known (Objective) and their feelings (Reflective) before considering issues (Interpretive) and decisions (Decisional).
Q-methodology	Investigating the different perspectives of participants on an issue by ranking and sorting a series of statements (also known as Q-sort).
SWOT Analysis	Reflecting on and assessing the Strengths, Weaknesses, Opportunities, and Threats of a particular strategy.
Stakeholder Mapping Analysis	The mapping and analysis of stakeholders provide information on key target groups and players who will be impacted by a proposed reform. It helps to predict whether they might support or block the implementation of the latter and thus to propose strategies to promote supportive actions and decrease opposing actions.
World Cafe	Hosting group dialogue in which the power of simple conversation is emphasized in the consideration of relevant questions and themes.

to expect to reach their goal within the time and resources available. The exercise of creating a TOC is really a management tool that can benefit planning of a surveillance strategy as well as evaluation of the strategies (cf. Case Study 1) or evaluating the impact of the evaluation process itself (cf. Case study 2).

15.2 IMPRESS Impact Assessment Method

The ImpresS method was developed by CIRAD to evaluate the impact of research projects [2]. This method is based on the theory of change and the participatory evaluation of the impact pathway. The ImpresS methodology mobilized a set of key concepts: case study research [4], impact pathway evaluation [3], and contribution analysis [5]. This choice relies on a scientific interest in unveiling the processes and mechanisms that lead to impacts in agricultural research. The evaluation followed participatory principles [6] to achieve a convergent vision among actors of the process being evaluated and its effects [7] and improve the quality of the evaluation by mobilizing different knowledge and perceptions [8, 9].

The ImpresS assessment consists of three phases:

- Describing the story of the process under evaluation: reconstructing with the actors the narrative of the innovation process, including a specific focus on capacity strengthening activities and interactions with public actors.
- Mapping the causal chain from inputs used by research, to research outputs, to outcomes, which are generated when actors used and transformed the outputs, and finally to impacts, which are the effects of this use using the impact pathway approach. First-level impacts, those on actors who directly or indirectly interacted with research and its partners, are differentiated from second-level impacts, corresponding to scaling processes.
- Characterizing and measuring of the impact indicators: each impact is characterized by a set of quantitative and qualitative indicators that account for the evolution occurring between the start of the innovation process and the evaluation. The sources of information for these indicators included ad hoc surveys, interviews, focus groups or secondary data.

Participatory approaches are implemented during each phase of the method, to engage and codevelop the impact pathway with all the relevant stakeholders involved in the innovation process (either as part of the development of the innovation or as being impacted by the innovation or influencing the innovation): (i) semi-structured individual interviews in the preparation/framing phase followed by a participatory stakeholder workshop to validate the framing and method to collect data; (2) data collection and impact measurement using semi-structured interviews, focus groups or surveys (3) validation of the results—participatory workshop with all the actors involved and identification of scenarios to initiate activities for missing outcomes if any.

Box 15.1 Useful definitions

What is an innovation?

- **Invention**: novelty developed by researchers
- **Innovation** = invention implemented by actors with an adaptation phase, and the aim to change things in place
  - Novel technique (hardware)
  - Novel knowledge and way of thinking (software)
  - Novel institution, organization (orgware)

Which differences between inputs/outputs and outcomes?

- **Inputs**: Intervention and resources which allows the research (e.g., previous knowledge)

- **Outputs**: Products/results from research
- **Outcomes**: Use of outputs by actors without research control

What is an impact?

- **Impact:** long-term effects induced by an intervention. This is what stays after the end of the intervention (research program for example)
- **Impact could be**:
  - Of different nature: economic, social, sanitary, political, etc.
  - At different level of actors: individual, groups, institutions
  - Positive or negative
  - Intentional or not
  - Direct or indirect
- **Impact could be** measured by indicators (quantitative or qualitative)

15.3 Application of Principles to Case Studies

15.3.1 Case Study 1: Evaluation of the Impact of the Development of a Cost-Effective Swine Influenza Surveillance Protocol in Vietnam

15.3.1.1 Introduction

The need for animal disease surveillance to improve animal and public health and prevent pandemic threats is now widely recognized. Efforts to develop and/or improve surveillance programs targeting zoonotic diseases are made all over the world especially in disease emergence hotspot areas, including Southeast Asia. However, there is an important financial pressure as funding is usually limited, especially in developing countries, and therefore the surveillance systems must be efficient at the lowest possible cost to ensure sustainability. Evaluation of surveillance systems is an essential step in this process of improving their performance and efficiency; evaluation must be done on a regular basis and the most relevant aspects to evaluate must be selected according to the surveillance objectives. In Vietnam, passive surveillance is present for diseases in swine such as porcine respiratory and reproductive syndrome virus (PRRSV), classical swine fever virus (CSF), and foot and mouth disease (FMD). Regarding influenza, a sentinel surveillance system for human influenza based on the testing of patients with ILI in selected healthcare practices, and a passive avian influenza system for surveillance in poultry are in place. However, there is no long-term surveillance activity for SIV; only sporadic research-based studies have been carried out. Such studies are usually costly and with low efficiency for virus isolation, and as they are not carried out in the long term, virus evolution cannot be monitored over long periods. Continuous systematic surveillance activities would remedy this issue. However, resources are limited in developing countries such as Vietnam, and the swine industry has usually a low interest for SIV as the disease causes often mild symptoms, especially in endemic countries, and low mortality, as compared to diseases considered of major economic importance such as PRRSV. In 2011, a study was implemented to identify the most cost-effective surveillance strategies to ensure sustainable surveillance of SIV in Vietnam. The ImpresS methodology was applied to the evaluation of the impact of the development of a cost-effective swine influenza surveillance protocol in Vietnam.

15.3.1.2 Story of the innovation

The development of a cost-effective SIV surveillance protocol was performed as part of a PhD research project in collaboration between CIRAD, the National Institute for Veterinary Research in Vietnam (NIVR), and the School of Public health and the Pasteur Research Center from Hong Kong University (HKU) (Fig. 15.3) (**INPUTS 2–4**) [10–14]. This study used previously developed methodologies (e.g., network analysis and risk assessment) to understand and quantify the movement of swine along the swine value chain with regard to the risk of SIV circulation in Vietnam the design SIV surveillance protocols to be tested in Vietnam (**INPUT 1** and **OUTPUTS 1–3**). The SIV isolation laboratory capacities were strengthened by the training of NIVR staff on isolation techniques using cell culture and fresh isolates (**OUTPUT 4**). Several surveillance pilot protocols were designed and implemented; they included surveillance in abattoirs, in a market, in sentinel farms, and a syndromic surveillance in the Red River Delta region (**OUTPUT 5**).

Cost-effectiveness of each surveillance protocol was evaluated based on the two main surveillance objectives, i.e., virus characterization and knowledge of SI epidemiology. The collective slaughterhouse surveillance was the protocol with the highest cost-effectiveness. Indeed, it allowed continuous virus isolation from pigs of different origins and had the capacity to provide estimates of SI seroprevalence and

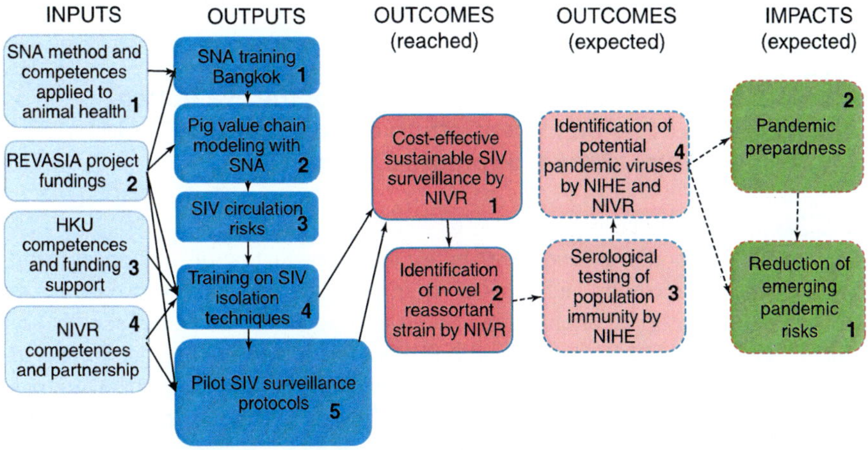

Fig. 15.3 Simplified impact pathway of swine influenza surveillance in Vietnam

serological identification of the circulating SIV lineages in the pig population. This protocol has been implemented monthly since 2013 and is now part of the routine surveillance activities by NIVR (**OUTCOME 1**). Every month, the NIVR laboratory samples pigs in the largest slaughterhouse in Hanoi and performs SIV virus isolation and serological testing on those samples. Positive isolates are then sent out to HKU for further sequencing to identify novel reassortant strains (**OUTCOME 2**). At the moment, this surveillance protocol is not able to reach its expected impacts related to the reduction of emerging pandemic risks linked to SIV in Vietnam (**expected IMPACT 1**) that should contribute to improving Vietnam pandemic preparedness (**expected IMPACT 2**). Indeed, the novel reassortants are not yet being tested again the Vietnam human population serum bank in collaboration with the National Institute for Hygiene and Epidemiology (NIHE) (**expected OUTCOME 3**); which will allow to identify potential pandemic viruses—i.e., viruses against which the population of Vietnam has no baseline immunity (**expected OUTCOME 4**).

15.3.1.3 Added value of the impact evaluation

This impact evaluation work has demonstrated the uptake of research outputs by decision-makers in Vietnam: the most cost-effective surveillance protocol has been adopted and slightly adapted by NIVR and has been implemented and running since 2013 outside of the research project. This ongoing surveillance protocol is providing valuable information to the NIVR researchers on the epidemiology and seasonal patterns of SIV but also the development of a swab and serum bank that could be used to test for other pathogens. NIVR has collaborated with Oxford Clinical Research Unit (OUCRU) to test samples for Japanese encephalitis virus; and with the International Livestock Research Institute (ILRI) to test for bacterial pathogens. Moreover, this work has also allowed identifying the limits of this SIV surveillance in terms of reaching its objectives and therefore impacts: additional activities in collaboration with the human health sector are still required to assess the risk of novel SIV pandemic threat in humans.

15.3.2 Case Study 2: Assessing the Impact of the Evaluation Process of Avian Influenza Surveillance Strategy in Vietnam: a Way to Promote Changes

15.3.2.1 Introduction

The ImpresS methodology has been applied to the evaluation of the impact using novel evaluation methods and tools to strengthen animal health surveillance in Vietnam. Participatory approaches have been used to describe in detail the history (Fig. 15.4); to map all the actors and collaborations involved (Fig. 15.5); and to codevelop a detailed impact pathway with all the actors (Fig. 15.6). This work has also allowed to identify different scenarios and missing activities to ensure in the near future the impact of the application of evaluation to strengthen animal health surveillance in Vietnam.

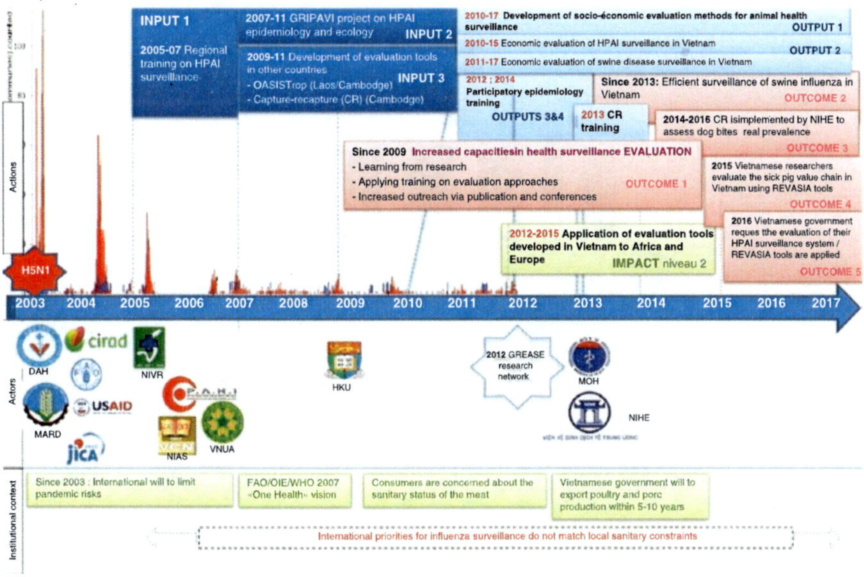

Fig. 15.4 Story of the improvement of animal health surveillance using innovative evaluation tools in Vietnam

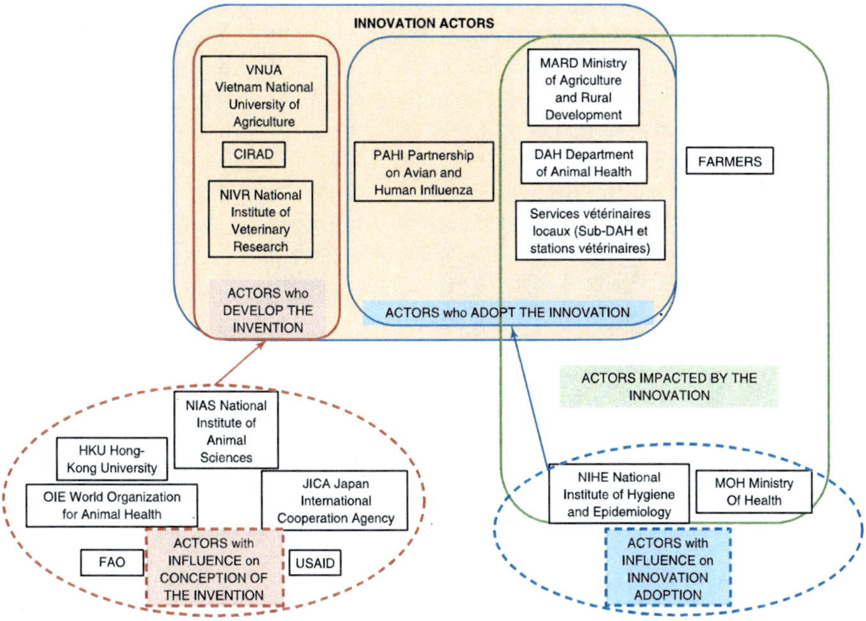

Fig. 15.5 Mapping of the actors involved in the strengthening of animal health surveillance using innovative evaluation approaches

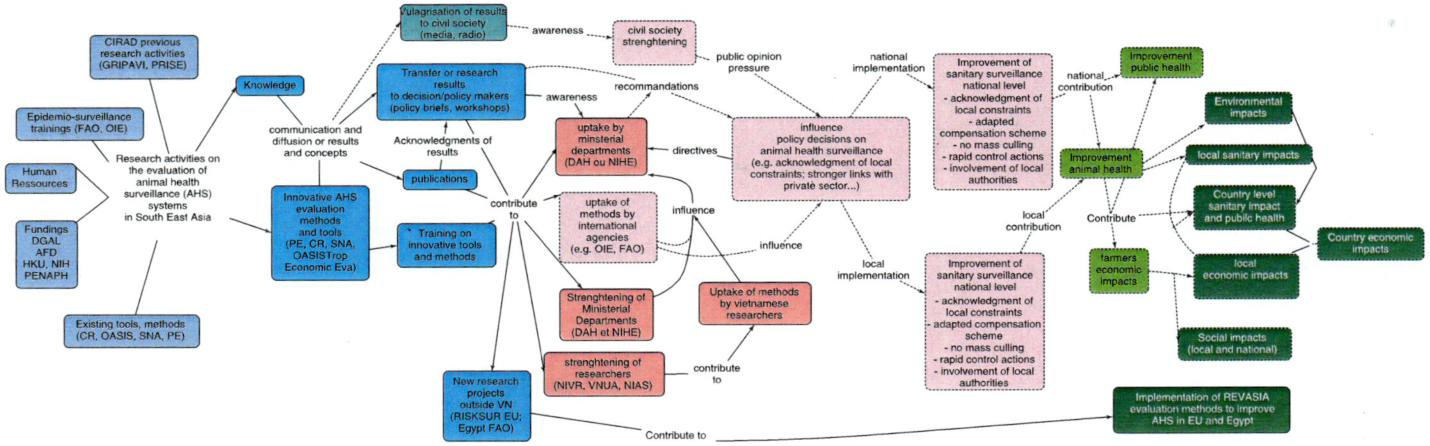

Fig. 15.6 Impact pathway on the strengthening of animal health surveillance using innovative evaluation approaches: INPUTS (light blue); OUTPUTS (dark blue); OUTCOMES (reached: dark pink; expected: light pink); IMPACTS level 1 (light green); IMPACTS level 2 (dark green); anything that has been implemented or reached is represented by the plain lines; anything that is still expected is represented by the dotted lines

15.3.2.2 Story of the Innovation Improving Animal Health Surveillance in Vietnam Using Evaluation Methods and Tools

In the context of the HPAI H5N1 avian influenza crisis in Asia in 2003, CIRAD's AGIRs unit carried out epidemiological surveillance training in Southeast Asia and implemented research projects on ecology and the epidemiology of the disease in the region (Fig. 15.4. INPUTS 1 and 2)

Phase 1: development and implementation of evaluation tools: From 2009 to 2011 (REVASIA-FRIA projects), tools for quantitative evaluation of the performance of surveillance systems (OASISTrop and CR method) are developed in Thailand, Laos, and Cambodia and will be applied in Vietnam later (INPUT 3) (Chap. 2). The NIVR and the Hanoi University of Agriculture (HAU now VNUA) are the historical partners of CIRAD in Vietnam in animal health; the DAH, a key political and technical player in surveillance systems, authorizes REVASIA implementation but does not take an active part in the development of innovation even if it remains its main beneficiary. From 2011 to 2015, pilot protocols for surveillance of swine influenza were implemented in Vietnam, in collaboration with the University of Hong Kong, NIVR and UNVUT (OUTPUT 1) (Baudon et al. [13, 14]). In 2012, participatory epidemiology (PE) tools are adapted to the economic evaluation of surveillance systems for animal diseases (pigs and poultry) in Vietnam, and in particular to evaluate the costs and societal benefits of surveillance systems (see Part III); the analysis of social networks (SNA) is adapted at the same time to the evaluation of health information flows (types of actors, types of contacts, types of information) (OUTPUT 2) (see Part IV).

Phase 2: adoption of the innovation, first OUTCOMES, first IMPACTS: From 2012 to 2016, the capacities of the researchers of the NIVR, VNUA, NIAS, of the University of Nong Lam (Ho Chi Minh), as well as agents of DAH and NIHE are strengthened with respect to monitoring system evaluation techniques (PE, CR, SNA) (OUTPUTS 3 and 4 and OUTCOME 1). In 2013, NIHE applied the CR method to the evaluation of rabies surveillance (OUTCOME 2). In 2014, the NIVR launched its swine influenza surveillance program following the results of the "swine flu" project; the program is still ongoing (OUTCOME 3). In 2012 and 2014, the PE tools developed in REVASIA are applied to the evaluation of surveillance in France, Belgium, and Germany (EU RISKSUR project), and in Egypt in collaboration with policy-makers and the FAO (IMPACT level 2). In 2015, VNUA (VD Ton) carries out a research project on the evaluation of the sick animals (pigs) sector in Vietnam using the SNA (SICKPIG) method (OUTCOME 4). In 2016, DHA and FAO contract the Royal Veterinary College (RVC) to evaluate the HPAI surveillance system in Vietnam. Timothée Vergne (trained in evaluation by CIRAD (Thesis) in the framework of REVASIA-FRIA) is in charge of the evaluation and applies the tools developed by CIRAD in REVASIA and in RISKSUR (OUTCOME 5). In 2016, the REVASIA research program includes a project cluster: REVASIA FRIA; REVASIA-Socio-Eco; SEA-PREID; Swine surveillance; SWEID.

Scenarios and Activities to Implement to Ensure the Impacts Reach Out

Three different scenarios were identified by the stakeholders to achieve the expected impacts:

i. *Influence of public policies at the national level:* the first step of this scenario is representing how research projects are implemented in the field in Vietnam; this research involves Vietnamese researchers, local authorities, and local beneficiaries (veterinarians and breeders). Currently (branch 2), the results are transferred to decision-makers (DAH, MARD) by means of scientific reports containing recommendations that can be directly taken into account to modify and improve the health surveillance (e.g., how to take into account local constraints to decrease the number of underreported cases of diseases). **The impact of this approach is limited by the involvement of policy-makers, and can be very limited if they do not contribute to the implementation of activities.**

   One possible alternative developed during the participatory discussions is the implementation of pilot research protocols at the national level to validate the results before recommendations can be made. These pilot studies can be directly implemented by the departments of the Ministry (DHA) to secure their confidence in the results or by Vietnamese researchers but at the request of the DAH and under its authority. The improvement of surveillance by a change of policy at the national level involves improved sanitary situation in the whole country, which favours efficiency and sustainability in the activities of disease control. However, the improvement of surveillance at the national level may also have a negative effect on local veterinarians (too much workload) and farmers (slaughter of animals) and must take into account local constraints to be effective and sustainable.

ii. *Influence of local public policies (provincial level)*: this scenario put forward the importance of local authorities in the implementation of surveillance activities and health control and their potential influence on activities at the national level. Indeed, in this scenario, the results obtained by the field research activities are presented to local authorities to help them to improve the local health surveillance system. If livestock production is a priority of the province, the People's Committee, the authority of the province, can directly take into account the scientific recommendations and influence the changes in the surveillance system of the Province. However the impact, which would be an improvement of the local health condition, might not be sustainable if the health condition is not also improved in the other provinces. However, if these changes result in a positive impact and an improvement in the health condition of the Province, this may influence the Ministry to test this type of change in other provinces, or neighboring provinces may decide to implement the same changes (snowball effect).

iii. Influence of public opinion: the third scenario proposes to sensitize civil society by widely disseminating scientific results in a popularized format via different media. However, this type of information must be first authorized by the MARD. Vietnam has many media; they are, however, much controlled by the central government. They have a dual role as mass organizations; on the one side, they are the spokespersons of the government, which finances and controls them, but, on the other side, they are also the spokespersons of the people. Another approach would be to use the Internet and social networks to inform consumers. Today, more and more Vietnamese have access to the Internet, particularly via their mobile phones. It is a neutral way for Vietnamese and social networks to play a major role in mobilizing the population around a social event. Another approach would be the dissemination of information by farmers' organizations but they remain marginal in Vietnam and still have a limited political influence.

15.3.2.3 Added Value of the Impact Evaluation

This work was critical to provide relevant and meaningful recommendations to the decision-makers to identify the changes required to ensure uptake of the evaluation tools and implementation of the evaluation recommendations to achieve the impacts.

It enabled us not only to evaluate the performances of the work implemented during the project but also to involve our partners and beneficiaries in the identification of actions to be implemented and activities to be planned to ensure achieving the impacts not yet reached (Cong 2016). Once more, public–private partnerships and the strengthening of these partnerships were critical, particularly at the local level, to ensure impact of animal health surveillance strategies. This work highlights the importance of evaluation to inform changes that need to be adopted in public animal health policies at the national level to ensure the sustainability and impact of the actions.

References

1. Faure G, Barret D, Blundo-Canto G, Dabat M-H, Devaux-Spatarakis A, Le Guerroué JL, Marquié C, Mathé S, Temple L, Toillier A, Triomphe B, Hainzelin E. How different agricultural research models contribute to impacts: evidence from 13 case studies in developing countries. Agric Syst. 2018;165:128–36. https://doi.org/10.1016/j.agsy.2018.06.002.
2. Barret D, Blundo-Canto G, Dabat M-H, Devaux-Spatarakis A, Faure G, Hainzelin E, Mathé S, Temple L, Toillier A, Triomphe B, Vall E. IMPRESS methodological guide; methodological guide to ex post impact evaluation of agricultural research in developing countries; 2018.
3. Douthwaite B, Kuby T, van de Fliert E, Schulz S. Impact pathway evaluation: an approach for achieving and attributing impact in complex systems. Agric Syst. 2003;78:243–65. https://doi.org/10.1016/S0308-521X(03)00128-8.
4. Yin R. Case study research: design and methods. 4th ed. Thousands Oaks, CA: Sage; n.d.
5. Mayne J. Addressing attribution through contribution analysis: using performance measures sensibly. n.d.;20.
6. Baron G, Monnier E. Une approche pluraliste et participative: 7; n.d..
7. Habermas J. The theory of communicative action, vol. 1. Boston: Beacon Press; 1984.
8. Calba C, Antoine-Moussiaux N, Charrier F, Hendrikx P, Saegerman C, Peyre M, Goutard FL. Applying participatory approaches in the evaluation of surveillance systems: a pilot study on African swine fever surveillance in Corsica. Prev Vet Med. 2015;122:389–98. https://doi.org/10.1016/j.prevetmed.2015.10.001.

9. Ridde V. Suggestions d'améliorations d'un cadre conceptuel de l'évaluation participative. Can J Program Eval. n.d.;23.
10. Baudon E, Chu DKW, Tung DD, Thi Nga P, Vu Mai Phuong H, Le Khanh Hang N, Thanh LT, Thuy NT, Khanh NC, Mai LQ, Khong NV, Cowling BJ, Peyre M, Peiris M. Swine influenza viruses in Northern Vietnam in 2013-2014. Emerg Microbes Infect. 2018;7:123. https://doi.org/10.1038/s41426-018-0109-y.
11. Baudon E, Fournie G, Hiep DT, Pham TTH, Duboz R, Gely M, Peiris M, Cowling BJ, Ton VD, Peyre M. Analysis of swine movements in a province in Northern Vietnam and application in the design of surveillance strategies for infectious diseases. Transbound Emerg Dis. 2017a;64:411–24. https://doi.org/10.1111/tbed.12380.
12. Baudon E, Peyre M, Peiris M, Cowling BJ. Epidemiological features of influenza circulation in swine populations: A systematic review and meta-analysis. PloS One. 2017b;12:e0179044. https://doi.org/10.1371/journal.pone.0179044.
13. Baudon E, Poon LL, Dao TD, Pham NT, Cowling BJ, Peyre M, Nguyen KV, Peiris M. Detection of novel reassortant influenza A (H3N2) and H1N1 2009 pandemic viruses in swine in Hanoi, Vietnam. Zoonoses Public Health. 2015;62:429–34. https://doi.org/10.1111/zph.12164.
14. Baudon EM. Sustainable surveillance strategies for the detection of swine influenza in Vietnam (Doctor of Philosophy). The University of Hong Kong, Pokfulam Road, Hong Kong SAR; 2015. https://doi.org/10.5353/th_b5736657.

Synthesis—Evaluate to Better Inform: A Way to Strengthening Health Surveillance Systems

16

Marisa Peyre and Flavie Goutard

Abstract

Over the past 15 years, innovative approaches and tools have been developed and applied to evaluate health surveillance systems, in Southeast Asia and in Europe mainly. This work has allowed to better understand the local constraints observed in different contexts and to draw generic recommendations to improve health surveillance on a global scale. Acceptability of the strategies by all actors has been acknowledged as a key issue to ensure success of the actions along with the integration of private networks and actors within the surveillance system. This work helped in raising awareness among researchers, public decision-makers and private actors on evaluation issues, moving away from it being perceived as a control (audit) action often carried out by experts external to the issues and with limited benefits in return. In this regard, integrated evaluation, taking into consideration technical but also socio-economic issues in surveillance, should be promoted. This way, evaluation could be used as a programming tool, and in a participatory way to codevelop solutions with field actors to better inform decision-making in both animal and one health surveillance strategies.

Keywords

Health surveillance · Evaluation · Integrated evaluation · Decision-making · Policy

M. Peyre (✉) · F. Goutard
CIRAD, UMR ASTRE, Montpellier, France

ASTRE, CIRAD, INRAE, University of Montpellier, Montpellier, France
e-mail: marisa.peyre@cirad.fr

M. Peyre et al. (eds.), *Principles for Evaluation of One Health Surveillance: The EVA Book*, https://doi.org/10.1007/978-3-030-82727-4_16

16.1 Introduction

Over the past 15 years, innovative approaches and tools have been developed and applied to evaluate health surveillance systems, in Southeast Asia and in Europe mainly. This work has allowed to better understand the local constraints observed in different contexts and to draw generic recommendations to improve health surveillance on a global scale. Socioeconomic and cultural constraints are impacting the decision of the actors of the surveillance system to declare or not declare a suspect case of disease and thus independently of the country development level. However, the origin and response to these constraints will vary according to the specific socioeconomic and cultural contexts of each country [1–5]. Similarities and differences are strongly related to the type and structuring level of the production and value chains of the livestock sector concerned [4].

Implementing innovative evaluation methods based on participatory approaches, under different epidemiological, socioeconomic, and cultural contexts, and targeting different systems and diseases have highlighted the great flexibility of these approaches. The added value of participatory approaches to evaluation, favoring comparative analysis between studies, and providing avenues for standardization and possible harmonization of the evaluation process between different contexts have been demonstrated [4, 6]. This work also highlighted major challenges in the field of animal and one health surveillance system evaluation, most of which have been addressed in this book and are synthesized in this chapter and, especially, how to account for socioeconomic constraints that impact health surveillance performances; how to ensure acceptability and stakeholder engagement; how to account for the critical role of private surveillance networks and how to advocate for an integrated approach to evaluation.

16.1.1 Accounting for Major Socioeconomic Constraints that Impact the Performance of Health Surveillance Systems

The official declaration of disease cases often leads to strong social and economic constraints to farmers and other local surveillance actors: uncertainties related to compensation, limited confidence in risk management skills by the official authorities, impact on sales opportunities, stigma in the community, stress related to slaughter and loss of genetic material, etc. [7–11]. Several alternative options to the official report of diseases are available: treatment of sick animals under the advice of private veterinarians or sellers of medicines/veterinary pharmacies; fast sale of healthy and/or sick animals; slaughter of sick animals [8, 10–12].

The structuring and the quality of the animal production and value chains impact the performances of the disease surveillance systems independently of the development level of the country [4]. The health information exchange networks and the socio-economic constraints of the different actors are closely linked to the level of structuring of the production chains, playing a determining role in the performance of the surveillance. These elements are critical and must be accounting for when making decisions about optimizing health surveillance systems. Organized commercial sector for sick animals have been identified in some low- and middle-income countries (LMIC) [12]. In addition to the animal and human health risks posed by these sick animal value chains, they also directly impact the performance of surveillance systems by reducing the benefits of the surveillance for its actors, and as a vicious circle, increasing further the health risk and further promoting their activity [12]. Additional studies are needed to understand further the motivations of actors in these sectors and to make relevant recommendations to limit their impacts.

The health information exchange networks and the socioeconomic constraints of the different actors are closely linked to the level of structuring of the production chains, playing a determining role in the performance of the surveillance. These elements are critical and must be accounted for when making decisions about optimizing health surveillance systems.

16.2 Acceptability: A Critical Issue to Ensure Stakeholder Engagement

Recent studies have highlighted a recurring lack of acceptability of surveillance systems by its actors, and its consequences in terms of underreporting both in LMIC and high-income countries (HIC) [13, 14]. Trust issues between field private actors and the health authorities strongly impact health surveillance performances, independently from the economic context and the development level of the country. Similar trust issues also exist within the official surveillance system process, involving conflicts of interest often linked to a dual public and private activity of the system's stakeholders [15]. Regulatory compliance in terms of health surveillance by farmers in HIC seems more prevalent than in LMIC, the control bodies being more present and organized in the former, forcing farmers to better comply with good practices. In LMIC, it is very clear that the priority for local veterinarians is to maintain a privileged relationship with the farmers and members of the community to which they belong [2, 7, 15] and not to maintain declaration at all cost.

16.3 Private Surveillance Networks: How to Integrate Them?

The private sector plays a central role in the surveillance and management of animal and zoonotic diseases at the local level. These private systems operate in parallel with official systems, due to the lack of public–private partnerships in the majority of situations in LMIC [16]. The situation could be different in HIC or in LMIC countries where the state gives a health mandate to the private sector to implement health surveillance, especially on nonpriority diseases, which allows the state resources to be concentrated on priority diseases and strengthen public–private collaborations. However, these public–private partnerships seem to lack transparency and cooperation and could themselves be strengthened [1]. This again highlights the issues of trust between the two sectors.

16.4 The Importance of an Integrated Evaluation Approach to Inform Decision

The work presented throughout this book and summarized here highlights the importance of an integrated evaluation of health surveillance systems—accounting for social, economic, and technical aspects—to ensure their efficiency, sustainability, and impact. This type of evaluation, favored by the SurvTool decision support tool, along with all the innovative methods presented here would allow to better address decision-makers' needs in order to promote meaningful evaluation and recommendations to improve the current systems [1, 17–19].

New or improved health surveillance systems (or components within these systems) ideally should be codeveloped with all the actors of the system, from the field actors who are at the source of the data to the decision-makers in charge of defining the national strategies. Companion modeling, described in the following section, seems to be an interesting approach to foster this co-construction [20].

16.5 Remaining Challenges and Future Perspectives to Further Improve Animal Health Surveillance Systems

16.5.1 Participatory Modeling to Build User-Centered Surveillance Systems—Adapted to the Socioeconomic Constraints of Its Actors

Conceptual models of interaction between social actors have been used to manage conflicting environmental resources using companion modeling approaches (ComMod) previously developed are also adapted to the issues involved in assessing the social impacts of surveillance [20].

These approaches offer remarkable potential for the codevelopment of surveillance systems adapted to the constraints of all its stakeholders. A pilot study performed in Vietnam to strengthen its HPAI one health surveillance system has demonstrated great potential to foster the co-construction by promoting intersectoral collaboration; as well as improving the understanding and commitment of actors to the issues of health surveillance in their country. More importantly, this pilot study has demonstrated the interest of stakeholders and their willingness to engage in this type of approach. This method has also been applied to manage health issues in Thailand, Laos, and Cambodia but not directly regarding health surveillance systems [20]. A similar approach based on participatory engagement of all the actors of the system has been implemented to successfully codevelop the ISIKHNAS surveillance system in Indonesia [21].

16.5.2 The Importance of Understanding the Utility of Health Programs (Surveillance and Control)

The utility of the system for its actors needs to be better understood to inform the development of improved health surveillance systems. When evaluated, the value of the systems has been characterized by its cost-effectiveness or cost–benefit that look at the balance between the cost of the system and its performances and/or its consequences at a given level [17]. These econometric analyses still neglect all too often the socioeconomic and socioecological aspects and only give a partial view of the agricultural system considered. Indeed, the issues of surveillance and control of animal health go far beyond the scope of health risk issues and require a more interdisciplinary approach. To answer this interdisciplinary challenge, the concept of utility, relating to the well-being economy, seems to be a field of investigation for research in animal health with a view to dialogue between epidemiology, economics, geography, and sociology.

Traditionally applied in areas such as human health or agriculture, the utility approach is concerned with decision-making in situations of uncertainty. The approach accounts for the attitude or preferences of individuals facing risks in specific socioeconomic and cultural contexts. Accounting for the diversity of the utilities of a surveillance system, the evaluation makes it possible to comprehend the different distribution of costs and benefits linked to animal health surveillance decision for the various actors concerned. It reveals the diversity of interests and therefore interest-bearing that the surveillance system favors. This characterization can foster a space for negotiation between these actors, and lead to a more inclusive governance of the monitoring system (and therefore to its better acceptability). There are various tools to measure these preferences, including the declared preference method but also multicriteria analysis methods associated for example with grading grids that allow weighting the different criteria [10, 22]. In their application, these approaches need to go beyond the health disciplinary field to consider the utility of animal health within its broader context of agriculture.

It would be interesting to evaluate the feasibility of developing and implementing this type of methodology to characterize the utility and value of animal health according to different scales of analysis: exploitation, territory, and sector. This would be an opportunity to account for the influence of animal health on the economy and the health of producers, the organization of agricultural soils and, more broadly, the agricultural economy and the public health of an area or region, a country. The aim would thus be to place livestock production in a broader systemic context in order to better understand breeders' adaptation to health crises and, through these processes, to analyze in a holistic manner the efficiency of livestock health programs. This type of approach does not exist at the moment and requires interdisciplinary collaboration that remains to be built.

16.6 From Policy to Field Implementation: The Need to Combine Top-Down and Bottom-Up Approaches

Health surveillance strategies are mostly defined at the national level, influenced by international standards and priorities, and applied in the field as a top-down approach (Fig. 16.1a). Improving surveillance through policy change at the national level implies improving the health situation at the national level and thus the effectiveness and sustainability of disease surveillance and control actions. However, as we have seen previously, promoting actions not relying on local constraints will not be implemented in the field. Indeed, the change in strategy can foster additional negative effects on local veterinarians and on farmers and must account for local constraints to be effective and sustainable.

Therefore, in practice, those national strategies are often adapted at each administrative level to account for local specificity and even further adapted by the farmers and the local actors of the system (e.g. veterinarians) to account for their socioeconomic constraints (Fig. 16.1) [7]. Too often those strategies are even not implemented at all and local private surveillance and disease management prevail (Fig. 16.1) [16]. Relying on health surveillance management at the local level would not be sufficient to ensure sustainability of the actions if the health situation does not improve also at the national level (boomerang effect). However, if these local changes demonstrate a positive impact and an improvement at the local level, this

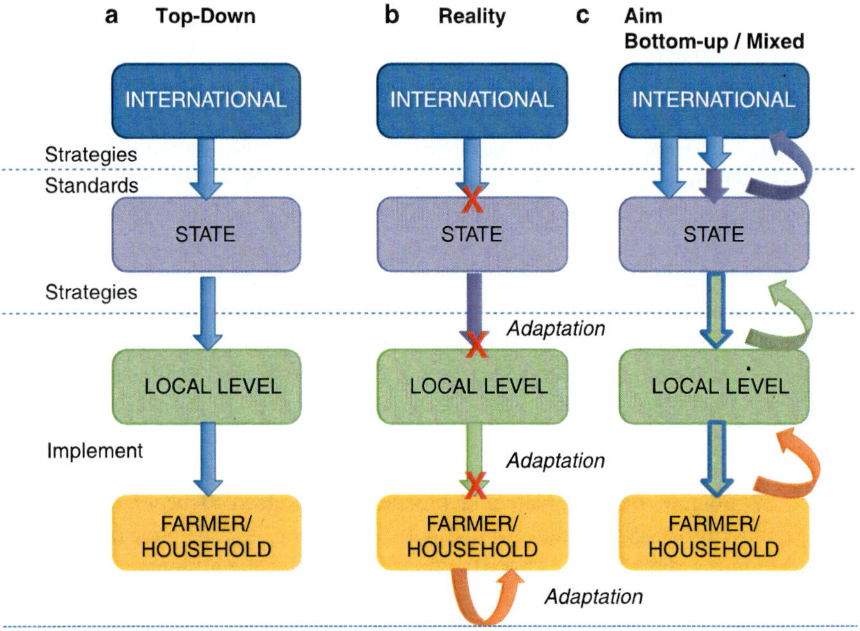

Fig. 16.1 Animal health surveillance strategies: top-down approach (**a**); field implementation (**b**); mixed approach (**c**)

may influence the national authorities to promote this type of change/action in other areas (snowball effect of a bottom-up approach). This could only work by ensuring strong collaboration between private and public actors involved in the system and by promoting a mixed approach: merging top-down and bottom-up strategies to ensure that the needs of all actors are accounted for and efficiency and sustainability of the system (Fig. 16.1c).

16.7 Public–Private Partnerships (PPP): At the Heart of Surveillance in Animal Health

The work presented in this chapter highlights the key role of the private sector in the management (surveillance and control) of animal diseases, with often limited interactions with national surveillance systems. It is essential to account for these issues and strengthen the links between private and public surveillance [15, 23]. In order to strengthen it, we propose to consider animal disease surveillance as a PPP where public and private actors share resources, responsibilities, and risks to meet a common goal and achieve shared benefits: the control of animal diseases.

The surveillance of animal diseases represents the continuous collection of data from private actors (breeders, private veterinarians) to inform public decision-makers (veterinary services) to act (household investigation, control measures, etc.). The private sector thus plays a central role in the surveillance and management of animal diseases at the local level, but with often limited interactions in practice with national surveillance systems.

As we have seen before, in the majority of situations in LMIC, private surveillance systems operate in parallel with formal systems, due to a lack of collaboration and limited trust between sectors (1). The situation is different in HIC where the state gives a mandate to the private sector to implement health surveillance; however, these PPPs sometimes lack transparency and cooperation and could themselves be strengthened (2). It is therefore essential to strengthen the links between private and public surveillance (3). Consideration of the constraints and needs of the actors involved in monitoring, which are not often accounted for, is essential for their commitment and the improvement of systems. Sustainability of the actions can only be ensured by the commitment of the actors of the system; there is a real need to reinforce the links, the communication and the trust between the private actors of the surveillance systems and the public actors. The challenges of these private–public partnerships must be correctly identified, characterized for each type of actors, in order to propose recommendations adapted to this strengthening of collaborations.

PPPs represent an interesting approach to solving complex problems in resource-constrained contexts, specifically with respect to surveillance and control of infectious diseases [24]. However, the development of these approaches on the ground is difficult; it is essential to identify the barriers and brakes to these initiatives in situ to promote good practices of implementation of PPPs [4]. A handbook on PPP best practices has been recently developed and helps in identifying the factors limiting the application of PPPs in the context of strengthening the management of animal health [25].

16.8 Conclusion

These 15 years of research in the evaluation of animal and zoonotic disease surveillance and control systems have addressed key issues in the functioning and operationalization of these systems, especially with regard to the drivers of underreporting and the optimization of resources allocated to these systems. This work also contributed to raising awareness of researchers, decision-makers, and private actors to evaluation issues, previously perceived essentially as a control (audit) action often carried out by experts external to the issues and with limited benefits in return. Evaluation could be used as a programming tool, and in a participatory way to codevelop solution with field actors to improve one health surveillance strategies and prevent emergence and spread of animal diseases and zoonotic risks.

References

1. Bisdorff B, Schauer B, Taylor N, Rodríguez-Prieto V, Comin A, Brouwer A, Dórea F, Drewe J, Hoinville L, Lindberg A, Martinez Avilés M, Martínez-López B, Peyre M, Pinto Ferreira J, Rushton J, Van Schaik G, Stärk KDC, Staubach C, Vicente-Rubiano M, Witteveen G, Pfeiffer D, Häsler B. Active animal health surveillance in European Union Member States: gaps and opportunities. Epidemiol Infect. 2017;145:802–17. https://doi.org/10.1017/S0950268816002697.
2. Goutard FL, Binot A, Duboz R, Rasamoelina-Andriamanivo H, Pedrono M, Holl D, Peyre MI, Cappelle J, Chevalier V, Figuié M, Molia S, Roger FL. How to reach the poor? Surveillance in low-income countries, lessons from experiences in Cambodia and Madagascar. Prev Vet Med. 2015;120:12–26. https://doi.org/10.1016/j.prevetmed.2015.02.014.
3. Peyre M, Choisy M, Sobhy H, Kilany WH, Gély M, Tripodi A, Dauphin G, Saad M, Roger F, Lubroth J, Jobre Y. Added value of avian influenza (H5) day-old chick vaccination for disease control in Egypt. Avian Dis. 2016;60:245–52. https://doi.org/10.1637/11131-050715-ResNote.
4. Peyre M, Pham H, Calba C, Schulz K, Delabouglise A, Goutard F, Roger F, Antoine-Moussiaux N. Animal health surveillance constraints in North and South: same-same but different? Proceedings of the 3rd international conference on animal health surveillance, Rotorua, New Zealand; 2017.
5. Peyrel M, Hendrikx P, Thanh HPT, Huu DD, Goutard F, Desvaux S, Roger F. Evaluation of surveillance systems in animal health: the need to adapt the tools to the contexts of developing countries, results from a regional workshop in South East Asia, pp 415–417; 2011.
6. Calba C, Goutard FL, Vanholme L, Antoine-Moussiaux N, Hendrikx P, Saegerman C. The added-value of using participatory approaches to assess the acceptability of surveillance systems: the case of bovine tuberculosis in Belgium. PLoS One. 2016;11:e0159041. https://doi.org/10.1371/journal.pone.0159041.
7. Delabouglise A, Antoine-Moussiaux N, Tatong D, Chumkaeo A, Binot A, Fournié G, Pilot E, Phimpraphi W, Kasemsuwan S, Paul MC, Duboz R, Salem G, Peyre M. Cultural practices shaping zoonotic diseases surveillance: the case of highly pathogenic avian influenza and Thailand native chicken farmers. Transbound Emerg Dis. 2017a;64:1294–305. https://doi.org/10.1111/tbed.12506.
8. Delabouglise A, Choisy M, Phan TD, Antoine-Moussiaux N, Peyre M, Vu TD, Pfeiffer DU, Fournié G. Economic factors influencing zoonotic disease dynamics: demand for poultry meat and seasonal transmission of avian influenza in Vietnam. Sci Rep. 2017b;7:5905. https://doi.org/10.1038/s41598-017-06244-6.
9. Pham HTT, Antoine-Moussiaux N, Grosbois V, Moula N, Truong BD, Phan TD, Vu TD, Trinh TQ, Vu CC, Rukkwamsuk T, Peyre M. Financial impacts of priority swine diseases to pig farm-

ers in red river and Mekong River delta, Vietnam. Transbound Emerg Dis. 2017a;64:1168–77. https://doi.org/10.1111/tbed.12482.
10. Pham HTT, Peyre M, Trinh TQ, Nguyen OC, Vu TD, Rukkwamsuk T, Antoine-Moussiaux N. Application of discrete choice experiment to assess farmers' willingness to report swine diseases in the Red River Delta region, Vietnam. Prev Vet Med. 2017b;138:28–36. https://doi.org/10.1016/j.prevetmed.2017.01.002.
11. Pham TTH. Economic evaluation of swine disease surveillance system in Vietnam (PhD). Bangkok, Thailand: Kasetsart University; 2016.
12. Hoang MN, Nguyen PT, Han HQ, Nguyen TD, Vu TD, Peyre M. Network analysis of the sick-pig commodity chain in Northern Vietnam: risk of disease dissemination. Rev D'élevage Médecine Vét Pays Trop. 2020;73:61–70. https://doi.org/10.19182/remvt.31872.
13. Calba C, Antoine-Moussiaux N, Charrier F, Hendrikx P, Saegerman C, Peyre M, Goutard FL. Applying participatory approaches in the evaluation of surveillance systems: a pilot study on African swine fever surveillance in Corsica. Prev Vet Med. 2015;122:389–98. https://doi.org/10.1016/j.prevetmed.2015.10.001.
14. Schulz K, Calba C, Peyre M, Staubach C, Conraths FJ. Hunters' acceptability of the surveillance system and alternative surveillance strategies for classical swine fever in wild boar—a participatory approach. BMC Vet Res. 2016;12:187. https://doi.org/10.1186/s12917-016-0822-5.
15. Figuié M, Peyre M-I, Binot A. Surveillance of infectious animal diseases in Southeast Asia. Promoting the multiplicity of information networks. Perspect Cirad. 2013:1–4. https://doi.org/10.19182/agritrop/00040.
16. Delabouglise A, Dao TH, Truong DB, Nguyen TT, Nguyen NTX, Duboz R, Fournié G, Antoine-Moussiaux N, Grosbois V, Vu DT, Le TH, Nguyen VK, Salem G, Peyre M. When private actors matter: information-sharing network and surveillance of Highly Pathogenic Avian Influenza in Vietnam. Acta Trop. 2015;147:38–44. https://doi.org/10.1016/j.actatropica.2015.03.025.
17. Antoine-Moussiaux N, Vandenberg O, Kozlakidis Z, Aenishaenslin C, Peyre M, Roche M, Bonnet P, Ravel A. Valuing Health Surveillance as an Information System: Interdisciplinary Insights. Front Public Health. 2019;7:138. https://doi.org/10.3389/fpubh.2019.00138.
18. Hennessey M, Kim S, Unger F, Nguyen-Viet H, Dang-Xuan S, Nguyen-Thi T, Häsler B. Exploring the potential of using nudges to promote food hygiene in the pork value chain in Vietnam. Prev Vet Med. 2020;181:105003. https://doi.org/10.1016/j.prevetmed.2020.105003.
19. Peyre M, Hoinville L, Njoroge J, Cameron A, Traon D, Goutard F, Calba C, Grosbois V, Delabouglise A, Varant V, Drewe J, Pfeiffer D, Häsler B. The RISKSUR EVA Tool (Survtool): a tool for the integrated evaluation of animal health surveillance systems. Prev Vet Med. 2019;104777 https://doi.org/10.1016/j.prevetmed.2019.104777.
20. Duboz R, Binot A. Animal and human health: tackling uncertainty through participatory modelling and simulation. Perspect Cirad. 2017:1–4. https://doi.org/10.19182/agritrop/00011.
21. Hutchison J, Mackenzie C, Madin B, Happold J, Leslie E, Zalcman E, Meyer A, Cameron A. New approaches to aquatic and terrestrial animal surveillance: the potential for people and technology to transform epidemiology. Prev Vet Med. 2019;167:169–73. https://doi.org/10.1016/j.prevetmed.2018.10.009.
22. Tran A, Roger F. Strengthening health decision-making at the territorial level: Operational support for spatial multi-criteria evaluation. Perspect Cirad. 2018:1–4. https://doi.org/10.19182/agritrop/00022.
23. Peyre M. Public-private partnerships: at the heart of animal health surveillance. Bull OIE. 2020;2019:19–20. https://doi.org/10.20506/bull.2019.3.3037.
24. Eloit M. Public–private partnerships: a winning strategy to sustainably improve national Veterinary Services. FR- Partenariats public–privé : une stratégie gagnante pour améliorer durablement les services vétérinaires nationaux -ES- Asociaciones público-privadas: una estrategia acertada para mejorar de manera sostenible los Servicios Veterinarios nacionales. Bull OIE. 2020;2019:1–2. https://doi.org/10.20506/bull.2019.3.3037.
25. World Animal Health Organisation (OIE). The OIE PPP Handbook: Guidelines for Public-Private Partnerships in the veterinary domain, OIE Eds. ed. Paris; 2019.

Glossary

Acceptability and engagement Willingness of persons and organizations to participate in the surveillance system, and the degree to which each of these users is involved in the surveillance process including the participation of stakeholders in the steering and technical committees. Could include an assessment of stakeholder awareness of the system and their understanding of it. Could also assess their beliefs about the benefits or adverse consequences of their participation in the system including the provision of compensation for the consequence of disease detection.

Active surveillance Also: Proactive surveillance; Investigator-initiated collection of animal health-related data using a defined protocol to perform actions that are scheduled in advance. Decisions about whether information is collected and what information should be collected from which animals are made by the investigator.

Advocacy Public support for or recommendation of a particular cause or policy.

Assessment The assessment of a surveillance system/component is the collection and analysis of data on the relevant surveillance attributes and/or criteria. It is a technical step within the evaluation process.

Assessment To determine, estimate, or judge the value of. An assessment provides technical results (either qualitative and/or quantitative), which may or may not be linked to a judgment on the validity/quality of those results.

Associated legislation and regulations A description of any legislation or regulations which act as the basis for determining the requirement for surveillance, including whether there are any compensation arrangements and any requirement for ethical approval.

Benefit Direct and indirect advantages produced by the surveillance system. This does not need to be limited to financial savings and better use of resources but can also include any losses avoided due to the existence of the system and the information it provides. These avoided losses may include improved animal production, maintenance of a structured network of actors able to react appropriately against a future threat, improved public health, increased understanding about a disease, maintained or increased trade, or improved ability to react in case of an outbreak of disease.

M. Peyre et al. (eds.), *Principles for Evaluation of One Health Surveillance: The EVA Book*, https://doi.org/10.1007/978-3-030-82727-4

Bias The extent to which a prevalence estimate produced by the surveillance system deviates from the value of the true prevalence . Bias is reduced as representativeness is increased.

Case definition # Clinical signs or syndrome (including death) # Indirect indicators (e.g., drug sales, production or performance information, abattoir sub missions) # Gross pathology # Laboratory test for pathogens or toxins # Laboratory test for host response (e.g., serology) # Specified diagnostic criteria (e.g., diagnostic codes (Veterinary Investigation Diagnosis and Analysis (VIDA)) code used in GB early warning surveillance system) # Risk factor(s).

Communication and dissemination An assessment of the methods used and ease of information exchange between people involved at all levels of the surveillance system (providers, analyzers, and users of surveillance data). Include an assessment of the data and information provided and of the timeliness and types of outputs produced. The efforts made to disseminate these outputs including the use of web-based systems should also be assessed. The methods used to provide feedback to data providers and to increase their awareness about hazards and surveillance activities should also be assessed. Internal communication and dissemination is directed at those working within the surveillance network or system. External communication and dissemination is directed at those outside the surveillance network or system (e.g., international organizations).

Contingent valuation A value is derived from the direct estimation of a good or service by the interviewee following a full description of its features. Hence, the good or service is valued as a whole.

Cost The evaluation should list and quantify each of the resources required to operate the surveillance system and identify who provides each resource. These resources could include time, personnel, financial input, and equipment.

Counterfactual Thinking about what did not happen but could have happened; with regard to surveillance, a counterfactual could be, e.g., a situation with an ideal surveillance system in place or with no surveillance at all.

Coverage The proportion of the population of interest (target population) that is included in the surveillance activity.

Cultural and Economic acceptability The traits of a society—its patterns of adaptation to the environment and its economic organization, social and political institutions, and beliefs system—will all affect the acceptance and performances of health surveillance strategies and innovations in health surveillance systems. The influence of these variables will have to be assessed in the context of each local culture.

Data analysis Whether appropriate methods are used for the analysis and interpretation of data at an appropriate frequency.

Data analysis method A description of the measures used to assess disease occurrence (e.g., incidence, prevalence, case numbers) and how the data are analyzed includes the spatial and temporal methods used, the frequency of analysis, and whether real-time and whether contextual information (e.g., the risk of introduction and the prior likelihood of disease) will be incorporated.

Data collection The use of appropriate data sources and collection methods including automation of data collection where appropriate and the existence of a case definition and a data collection protocol.

Data completeness and correctness The proportion of data that were intended to be collected that actually was collected and the proportion of data entries that correctly reflect the true value of the data collected.

Data management methods A description of how data is managed, e.g., whether a central relational database is used and the methods used to ensure confidentiality and security of information.

Data storage and management Appropriate use and documentation of data management systems for processing information, including data processing protocols, and effective use of data verification procedures and of data storage and back-up procedures.

Design prevalence A standard hypothetical prevalence of disease specified at the herd (herd design prevalence, P*H) or at the animal level (P*A) against which to measure surveillance sensitivity. Source: http://www.ncbi.nlm.nih.gov/pubmed/22305852 Cameron, 2012: PVM 2015, p. 280–286. The definition is based on the concept that if a particular pathogen is present, it is present in less than a specified proportion of the population at a given level of statistical confidence.

Discrete choice experiment The value is derived statistically from a series of choices between goods showing distinct features and prices. Conjoint analysis is mobilized to quantify the trade-offs made in his/her choices by the interviewee between the different features of the good or service and its price.

Disease focus: General Surveillance that is not focused on specific hazards and that uses general tests (e.g., clinical examination or gross pathology).

Disease focus: Hazard-specific Surveillance that is focused on one or more predefined hazards; often using diagnostic tests for the detection of particular pathogens (e.g., molecular diagnostic tests).

Dissemination method A description of the methods used for disseminating surveillance information during and after surveillance including whether web-access is possible and the methods used for data sharing.

Early warning surveillance Also: epidemiological watch, epidemiovigilance; Surveillance of health indicators and diseases in defined populations to increase the likelihood of timely detection of undefined (new) or unexpected (exotic or re-emerging) threats. These are surveillance systems for the early detection of these threats.

Economic efficiency Whether the surveillance system produces the desired effect without wasting resources. Three levels of economic efficiency can be defined: # Optimization: maximizing the net benefit to society achieved by the allocation of scarce resources to animal health surveillance and intervention to avoid losses resulting from animal diseases # Acceptability: ensuring that the benefits generated by a mitigation policy at least cover its costs; this is commonly assessed using cost-benefit analysis # Cost-minimization: ensuring that a technical target for disease mitigation (e.g., time to detection) is achieved at minimum cost without quantifying the benefit in monetary terms; this can be assessed using cost-effectiveness or least-cost analysis.

Effectiveness Is the capability of producing a desired result. When something is deemed effective, it means it has an intended or expected outcome.

Efficacy Is the capacity to produce an effect. In medicine, efficacy indicates the capacity for beneficial change (or therapeutic effect) of a given intervention. When talking in terms of efficacy vs. effectiveness, effectiveness relates to how well a treatment works in the practice of medicine, as opposed to efficacy, which measures how well treatment works in clinical trials or laboratory studies.

Efficiency The extent to which a resource is used for the intended purpose. Efficiency describes the extent to which time, effort, or cost is well used for the intended task or purpose. It is often used with the specific purpose of relaying the capability of a specific application of effort to produce a specific outcome effectively with a minimum amount or quantity of waste, expense, or unnecessary effort.

Efficiency assessment of a program Cost-benefit or cost-effectiveness analysis assesses the efficiency of a program. Evaluators outline the benefits and cost of the program for comparison.

Enhanced passive surveillance Observer-initiated provision of animal health-related data with active investigator involvement, e.g., by actively encouraging producers to report certain types of disease or by active follow-up of suspect disease reports.

Epidemiological watch See: Early warning surveillance

Epidemiovigilance See: Early warning surveillance

Evaluation The evaluation of a surveillance system/component is the determination of its merit by confronting the results of the assessment with targets set by the stakeholders, standard criteria, or a counterfactual system. The outcome of an evaluation is a judgment and/or recommendations placed in the overall surveillance context. An evaluation can be performed at any development stage of the surveillance system. Ideally, an evaluation is conducted in regular intervals in line with the policy cycle, by internal and/or external evaluators. One, several, or all components in the surveillance system and any number of attributes and/or criteria can be considered, depending on the question and the context of the evaluation.

Evaluation question An evaluation should be done with a clear objective, which comes with one or multiple clearly formulated question. The evaluation question(s) ensure framing the evaluation process exactly to the needs and to ensure saving resources.

Event-based (media-based, digital) surveillance Surveillance that complements indicator-based surveillance by continuously scanning the Internet and other communication media to detect information that might lead to the recognition of emerging threats. It uses unstructured data which need to be studied and verified and which cannot be summarized as an indicator.

False alarm rate Proportion of negative events (e.g., non-outbreak periods) incorrectly classified as events (e.g., outbreaks). This is the inverse of the specificity but can be more easily understood than specificity.

Flexibility Ability to adapt to changing information needs or operating conditions with little additional time, personnel or allocated funds. Flexible systems can accommodate new health hazards, changes in case definitions or technology, and variations in funding or reporting sources.

General surveillance Surveillance that is not focused on specific hazards and uses general tests (e.g., clinical examination or gross pathology). Syndromic surveillance is a form of general surveillance.

Gold standard The "ideal" surveillance system/component, of superior quality which serves as a point of reference against which other surveillance systems/components may be compared.

Guidance pathway (evaluation question) A step-by-step approach which guides the user in defining the evaluation question(s) relevant to his needs—a guidance pathway to define relevant evaluation questions in surveillance is available in Survtools (https://survtools.org)

Hazard A biological, chemical, or physical agent in, or a condition of, an animal or animal product with the potential to cause an adverse health effect. Source: http://www.oie.int/index.php?id=169&L=0&htmfile=glossaire.htm OIE Terrestrial Animal Health Code

Hazard situation Endemic, sporadic, free, exotic, re-emerging, new, situation varies. Source: RISKSUR

Hazard-specific surveillance Surveillance that is focused on one or more predefined hazards (disease, condition, biological, chemical or physical agent, or event); often this form of surveillance uses diagnostic tests for the detection of particular pathogens (e.g., molecular diagnostic methods).

Impact Indicates the changes that have been made based on the results of the surveillance providing a measure of the usefulness of the surveillance system in relation to its aims. This should include details of actions taken as a result of the information provided by the surveillance system (e.g., changes in protocols or behavior, changes in mitigation actions, and especially changes in disease occurrence).

Impact assessment A process aimed at structuring and supporting the development of policies. It identifies and assesses the problem at stake and the objectives pursued. It identifies the main options for achieving the objective and analyzes their likely impacts in the economic, environmental, and social fields. It outlines advantages and disadvantages of each option and examines possible synergies and trade-offs.

Impact evaluation (assessing effectiveness) The impact evaluation determines the causal effects of the program. This involves trying to measure if the program has achieved its intended outcomes. Assesses the changes that can be attributed to a particular intervention, such as a project, program, or policy, both the intended ones, as well as ideally the unintended ones. In contrast to outcome monitoring, which examines whether targets have been achieved, impact evaluation is structured to answer the question: how would outcomes such as participants' well-being have changed if the intervention had not been undertaken? This involves counterfactual analysis, that is, "a comparison between what actually happened and what would have happened in the absence of the intervention." Impact evaluations seek to answer cause-and-effect questions. In other words, they look for the changes in outcome that are directly attributable to a program

Impartiality Considering all stakeholders in the evaluation process; ensuring relevant links between evidence-based findings and recommendations produced.

Indicator-based surveillance Traditional disease surveillance which relies on the collection of data about the occurrence of predefined diseases or conditions and which uses agreed-upon case definitions; these data are analyzed to produce indicators that point towards the existence of a threat. Indicator-based surveillance may be hazard specific or general and includes the use of clinical or other data for syndromic surveillance.

Laboratory management Whether testing is carried out using appropriate methods with quality assurance scheme and timely and accurate delivery of results.

Management also: personnel and organizational structure. Name of organization(s) and expertise of the personnel managing the surveillance activity and description of the organizational structure.

Marginal product The increment of product (here, surveillance information) that results from an increment of (surveillance) resources.

Monitoring The systematic, continuous or repeated, measurement, collection, collation, analysis, and interpretation of animal health and welfare-related data in defined populations when these activities are not associated with a predefined risk mitigation plan although extreme changes are likely to lead to action.

Multi-objective Surveillance activities where samples collected for one disease agent are analyzed for more than one purpose or for other disease agents, either in parallel or at a later stage. Source: RISKSUR http://www.fp7-risksur.eu/sites/default/files/documents/Deliverables/RISKSUR%20D1.1%20Research%20Brief.pdf (Deliverable 1.1).

Multiple utility Whether the system captures information about more than one hazard.

Organization and management An assessment of organizational structures include whether the objectives are relevant and clearly defined and the existence of steering and technical committees whose members are representative of the surveillance stakeholders. The members of these committees should have appropriate expertise, clearly defined roles and responsibilities; these member should hold meetings (with minutes taken and kept)regularly to oversee the function of the system.

Origin of data: Active See: Active surveillance

Origin of data: Enhanced passive See: Enhanced passive surveillance

Origin of data: Passive See: Passive surveillance

Participation, basis of # Voluntary # voluntary recruitment with mandatory participation # mandatory.

Participatory surveillance Participatory surveillance explores traditional information networks by using participatory rural appraisal methods such as ranking, scoring, and visualization techniques to conduct risk-based, hazard-specific surveillance. The approach uses semi-structured interviews with key informants. This enables communities to provide their knowledge regarding health events, risks, impacts, and control opportunities by gathering qualitative health data from defined populations. The analysis of participatory data emphasizes the comparison of information obtained from multiple informants; the method uses a variety of techniques to obtain the most likely interpretation of events. The objective is to enhance sensitivity by identifying cases based on a clinical case definition; these may then be evaluated and confirmed using either rapid tests in the field or laboratory diagnostics. Conventional epidemiological investigation techniques can be used to evaluate and confirm outbreaks detected by participatory surveillance as part of trace-back and trace-forwards activities.

Passive surveillance Observer-initiated provision of animal health-related data (e.g., voluntary notification of suspect disease) or the use of existing data for surveillance. Decisions about whether information is provided, and what information is provided from which animals is made by the data provider.

Pattern of disease occurrence: Endemic The constant presence of a disease in the population of interest.

Pattern of disease occurrence: Exotic A previously defined (known) disease that crosses political boundaries to occur in a country or region in which it is not currently recorded as present.

Pattern of disease occurrence: New Also: emerging; A previously undefined (unknown) disease or condition, which might result from the evolution or change in an existing pathogen or parasite resulting in a change of strain, host range, vector, or an increase in pathogenicity. This might also be due to the occurrence of any other previously undefined condition.

Pattern of disease occurrence: Re-emerging A previously defined (known) disease that is currently either absent or present at a low level, in the population in a defined geographical area that reappears or significantly increases in prevalence.

Pattern of disease occurrence: Sporadic A known disease which occurs intermittently in an irregular or haphazard pattern.

Performance monitoring and evaluation Whether performance indicators are routinely used to monitor system performance and periodic external evaluations are used to assess the system outputs in relation to its objectives.

Policy analysis Determining which of various alternative policies will most achieve a given set of goals in light of the relations between the policies and the goals. However, policy analysis can be divided into two major fields. Analysis **of** policy is analytical and descriptive—i.e., it attempts to explain policies and their development. Analysis **for** policy is prescriptive—i.e., it is involved with formulating policies and proposals (e.g., to improve social welfare). The area of interest and the purpose of analysis determines what type of analysis is conducted. A combination of policy analysis together with program evaluation would be defined as policy studies.

Policy purpose Describes how surveillance information is used by policymakers to inform decisions about how best to support policy objectives such as maintaining a healthy and sustainable food and farming industry, protection of the livelihood of producers, other value chain stakeholders and public health and to support national economic development. The specific decisions that surveillance information can assist policymakers with are: # Management of outbreaks: whether additional control measures are required to limit the spread of an emerging or exotic disease outbreak # Informing trade: whether to permit import or support export of animals or animal products. This decision should be based on evidence about the prevalence and distribution of disease and about the risk of disease transmission through the commodity being traded. The purpose being to protect the indigenous population and facilitate access to international markets # Prioritization: how to prioritize surveillance and control measures for different health hazards. The prioritization should be based on the level of hazard occurrence and impact on animal health and welfare, public health, trade, and the wider economy; the prioritization should use information about the relative importance of hazards # Informing control: whether existing control measures should be maintained, stopped, or changed to improve the efficiency of surveillance and risk mitigation. This may include providing reassurance about the absence of specific existing or new diseases (which could threaten animal health or welfare or public health) to confirm that risk mitigation is not required.

Portfolio A portfolio considers multiple items between which a resource allocation decision has to be made.

Precision How closely defined a numerical estimate is. A precise estimate has a narrow confidence interval. Precision is influenced by prevalence, sample size, and surveillance system quality.

Proactive surveillance See: Active surveillance

Process effectiveness/quality The surveillance system organization according to best practices

Program evaluation A systematic method for collecting, analyzing, and using information to answer questions about projects, policies, and programs, particularly about their effectiveness and efficiency. In both the public and private sectors, stakeholders often want to know whether the programs they are funding, implementing, voting for, receiving, or objecting to are producing the intended effect. While program evaluation first focuses around this definition, important considerations often include how much the program costs per participant, how the program could be improved, whether the program is worthwhile, whether there are better alternatives, if there are unintended outcomes, and whether the program goals are appropriate and useful. Program evaluation may be conducted at several stages during a program's lifetime. Each of these stages raises different questions to be answered by the evaluator, and correspondingly different evaluation approaches are needed. Rossi, Lipsey, and Freeman (2004) suggest the following kinds of assessment, which may be appropriate at these different stages: Assessment of the need for the program; Assessment of program design and logic/theory; Assessment of how the program is being implemented (i.e., is it being implemented according to plan? Are the program's processes maximizing possible outcomes?); Assessment of the program's outcome or impact (i.e., what it has actually achieved); Assessment of the program's cost and efficiency.

Reactive surveillance See: Passive surveillance

Recommendations The suggestion or proposal as to the best course of action, especially one put forward by an authoritative body. Recommendations on how to improve health surveillance strategies and systems are the major outcomes of health surveillance evaluations. The recommendations should follow best evaluation practices, including impartiality, independence, and transparency.

Repeatability How consistently the study results can be reproduced over time.

Representativeness The extent to which the features of the population of interest are reflected by the population included in the surveillance activity. These features may include herd size, production type, age, sex or geographical location or time of sampling (important for some systems, e.g., for vector-borne infection).

Requirement Input-based standards prescribe the surveillance activities to be carried out (i.e., sampling strategy, sample size, choice of test, and frequency of testing), assuming that the population properties of herds are homogeneously distributed. Output-based standards prescribe what surveillance has to achieve, thus providing flexibility required to find the most effective surveillance approach for the specific population under surveillance. Source: http://www.ncbi.nlm.nih.gov/pubmed/22305852 Cameron, 2012: PVM 2015, p. 280–286

Resource availability An assessment of the financial and human resources available for implementing the surveillance activity including the expertise and capability of personnel.

Risk The likelihood of the occurrence and the likely magnitude of the biological and economic consequences of an adverse event or effect to animal or human health. Source: http://www.oie.int/index.php?id=169&L=0&htmfile=glossaire.htm OIE Terrestrial Animal Health Code

Risk factor assessment The evaluation of the likelihood and the biological and economic consequences of entry, establishment, and spread of a hazard within the territory of a country. Source: http://www.oie.int/index.php?id=169&L=0&htmfile=glossaire.htm OIE Terrestrial Animal Health Code

Risk factors # geography # animal # management # environmental or other factors # + free text to describe. Source: RISKSUR

Risk-based analysis Use of prior or additional information about the probability of hazard occurrence, including contextual information and prior likelihood of disease to revise conclusions about disease status.

Risk-based prioritization Determining which hazards should be selected for surveillance based on information about the probability of their occurrence and the extent of biologic and/or economic consequences of their occurrence.

Risk-based requirement Use of prior or additional information about the probability of hazard occurrence to revise the surveillance intensity required to achieve the stated surveillance purpose.

Risk-based sampling Designing a sampling strategy to reduce the cost or enhance the accuracy of surveillance by preferentially sampling strata (e.g., age groups or geographical areas) within the target population that are more likely to be exposed, affected, detected, become affected, transmit infection, or cause other consequences (e.g., large economic losses or trade restrictions).

Risk-based surveillance Use of information about the probability of occurrence and the magnitude of the biological and/or economic consequence of health hazards to plan, design, and/or interpret the results obtained from surveillance systems. Risk-based surveillance can include one or several of the following four approaches: # Risk-based prioritization # Risk-based requirement # Risk-based sampling # Risk-based analysis

Sample type(s) # blood / plasma / serum # animal swab, tissue # carcass # feces # urine # semen # milk / colostrum # environmental sample # clinical surveillance # postmortem <h6> Source: RISKSUR</h6>

Sampling strategy Use of appropriate sampling strategies including the use of risk-based approaches (i.e., risk-based requirement calculation or risk-based sampling) and pooled sampling where appropriate. The basis of the risks used in the design of the risk-based sampling strategy should be assessed.

Scope of surveillance activity: Component A single surveillance activity (defined by the source of data and the methods used for its collection) used to investigate the occurrence of one or more hazards in a specified population.

Scope of surveillance activity: Portfolio A range of surveillance components (and the associated organizational structures) used to investigate the occurrence of more than one hazard in a specified population.

Scope of surveillance activity: System or network A range of surveillance components (and the associated organizational structures) used to investigate the occurrence of a single hazard in a specified population.

Sensitivity Sensitivity of a surveillance system can be considered on three levels: # Surveillance sensitivity: Case detection # Surveillance sensitivity: Outbreak detection # Surveillance sensitivity: Presence

Sentinel surveillance The repeated collection of information from the same selected sites or groups of animals (e.g., veterinary practices, laboratories, herds, or animals) to identify changes in the health status of a specified population over time. These sentinels should act as a proxy for the larger population of interest; they may be selected on the basis of risk but can also be selected randomly or on the basis of convenience or compliance.

Simplicity Refers to the surveillance system structure, ease of operation, and flow of data through the system.

Stability and sustainability The ability to function without failure (reliability), the ability to be operational when needed (availability) and the robustness and ability of the system to be ongoing in the long term (sustainability).

Stakeholders Also: owners and beneficiaries. Name of organization(s) paying for the surveillance activity and identification of beneficiaries.

Study design # Case reporting (voluntary or mandatory) # Survey # Continuous collection # Participatory # Sentinel # Event-based (media-based).

Surveillance The systematic, continuous or repeated, measurement, collection, collation, analysis, interpretation, and timely dissemination of animal health and welfare-related data from defined populations. These data are then used to describe health hazard occurrence and to contribute to the planning, implementation, and evaluation of risk mitigation actions.

Surveillance component A specific activity undertaken within a surveillance system (e.g., event-based surveillance in farms; active sampling of birds in slaughterhouses; active sampling of birds in live bird markets, etc.).

Surveillance context The epidemiological, social, economic, and political situation(s) within which the surveillance is undertaken and that could potentially affect its performances; the surveillance context could differ within different administrative levels within one country.

Surveillance objective States those goal(s) that when met will result in the collection and analysis of data in order to achieve the purpose of the system (http://www.fp7-risksur.eu/terminology/faq#References).

Surveillance purpose Describes why surveillance is necessary and what it will accomplish (http://www.fp7-risksur.eu/terminology/faq#References).

Surveillance sensitivity: Case detection The proportion of individual animals or herds in the population of interest that have the health-related condition of interest and that the surveillance system is able to detect.

Surveillance sensitivity: Outbreak detection The probability that the surveillance system will detect a significant increase (outbreak) of disease. This requires a clear definition of what constitutes an outbreak.

Surveillance sensitivity: Presence The probability that disease will be detected if present at a certain level (prevalence) in the population.

Surveillance system The network of actors engaged in health surveillance activities: sharing information and taking relevant actions as defined in the surveillance strategy and different surveillance component protocols.

Sustainability The ability to be maintained over time.

Syndromic surveillance Surveillance that uses health-related information (clinical signs or other data) that might precede or substitute for formal diagnosis. This information may be used to indicate a sufficient probability of a change in the health of the population to deserve further investigation or to enable a timely assessment of the impact of health threats which may require action. This type of surveillance is not usually focused on a particular hazard and so can be used to detect a variety of diseases or pathogens including new (emerging) diseases. This type of surveillance is particularly applicable for early warning surveillance.

Target value The Target Value of a process is the numerical aim of the process that is preferred for the quality characteristic of interest; e.g., a surveillance system could have a target value for its sensitivity set at 90%.

Technical effectiveness Technical efficiency is the effectiveness with which a given set of inputs is used to produce an output. A surveillance system is said to be technically efficient if it reaches its maximum outputs (e.g., performances) from the minimum quantity of inputs, such as labor, capital, and technology.

Timeliness Timeliness can be defined in various ways: Usually defined as the time between any two defined steps in a surveillance system. The time points chosen are likely to vary depending on the purpose of the surveillance activity.

For outbreak detection this can be defined using various time points (e.g., the time between exposure to the infectious agent and the initiation of risk-mitigation measures or the time between when disease could have been detected and reported and the time when it actually was reported). For planning purposes, timeliness can also be defined as whether surveillance detects changes in time for risk-mitigation actions to reduce the likelihood of further spread. One way of measuring this would be to assess the number of cases present in the population when disease was detected. The precise definition of timeliness chosen should be stated as part of the evaluation process.

Training provision Provision of adequate initial training and an ongoing program of training for those implementing the surveillance system.

Transparency All stakeholders aware of the evaluation aim and detail process.

Unit of interest Units selected for sampling in surveillance activity (level of sampling), e.g., animal, farm, batch, village